CONTENTS

1. **Psychological aspects of dental care** 1
I. G. Chestnutt

2. **History and examination** 11
I. G. Che...

3. **Law, e... quality... care**
J. A. D. ...

4. **Dental radiology** 33
P. P. Nixon

5. **Drug prescribing and therapeutics** 59
D. Stenhouse

6. **Analgesia, sedation and general anaesthesia** 91
D. Stenhouse, J. Leitch

7. **Dental materials** 115
J. Rees, A. J. Paterson

8. **Preventive and community dental practice** 149
I. G. Chestnutt

9. **Paediatric dentistry** 167
B. L. Chadwick

10. **Periodontology** 197
I. G. Chestnutt

11. **Operative dentistry** 231
J Rees, A. J. Paterson

12. **Removable prosthodontics** 299
A. J. Paterson

13. **Orthodontics** 341
... Buchanan

... 1

... e 439

16. **General medicine of relevance to dentistry** 489
J. Gibson

17. **Emergencies in dentistry** 521
J. Gibson

Appendix A: Further reading 534

Appendix B: Useful websites 537

Appendix C: Average dates of mineralization and eruption 540

Appendix D: Tooth notation 542

Appendix E: Infection control 542

Appendix F: Normal laboratory values of relevance to medicine 544

Index 547

...issioning Editor: Michael Parkinson
...pment Editor: Janice Urquhart
Manager: Emma Riley
Direction: Erik Bigland
...tions Manager: Merlyn Harvey
...tor: Robert Britton

Clinical Dentistry

Comm
Devel
Projec
Design
Illustra
Illustra

Clinical Dentistry

EDITED BY

Ivor G. Chestnutt BDS MPH PHD FDS (DPH) RCS (Edin) DDPHRCS (Eng) FDS RCS(Eng) FDS RCPS(Glasg) MFPH
Professor and Honorary Consultant in Dental Public Health, School of Dentistry, Cardiff University, Cardiff, UK

John Gibson PHD BDS MB CHB FDS (OM) RCPS (Glasg) FFDRCS (Irel) FDSRCS (Edin)
Consultant and Honorary Clinical Senior Lecturer in Oral Medicine, Dundee Dental Hospital and School, Dundee, UK

THIRD EDITION

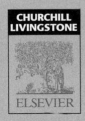

EDINBURGH LONDON NEW YORK OXFORD PHILADELPHIA ST LOUIS SYDNEY TORONTO 2007

CHURCHILL LIVINGSTONE
ELSEVIER

© Harcourt Publishers Limited 2002
© 2007, Elsevier Limited. All rights reserved.

The right of Dr … … … and … … Gibson to be identified as editors of this work has been asserted by them in accordance with the Copyright, Designs and Patents Act 1988.

No part of this publication may be reproduced, stored in a retrieval system, or transmitted in any form or by any means, electronic, mechanical, photocopying, recording or otherwise, without the prior permission of the Publishers. Permissions may be sought directly from Elsevier's Health Sciences Rights Department, 1600 John F. Kennedy Boulevard, Suite 1800, Philadelphia, PA 19103-2899, USA: phone: (+1) 215 239 3804; fax: (+1) 215 239 3805; or, e-mail: *healthpermissions@elsevier.com*. You may also complete your request on-line via the Elsevier homepage (*http://www.elsevier.com*), by selecting 'Support and contact' and then 'Copyright and Permission'.

First edition 1998
Second edition 2002
Third edition 2007

ISBN-13: 9780443102110
   Reprinted 2007
International edition ISBN-13: 9780443102127

British Library Cataloguing in Publication Data
A catalogue record for this book is available from the British Library

Library of Congress Cataloging in Publication Data
A catalog record for this book is available from the Library of Congress

Note
Knowledge and best practice in this field are constantly changing. As new research and experience broaden our knowledge, changes in practice, treatment and drug therapy may become necessary or appropriate. Readers are advised to check the most current information provided (i) on procedures featured or (ii) by the manufacturer of each product to be administered, to verify the recommended dose or formula, the method and duration of administration, and contraindications. It is the responsibility of the practitioner, relying on their own experience and knowledge of the patient, to make diagnoses, to determine dosages and the best treatment for each individual patient, and to take all appropriate safety precautions. To the fullest extent of the law, neither the Publisher nor the Editors assume any liability for any injury and/or damage to persons or property arising out or related to any use of the material contained in this book.
The Publisher

ELSEVIER   your source for books,
journals and multimedia
in the health sciences

www.elsevierhealth.com

The
publisher's
policy is to use
paper manufactured
from sustainable forests

Printed in China

CONTENTS

1. **Psychological aspects of dental care**   1
   I. G. Chestnutt

2. **History and examination**   11
   I. G. Chestnutt

3. **Law, ethics and quality dental care**   19
   J. A. D. Cameron

4. **Dental radiology**   33
   P. P. Nixon

5. **Drug prescribing and therapeutics**   59
   D. Stenhouse

6. **Analgesia, sedation and general anaesthesia**   91
   D. Stenhouse, J. Leitch

7. **Dental materials**   115
   J. Rees, A. J. Paterson

8. **Preventive and community dental practice**   149
   I. G. Chestnutt

9. **Paediatric dentistry**   167
   B. L. Chadwick

10. **Periodontology**   197
    I. G. Chestnutt

11. **Operative dentistry**   231
    J Rees, A. J. Paterson

12. **Removable prosthodontics**   299
    A. J. Paterson

13. **Orthodontics**   341
    I. B. Buchanan

14. **Oral and maxillofacial surgery**   381
    J. McManners

15. **Oral medicine**   439
    D. H. Felix

16. **General medicine of relevance to dentistry**   489
    J. Gibson

17. **Emergencies in dentistry**   521
    J. Gibson

Appendix A: Further reading   534

Appendix B: Useful websites   537

Appendix C: Average dates of mineralization and eruption   540

Appendix D: Tooth notation   542

Appendix E: Infection control   542

Appendix F: Normal laboratory values of relevance to medicine   544

Index   547

PREFACE TO THE THIRD EDITION

Nothing cheers an author more than to see his or her own textbook being used by the target audience! So it has been delightful to see more and more undergraduate dental students, vocational dental practitioners, general professional trainees, dental surgeons in primary care and in the hospital service, as well as dental care professionals in-training and post-qualification using this readily accessible little book.

The staff at Elsevier have been delighted at the success of the Second Edition at home and overseas, making the Pocketbook their best selling dental book! It was inevitable, therefore, that a Third Edition would be requested. We thank Michael Parkinson and Janice Urquhart for their support and advice throughout this project.

For this Third Edition we have, once again, expanded the size and quality of authorship. We welcome to the team Professor Jeremy Rees and Mr. John Cameron, both bringing additional expertise in the areas of restorative dentistry and dento-legal practice respectively.

In updating this edition, each author has addressed significant change within his or her areas of expertise and we are grateful to them for their enthusiasm and great industry. As with the Second Edition, we believe that this new edition has been invigorated and enhanced. Our aims and objectives remain the same – to educate and inspire each member of the dental team, whether in-training or post-qualification.

2006

Happy reading!
I. G.C. Cardiff
J. G. Edinburgh

PREFACE TO THE FIRST EDITION

The primary objective of this pocketbook is to provide a readily accessible source of information when it is most needed, as an aide-memoire prior to carrying out clinical tasks or to enable students (at undergraduate and postgraduate level) to apprise themselves of important details prior to tutorials and seminars.

The authors of this text are experienced clinicians and teachers within their individual specialties and emphasis has been given to information of practical clinical significance. Descriptions of rarely encountered conditions and situations have been kept deliberately to a minimum.

In a publication of this nature, information must be presented in a concise and at times didactic fashion. For those who read this text and feel it could only result in superficial learning, we have deliberately included sufficient basic information to permit examinations to be passed. However, the desire of an educationalist is always to promote deep learning and the layout and content of the text are intended to motivate and guide the reader to the appropriate parts of more substantive texts, many of which have proven both inspirational and motivational for the editors and contributors of this book throughout their careers.

Glasgow 1998

I.G.C.
J.G.

CONTRIBUTORS

I. B. Buchanan BDS MSc MOrthRCS (Eng) FDSRCS (Edin) FDSRCPS (Glasg)
Consultant in Orthodontics, Glasgow Dental Hospital and School, Honorary Clinical Senior Lecturer in Orthodontics, University of Glasgow, Glasgow, UK

J. A. D. Cameron BDS DGDP LLB (Hons)
Independent Dento-legal Adviser, Solutions in Dentistry, Edinburgh, UK

B. L. Chadwick BDS MScD PhD FDSRCS (Edin)
Professor and Honorary Consultant in Paediatric Dentistry, School of Dentistry, Cardiff University, Cardiff, UK

I. G. Chestnutt BDS MPH PHD FDS (DPH) RCS (Edin) DDPHRCS (Eng) FDS RCS (Eng) FDS RCPS (Glasg) MFPH
Professor and Honorary Consultant in Dental Public Health, School of Dentistry, Cardiff University, Cardiff, UK

D. H. Felix BDS MB ChB FDSRCS (Eng) FDSRCPS (Glasg) FDSRCS (Edin)
Consultant in Oral Medicine, North Glasgow University Hospitals NHS Trust, Honorary Clinical Senior Lecturer in Oral Medicine, University of Glasgow; Associate Dean for Postgraduate Dental Education, NHS Education for Scotland

J. Gibson PHD BDS MB CHB FDS (OM) RCPS (Glasg) FFDRCS (Irel) FDSRCS (Edin)
Consultant and Honorary Clinical Senior Lecturer in Oral Medicine, Dundee Dental Hospital and School, Dundee, UK

J. Leitch DDS BDS FDSRCS (Eng) FDSRCS (Edin) FDSRCPS (Glasg) DipConSed
Clinical Lecturer in Oral Surgery/Sedation, University of Glasgow Dental School, Glasgow, UK

J. McManners BDS MB ChB FDSRCS (Eng) FDSRCPS (Glasg) FRCS (Edin)
Consultant in Oral and Maxillofacial Surgery, Falkirk and District Royal Infirmary NHS Trust, Falkirk, UK

P. P. Nixon BDS FDSRCS(Eng) DDRRCR
Consultant in Dental and Maxillofacial Radiology, Liverpool University Dental Hospital, Liverpool, UK

A. J. Paterson BDS (Hons) FDSRCPS (Glasg) DRDRCS (Edin) MRDRCS (Edin)
Specialist in Restorative Dentistry and Prosthodontics, Private Dental Practice, Glasgow; Consultant in Restorative Dentistry, North Glasgow Hospitals University NHS Trust, Glasgow, UK

J. Rees BDS MScD FDSRCS(Edin) PhD
Professor of Restorative Dentistry, School of Dentistry, Cardiff University, Cardiff, UK

D. Stenhouse DDS BDS (Hons) FDSRCPS (Glasg)
Senior Lecturer and Honorary Consultant in Oral Surgery, University of Glasgow Dental School, Glasgow, UK

CHAPTER 1

PSYCHOLOGICAL ASPECTS OF DENTAL CARE

Introduction   2

Social and psychological influences on dental care   2

Communication   3

Behaviour change   4

Anxiety   7

Pain   9

Reference   10

INTRODUCTION

Above all else, the practice of dentistry involves working with people. Whilst a high degree of technical skill and judgement is required, an understanding of how social and psychological factors impact on oral health is crucial.

Dental disease and the provision of dental treatment are influenced heavily by patients' beliefs, attitudes and values. The aetiology of many dental diseases (e.g. dental caries, periodontal disease and mouth cancer) is influenced greatly by behavioural and lifestyle factors. Furthermore, changes in oral and systemic physiology, induced by psychological states, play an important role in conditions such as functional disorders of the masticatory system and chronic orofacial pain.

An appreciation of psychological factors enables the practitioner to:

● communicate more effectively
● understand causes of anxiety
● understand the nature of pain
● motivate patients and influence behaviour change.

This chapter will discuss the influence of psychological factors on dental care.

SOCIAL AND PSYCHOLOGICAL INFLUENCES ON DENTAL CARE

Oral health is a standard of health of the oral and related tissues which enables an individual to eat, speak and socialize without active disease, discomfort or embarrassment and which contributes to general well-being.

Dentists' perceptions of oral disease differ markedly from that of many of their patients, for whom oral health may be a low priority. Not everyone who has disease will seek professional care, nor does the presence of disease imply an absolute need for treatment. Whilst a high proportion of people in the general population would benefit from dental treatment (as judged by clinical criteria), the frequency with which patients choose to visit the dentist varies. Some choose not attend on a regular basis, but seek treatment only when in trouble. Thus, there is a difference between the *need* for dental treatment and the *demand* for it.

Although the general public's perception of dentistry has improved in recent times, some still view a visit to the dentist as a negative experience, and the decision to attend will be influenced by many factors.

These include:

- value placed on oral health by patient
- perceived ability to influence the maintenance of oral health or outcome of disease
- worsening of symptoms – patients may accept intermittent pain and seek care only when pain becomes constant or intolerable
- perceived seriousness of a disease – may encourage or discourage attendance. Some patients will deny the existence of a disease if it is thought to be very serious (e.g. cancer)
- access to dental care – influenced not only by geographic location of the dentist but also by factors such as availability of public transport
- disruption of daily life – attendance may involve having to take time off work, arrange a childminder, etc.
- financial implications – cost may be a barrier, even to those who can afford to pay
- advice from family and friends – can have positive or negative influences.

In the past, an emphasis on restorative care has forced dental decay, restorations and tooth loss to be viewed by some patients as an inevitable consequence of ageing.

 In common with health in general, oral health is influenced markedly by social class and is related to income, education, living and working conditions.

COMMUNICATION

The ability to communicate effectively is an essential skill and is necessary when:

- eliciting a history from a patient
- explaining proposed treatment and the merits of available options
- managing anxious patients – reducing anxiety requires skilled communication
- encouraging behaviour change.

Successful dental practice requires the development of a relationship between dentist and patient. Patients frequently place as much emphasis on the dentist's personality and clinical manner as on their technical skill; *how* something is said can therefore be as important as *what* is said. The use of good communication skills will greatly enhance patient satisfaction and compliance with advice. As the professional partner in the relationship, the responsibility for good communication lies with the dentist.

Factors inhibiting good communication include:

- difference in social class between dentist and patient
- priorities of the clinician may differ markedly from those of the patient
- supine dentistry places the patient in a passive (and often threatened) position
- technical language is not understood by patients
- 'lay theories of disease' (e.g. 'soft teeth' lead to caries) – patients may have their own concept of a particular problem and be reluctant to accept the correct scientific explanation
- time pressures may lead to information being presented too quickly for the patient to understand
- anxiety hinders ability to absorb information.

NON-VERBAL COMMUNICATION

Non-verbal communication is also very important in the context of providing dental care. This applies not only to the environs of the dental surgery and the postures, gestures and expressions of the clinician but also to the patient's reaction. Much information can be gained from observation of the patient and may give an indication of a patient's true feelings.

COMMUNICATION WITHIN THE DENTAL TEAM

Good communication skills are important, not only in dealing with patients but also in managing the dental team. As leader, it is the dentist's responsibility to communicate effectively with members of the practice staff – dental nurse, hygienist, therapist, receptionist and technician. Effective transfer of information is essential to the efficient operation of any organization.

BEHAVIOUR CHANGE

Prevention of the major dental diseases is possible if patients can be persuaded to adopt appropriate changes in behaviour and lifestyle. However, persuading and enabling patients to adopt and maintain healthy behaviour is a complex process.

Before behaviour can be changed, patients must:

- want to change
- believe they *can* change
- believe change will have the desired effect
- possess or be provided with the knowledge and skills to permit change.

THE PROCESS OF BEHAVIOUR CHANGE

It is recognized that changing behaviour is a complex process, involving different stages. The most commonly used model to explain behaviour change is the so-called 'stages of change model' which describes four stages: precontemplation, contemplation, action and maintenance.[1] This theory of behaviour change is explained below and discussed further in the context of helping patients give up smoking in Chapter 8 (Figure 8.3).

The stages of change model
Precontemplation
In this stage patients are not thinking about behaviour change.

Contemplating change
To promote behaviour change, patients must be made aware of alternatives to their present behaviour because, without information, patients will be unable to contemplate change. However, simply providing information (e.g. 'brush your teeth twice daily') is frequently insufficient to induce patients to adopt this habit.

In providing information it is necessary to:

- establish a current knowledge base (e.g. has the patient ever been shown previously how to brush?)
- establish the patient's current practice (e.g. how frequently do they brush at present?)
- provide an explanation of why behaviour change is necessary and desirable.

Written information (e.g. in the form of a leaflet) may be helpful but it should be personalized to the patient and appropriate to reading ability, level of understanding, account for linguistic and cultural factors. Be aware of the relatively high prevalence of illiteracy in the general population.

Information overload should be avoided. Changes should be introduced gradually. Having made choices explicit, it is often better if the patient then actively chooses to translate knowledge into action.

Taking action

An important step in encouraging behaviour change involves setting *goals*. This provides both patient and clinician with markers to gauge success. Differences in emphasis between dentist and patient should be borne in mind when setting goals – e.g. the dentist may be more concerned with aetiological factors of disease whereas patients may be more concerned about factors such as fresh breath or an attractive smile.

Targets for behaviour change should be:

Achievable Setting targets outwith the patient's ability will lead to failure and disillusionment.

Realistic If patients are to change behaviour, they must believe the actions required will have a positive benefit for them.

Important to the patient Identify and emphasize factors perceived as important to the patient, e.g. aesthetics.

Measurable Enables progress to be determined. Success will act as positive reinforcement.

Positive Targets should be positive – e.g. if encouraging avoidance of between-meal sugar consumption, occasions when snacks were avoided should be recorded rather than those occasions when snacks were taken.

Time related Enables progress to be measured.

Specific Avoid non-specific advice such as 'brush your teeth better'.

Health locus of control

The likelihood of an individual patient adapting to a preventive behaviour is influenced by many factors. An important concept is the patient's *perception* of factors influencing health outcomes. This is known as the health locus of control (HLOC), and three components have been described:

Internal HLOC The belief that by taking certain actions, health outcomes can be influenced. Therefore patients with a high internal HLOC will, for example, believe that regular toothbrushing with a fluoride toothpaste will prevent dental caries.

Powerful others HLOC The belief that, whilst health outcomes can be influenced, control lies with powerful others such as dentists. Such patients may therefore view regular dental attendance as important, but be less inclined to believe that health outcomes can be influenced by their own actions.

Chance HLOC The belief that health outcomes are largely a matter of chance or fate and that little can be done to influence the inevitable.

It should be noted that HLOC is a belief system and describes what patients actually believe rather than what they do.

Another important factor influencing patients' attitude to behaviour change is their perception of the future. Some patients are more willing to make sacrifices now in return for future benefits. The consequences of dental disease are long term and in the future. The rewards of sugar consumption are immediate! Furthermore, patients frequently do not experience the consequences of poor behaviours until it is too late.

MAINTAINING CHANGE

Maintenance of behaviour change is difficult. The clinician's role is ongoing. Reinforcement and encouragement is required to prevent relapse. Rewards (e.g. provision of sticky badges to children on successful completion of a toothbrushing programme) can be useful in promoting change. However, in the longer term the ultimate aim is to integrate positive behaviour into patients' everyday lifestyles to the point where they become habitual.

RELAPSE

Failure to encourage patients to change their behaviour can be frustrating and it is tempting to ascribe a patient's failure to comply with instructions as lack of motivation. It should be remembered that members of the dental team see their patients for a very brief period of time and are often faced with changing the habits of a lifetime. Behaviour change is cyclical in nature with patients frequently experiencing relapses and setbacks before achieving their goal (Figure 8.3).

Change – bearing in mind the principles outlined in this section – requires realistic goals, positive incentives, long-term follow-up, support and encouragement.

ANXIETY

Most patients are likely to be anxious to a greater or lesser extent at the prospect of dental treatment. This can vary from mild apprehension to anxiety sufficient to prevent the patient seeking care.

Anxiety may relate to the prospect of dental treatment in general or may be more specific and relate to fear of an individual object (e.g. needle) or procedure such as tooth extraction.

There are many possible causes of anxiety. Principal factors include:

Fear of pain Anxiety may affect pain threshold.

Uncertainty Fear of the unknown; anxious patients are pessimistic and 'expect the worst'.

Previous experience Many anxious patients ascribe their anxiety to previous 'bad experiences'. These frequently relate to the personal characteristics of a dentist. Parents can pass on their own anxiety to children.

Preparedness Some patients are 'innately' anxious. This is related to personality and such individuals are anxious in all sorts of situations, particularly those they have not previously encountered.

MEASURING ANXIETY

Questionnaires are available which can be used to measure anxiety. The patient is asked a series of questions related to potential threatening situations. Answers are scored according to severity and can be used to quantify anxiety. One of the best known is the *Dental Anxiety Scale*.

REDUCING ANXIETY

The ability to cope with anxious patients and to help alleviate anxiety is crucial in the practice of dentistry. Behaviour management techniques for use in dealing with anxious patients are discussed on page 170. The emphasis should be on helping patients acquire the skills necessary to cope with dental treatment.

Other factors which may help alleviate anxiety include:

- friendly and understanding attitude of the dental team
- welcoming environment – sights and smells are frequently cited as causes of anxiety
- communication during treatment – warn patients before reclining chair, blowing air from 3-in-1 syringe, etc. Explain the sensations that the patient is likely to experience
- decrease vulnerability – anxious patients feel vulnerable when supine. Instructions such as 'raise your hand if you want me to stop' help patients feel they have some control

- be honest and don't make unrealistic promises. Explain that a procedure may be slightly uncomfortable. Warn patients about what to expect postoperatively. This provides reassurance and may have a positive effect on pain threshold, etc.
- address anxieties directly. If a patient looks anxious, ask what is worrying them and take time to discuss and explain.

PAIN

An understanding of pain is important as it impinges on a dentist's daily activities in the following ways:

- pain is a common symptom of dental disease
- pain will be the precipitating factor that leads many patients to seek care
- pain may be experienced during treatment or as a consequence of treatment
- fear of pain may prevent patients seeking treatment.

THE NATURE OF PAIN

Pain is a complex phenomenon involving physiological, psychological and situational factors. The Gate Theory of Pain acknowledges that experience of pain results not only from physical sensations but also from emotional and evaluative reactions to these sensations. Therefore:

- pain does not always correlate with physical damage or demonstrable organic disease and is influenced by higher centres in the central nervous system
- reaction to pain is influenced by cultural and emotional factors
- pain is a highly personal experience
- patients will express the sensation of pain differently – i.e. there is a difference between pain sensation and pain behaviour. Thus it is not always possible to determine how much pain an individual is experiencing from observation alone
- reaction is influenced by the setting in which the pain is experienced. Thus in the dental surgery patients may confuse other sensations with pain, especially if anxious
- pain is influenced by anxiety
- previous experience of pain influences subsequent exposure: pain during a given procedure may lead to the expectation that it

will be more painful in future and will actually be perceived as
more painful
● variation in individual situational factors means that what is
painful to one person will not be to another.

> ⚠ **It is important that pain is not dismissed simply because
> there is no obvious organic cause. However, pain should
> not be deemed to be psychological in origin until all possibilities
> of an organic source have been investigated thoroughly and
> eliminated.**

PSYCHOLOGICAL APPROACHES TO PAIN CONTROL

The manner in which analgesic agents are prescribed has an
important influence on their effectiveness. In addition to their
pharmacological effect, much of the positive effect of drugs stems
from the patient's *belief* in their efficacy: the *placebo effect*.

Psychological approaches to influencing patients' pain include
many of those useful in reducing anxiety (p. 8). Anxiety and pain
are positively related. Anxious patients are much more likely to
experience pain and in turn pain is likely to increase anxiety.

Techniques available include:

Distraction Involves shifting the patient's attention during
treatment. Suggested techniques include provision of
audiotapes, pictures on the ceiling of the surgery to be viewed
when the patient is reclined to prevent patient from focusing on
potentially painful stimulus.

Enhancing control Advise patient to raise a hand if they want to
stop (p. 8).

Effective communication Explain the sensations the patient is likely
to experience. Avoid suggestive words such as 'pain' and 'drill'.

Hypnosis Useful in some patients. Provides a sense of calm and
well-being, thereby reducing anxiety (p. 113).

REFERENCE

1. Prochaska JO, Diclemente CC 1983 Stages and process of self-
   change of smoking: toward an integrative model of change.
   Journal of Consulting Psychology 51:390–5

CHAPTER 2

HISTORY AND EXAMINATION

History 12
Examination 15
Diagnosis 16
Treatment planning 16

HISTORY

This chapter outlines the general principles of taking a history, conducting an examination and, having made a diagnosis, formulating a treatment plan. Details relating to specific clinical circumstances are expanded in subsequent chapters.

THE PURPOSE OF A HISTORY

Taking a good history is an essential first step in the diagnosis and management of any dental condition. The aim is to establish a rapport with the patient and to obtain an accurate account of individual concerns and circumstances which, following examination, will enable a diagnosis to be made and a treatment plan formulated. Whilst numerous schemes for obtaining a history have been described, information is gained with maximal efficiency by following a routine and systematic mode of enquiry.

PRESENTING COMPLAINT

Any history should begin with an invitation to the patient to explain the main problem or reason for attending, to: • indicate what is worrying the patient • help establish rapport by showing empathy.

Patients are often poor historians; thus there is a need to direct the history by asking specific questions related to the history of the presenting complaint. If there is more than one complaint, try to establish the patient's main concern. Avoid leading questions.

HISTORY OF PRESENTING COMPLAINT

Having established the patient's main concern, enquiry into the history of the problem provides valuable clues. The presenting complaint should be recorded by using the patient's own terms as much as possible. It is also necessary to establish the nature of the problem, e.g. is it: • pain, discomfort or merely an abnormal feeling? • an aesthetic problem? • altered function? • bleeding or exudate? • swelling? • halitosis?

Determine • When was the problem first noticed? • Is it continuous or intermittent? • If intermittent, how frequently does it occur? • Are there any initiating or relieving factors? • Is the problem becoming worse, better, or about the same? • Where exactly is the problem?

If *pain* is described as the main problem, the following must be established:

Location Specific tooth or generalized.
Initiating or relieving factors Hot/cold, worse on biting, worse on bending forwards.
Character Dull, sharp, throbbing, shooting.
Severity For example causing sleep loss, relieved by mild analgesics.
Spread/radiation To adjacent structures, referred pain.

The diagnosis of pulpal pain is discussed in detail on page 232.

 Remember, pain thresholds vary greatly between individuals.

PREVIOUS DENTAL HISTORY

Establish • Previous episodes of similar nature • Regular/irregular dental attender • When patient last received dental treatment • Attitude to dental treatment – anxious, relaxed.

PREVIOUS MEDICAL HISTORY

Knowledge of a patient's general health is essential and should be obtained before examination. It is best obtained by questionnaire (Table 2.1). This emphasizes the routine nature of enquiry into medical history as some patients fail to appreciate the relevance of general health to dental treatment. Elderly patients and those with language or literacy problems may need help in completing the questionnaire. Clarify any areas of uncertainty. This part of the history should be updated routinely at each patient visit.

Even when a questionnaire has been completed with no positive response, it is worth asking a general screening question of the patient such as, 'Are you generally fit and well?' or 'Are you attending any doctors or clinics or taking any medicines or tablets?' It is the clinician's responsibility to ensure that an accurate medical history has been obtained prior to commencing an examination.

SOCIAL HISTORY

Questions here relate to factors likely to influence dental disease or availability for treatment. Thus it is desirable to establish: • patient's

TABLE 2.1 Relevant questions in a medical history

Details	YES	NO
Do you feel generally healthy?	☐	☐
Have you had rheumatic fever or infective endocarditis?	☐	☐
Have you had hepatitis or jaundice?	☐	☐
Do you have any heart problems such as angina, heart murmur, replacement valve or have you suffered a heart attack?	☐	☐
Do you have high blood pressure?	☐	☐
Do you suffer from bronchitis, asthma or any other chest condition?	☐	☐
Do you have diabetes?	☐	☐
Do you have arthritis?	☐	☐
Have you ever had any infectious diseases such as hepatitis, HIV, TB or other infectious disease?	☐	☐
Are you receiving any tablets, creams or ointments from your doctor?	☐	☐
Are you using any tablets, creams, ointments, powders or medicines bought 'over the counter' in a pharmacy or shop?	☐	☐
Are you taking, or have you taken steroids in the last 2 years?	☐	☐
Are you allergic to any medicines, food or materials (e.g. latex)?	☐	☐
Do you suffer from epilepsy or are you prone to fainting attacks?	☐	☐
Have you ever bled excessively following a cut or tooth extraction?	☐	☐
Are you pregnant?	☐	☐
Have you been hospitalized? If yes, what for and when?	☐	☐
Are you attending any other hospital clinics or specialists?	☐	☐
Do you smoke?	☐	☐
Who is your doctor?		

age • occupation • marital circumstances • dependants • smoking habit • alcohol consumption.

 A good history should help considerably towards a diagnosis even before physical examination of the patient is carried out.

EXAMINATION

At this stage it is necessary to make the transition from questioning the patient to physical examination. Give reassurance as this is a troublesome moment for anxious patients.

Examination essentially begins when patients enter the surgery as much can be learned from their general demeanour. Do they look fit and well? Are they relaxed or apprehensive? The first few minutes of a consultation are important in establishing a rapport and communication between dentist and patient.

EXTRAORAL EXAMINATION

Look for • General appearance of patient. • Swellings of the face and neck. • Skeletal pattern. • Lip competency.
• temporomandibular joint (TMJ) problems.

Palpate • Lymph nodes. • TMJ. • Muscles of mastication.

INTRAORAL EXAMINATION

It is reassuring to the patient to look initially at the presenting complaint as this emphasizes your role as a caring professional.

Follow this by a systematic, detailed examination and note:
• condition of soft tissues, taking care to include lingual sulcus, floor of mouth, retromolar regions and record abnormal appearance, swelling, sinuses • teeth present, missing, unerupted • general state of the dentition • oral hygiene status • presence and site of restorations and carious lesions • presence and age of dentures • non-carious tooth surface loss, wear facets and 'high spots' • periodontal condition • path of closure of the mandible, premature contacts, overerupted teeth, intercuspal relationship, overbite, overjet • relation of the teeth in function – contacts on lateral and protrusive movements of the mandible.

DIAGNOSIS

PROVISIONAL DIAGNOSIS

From the history and examination a *provisional diagnosis* is made.
This provisional diagnosis may be part of a *differential diagnosis* –
whereby the most probable diagnosis is listed first, followed by
other possible diagnoses. However, special tests or investigations
may be required to confirm the diagnosis.

SPECIAL TESTS AND INVESTIGATIONS

Radiographs Should be used only to obtain additional information
   to supplement clinical findings. Principles governing the taking
   of radiographs are detailed in Chapter 4.
Sensitivity (vitality) tests Rely on stimulation of pulp either by
   application of thermal stimuli (e.g. ethyl chloride) or electrical
   stimuli. Measures response of pain receptors rather than testing
   blood flow. Can be complicated in multirooted or heavily
   restored teeth.
Study models Used to study occlusal relationships, design of
   bridges, partial dentures.
Biopsy Allows histological examination of tissues (p. 398).
Blood tests Important for some conditions (e.g. oral ulceration) and
   in patient management (e.g. INR for patients on warfarin).

DIAGNOSIS

From the history, examination and special tests, a *definitive
diagnosis* should be reached and *recorded in the patient's case
record*. Obviously there may be more than one definitive diagnosis
in the same patient, e.g. dental caries, periodontal disease,
toothbrush abrasion, and each should be clearly recorded.

TREATMENT PLANNING

The purpose of a treatment plan is to provide a work schedule. The
following principles apply:

1. Relieve pain. It is crucial that any patient presenting in pain
   receives treatment aimed at pain relief.
2. Extract teeth of hopeless prognosis. However, extraction of
   asymptomatic teeth may be delayed, especially if patient is

anxious (further treatment may improve confidence). Delaying extraction of anterior teeth may obviate the need for partial denture/bridge until oral hygiene has been improved.

3. Provide preventive advice.
4. Improve periodontal condition.
5. Restore carious teeth.
6. More advanced treatment procedures – endodontics, crowns, bridges, partial dentures.
7. Recall maintenance – the schedule for recall should be judged by disease risk status of the patient. The National Institute for Health and Clinical Excellence (NICE) has issued guidance on the frequency of recall for dental examination (p. 164).

FACTORS INFLUENCING TREATMENT PLANNING

Many factors influence treatment options available in individual circumstances. Frequently a compromise must be achieved between what the patient wants and what is technically feasible. Factors influencing treatment include:

Patient-related factors • complicating medical history • patient anxiety • inability/unwillingness to maintain adequate standards of plaque control • inability to afford time required for proposed treatment.

Dentist-related factors • treatment options may depend on ability of dentist • access to specialist services.

Cost-related factors • treatment available may depend on what patient can afford • availability of planned procedures under the health care system or insurance scheme covering patient's treatment.

Other factors in treatment planning • Don't comment definitively on treatment until examination, special tests and diagnosis are complete • Formulation of a treatment plan requires consultation with patient to select the most appropriate and acceptable plan • In any complex treatment schedule build in contingency plans; allow for 'what if?' • Good oral hygiene and adherence to preventive advice is of prime importance • Work on one segment (e.g. quadrant) of the mouth at a time • In anxious patients, carry out simplest treatment first.

CHAPTER 3

LAW, ETHICS AND QUALITY DENTAL CARE

Ethical and medico-legal considerations associated with dental care   20

Quality dental care   25

Clinical governance   25

Clinical audit   26

Evidence-based dentistry   28

Clinical effectiveness   28

Continuing professional development and lifelong learning   29

Significant event analysis   30

Complaints   30

Underperformance   31

Conclusion   31

Reference   32

ETHICAL AND MEDICO-LEGAL CONSIDERATIONS ASSOCIATED WITH DENTAL CARE

Patients have a right to expect that those providing dental care and treatment will do so safely, legally, appropriately and with a suitable degree of skill, attention and care. In the United Kingdom and most other jurisdictions there is a requirement for dentists and other members of the dental team to be registered with the regulatory authority. They must also hold adequate indemnity or liability insurance so that patients can be compensated in the event of mishap. In the United Kingdom the practice of dentistry is defined within the Dentists Act 1984. Illegal practice can result in prosecution under the criminal law. It is essential therefore that all members of the dental team understand their regulatory requirements and abide by them.

LEGISLATION

Dentistry in the United Kingdom is governed by the Dentists Act 1984 and the regulatory authority is the General Dental Council. If the Council considers that patients could be placed at risk by a registrant, it has the power to withdraw that individual's licence to practise or impose restrictions on their practice.

In addition to the Dentists Act, legislation impinges on virtually all aspects of dental practice and it is beyond the scope of this book to detail the implications of each individual Act or item of secondary legislation. Examples of legislation of particular significance in dental practice are given in Table 3.1. All dentists and Dental Care Professionals (DCPs, p. 165) should be aware of the implications of such legislation. Employment legislation also applies to those employing and directing dental personnel.

ETHICAL GUIDANCE

In 1998, the General Dental Council replaced their previous ethical guidance publication, *The Red Book*, with a much more prescriptive guidance *Maintaining Standards*. This was, in turn, replaced on 1 June 2005 with a much less prescriptive guidance called *Guidance for Dental Professionals*. This is likely to form the basis for establishing contemporaneous standards for many years to come.[1]

Irrespective of any published guidance, all those involved in patient care have an ethical duty:

● to do good, not harm
● to always act in their patient's best interests

TABLE 3.1 Legislation of relevance to dental practice
Ionising Radiation (Medical Exposure) Regulations 2000
Freedom of Information Act 2000
Freedom of Information (Scotland) Act 2002
Data Protection Act 1998
Health Act 1999
Health and Social Care Act 2001
Smoking Health and Social Care (Scotland) Act 2005
Cosmetic Product Regulations 1996 (as amended)
Various NHS Acts and Regulations
Health and Safety legislation
Employment legislation
Discrimination legislation

- to put their patient's best interests above their own
- to attempt, if possible, to relieve their patient's pain and suffering
- to ensure that they have sufficient knowledge by way of training and enquiry of the patient or others associated with that patient's care or well-being to ensure that they are acting in their patient's best interests
- to be honest.

DUTY OF CARE

A patient has a right to expect that any treatment or care that they receive from dentists or DCPs, holding themselves out to have a particular skill, will be provided safely and to a standard that would be adjudged reasonable by those holding themselves out to have that particular skill. In other words not the best, nor indeed the worst but reasonable skill and care, as judged by one's peers. A general dental practitioner would not be expected to have the same skill as a consultant but would be expected to know their own limitations and when it is appropriate to refer.

It is necessary for all practices to have robust, tested, cross-infection control protocols, procedures and policies in place (Appendix E).

A failure to fulfil one's duty of care to a patient with recoverable damage resulting (known in law as 'causation') is the basis for a claim by a patient in negligence.

CONFIDENTIALITY

All members of the dental team are bound by an ethical duty of confidentiality. It is essential that all staff have confirmed that they understand the need for confidentiality and have agreed to abide by the practice confidentiality protocol.

CONSENT

UK law holds integrity of the body in high regard. Treatment without a patient's consent could be regarded as trespass to the person or assault (dependent upon the jurisdiction) even if the treatment was appropriate, carried out with appropriate skill and in the patient's best interests.

The law permits a presumption of capacity regarding adults, in the absence of contrary information. Adults with capacity to consent have a right to refuse any treatment. Those providing care must be mindful of this and also of the requirements in their own jurisdiction when treating minors, infants or those unable to consent for themselves.

Regulatory authorities and employers may require practitioners to obtain written consent for treatment or particular types of treatment. The General Dental Council has defined that within the UK written consent is required for sedation and general anaesthesia. The prudent practitioner should also ensure that complex irreversible forms of treatment also receive written consent.

As a result of recent judgements, UK law is moving towards a doctrine of 'informed consent', but is still not as prescriptive as in certain states in the USA. The requirement in the UK is for patients to be given sufficient information, with regard to benefits, risks and possible complications, that they can come to a rational decision as to whether they wish to have the treatment carried out.

It is essential, therefore, that the patient's clinical record indicates clearly that a process of consent has been undertaken and that patients have been given sufficient information to come to a rational decision without any duress placed upon them.

CONTRACTUAL CONSIDERATIONS

Dental care and treatment can be carried out under different contractual regimes and it is incumbent upon the healthcare professional to ensure that the patient is fully aware of the nature of that contract. Healthcare professionals need to know the obligations that contracts place upon them. It is an implied term of any contract within the UK that the contract will be carried out with reasonable skill and care. Much dental treatment in the UK is carried out by practitioners in contract with a health authority providing care under a contract of employment (e.g. hospital and community employees), a contract under the general dental services or under a personal dental service type contract.

Under such contracts, the contract holder will have contractual duties and be subject to Terms of Service as laid down by the health authority who are parties to those contracts. Failure to comply might result not only in a breach of contract claim but also in implementation of disciplinary measures by the health authority under the contractual terms.

Although the patient and dentist may not have a direct contract between each other when treated under the National Health Service (NHS) general dental services or personal dental services, patients may still have contractual redress under third party rights in addition to claims in negligence or trespass. Third party funders, other than health authorities, may also prescribe contractual terms that require adherence by those carrying out patient care.

Those receiving private dental care will be in direct contract with the other contracting party, generally the dentist responsible for the patient's care. As well as the implication that any treatment will be of satisfactory quality, a patient may consider that remarks, comments or statements made by the practitioner form an express term of the contract (e.g. 'you will be able to eat better,' or 'you will look fantastic'), facilitating a possible potential claim for breach of contract.

REFERRAL

It is incumbent upon all practitioners to accept the limitations of their own skill and refer appropriately when required. As well as the act of referring, the practitioner should refer to an appropriate person and provide that person with sufficient information, in writing, for them to consider the urgency of that referral and whether it is appropriate for them to accept the referral. Particular attention must therefore be paid to furnishing those to whom practitioners refer with adequate referral letters.

It may be held out to be a misrepresentation for a dentist to profess that they have skills or abilities that their training and experience would not support when reviewed by peers. Dentists professing to have particular skills with regard to the provision of cosmetic treatments, particularly outwith the mouth or perioral region or outwith the practice of dentistry, may find themselves challenged by the regulatory authorities or the law in this regard.

TREATMENT

It is essential that treatment carried out is likely to be considered necessary when subjected to analysis by one's peers and would be considered appropriate treatment of a contemporaneous standard and in accordance with current treatment rationales. Any treatment which might be construed as outwith 'the norm' will require justification both in the clinical record and with reference to research and the practitioner's own review process. Similar caution and readily accessible justification must be apparent when treatment is carried out that could be construed as being of doubtful benefit to the patient.

Given a practitioner's ethical duty, the treatment must be considered appropriate and effective particularly with regard to the patient's presenting complaint and the need to deal expeditiously with any pain, suffering or potentiality for pain or suffering. A detailed appraisal of current acceptable operative techniques is readily available from up-to-date textbooks, journals, the Internet and similar sources.

RECORD KEEPING

Clinical records

The value of full, contemporaneous clinical records cannot be overstated. The making and retention of adequate contemporaneous records is a requirement of all dental care contracts. Clinical records also form the basis for establishing appropriate treatment planning, the completion of an adequate consenting process as well as the provision of adequate care in all circumstances.

Given the significance that may subsequently be placed upon the clinical record if a patient complains or queries their treatment, a full charting of both the restorations and teeth present as well as those requiring treatment or observation is desirable.

Periodontal assessment and appropriate charting is required. The record should also contain:

- advice and warnings issued
- a record of failure by the patient to comply with advice
- notes of missed or broken appointments.

A positive record regarding a patient's presenting condition, even if unremarkable, shows that any complaints have been addressed satisfactorily. An actual note in the clinical record supporting that a patient presented with no complaints is far more powerful than attempting to construe that no record of a complaint within the written note is indicative of no presenting problem.

Whoever writes the record, the clinician with ultimate responsibility for the patient's dental care will hold primary responsibility for any omissions or inadequacies.

Addenda can be added to notes subsequently, in light of ensuing events, but the record should never be altered or erased after the event. In the UK and Europe, given current consumer legislation, clinical records should be retained for at least 11 years after a patient last attended or after they reached the age of majority (18 in England, Wales and Northern Ireland, 16 in Scotland).

An adequate clinical governance protocol governing precisely how each item of treatment, examination or review is carried out will reduce the amount of information that is required to be written on the patient's record on each occasion (p. 29).

Records should be kept safely and access only given to those who are entitled to access them and who are bound by confidentiality agreements. Where records are held electronically, right of access to entries must be controlled securely and computerized records should be password protected. In the UK patients have rights to access their records and have the contents explained to them under the Data Protection Act 1998.

Other records

Records must be kept to comply with requirements for Continuing Professional Development (CPD), clinical audit, peer review, etc. Records demonstrate compliance with Health and Safety, employment, radiation and fire legislation; they are also a statutory requirement. Additionally, documentation will be required to be available when practices are inspected by contracting health authorities. The Freedom of Information Act further requires any dental practice providing NHS care in the UK to have a Publication Schedule available demonstrating what documentation is available from the practice for inspection.

QUALITY DENTAL CARE

Currently much emphasis is being placed on improving the quality of healthcare provision. This section describes some of the terms and definitions that have been introduced to describe quality issues. Whilst some of the terms are new, many of the concepts are not.

CLINICAL GOVERNANCE

Introduced in the 1998 White Paper *A First Class Service – Quality in the New NHS*. Many definitions have been suggested, including:

A framework through which NHS organizations are accountable for continuously improving the quality of their services and safeguarding high standards of care by creating an environment in which high standards of care will flourish. Or:

Corporate responsibility for the delivery of quality healthcare.

CLINICAL AUDIT

Clinical audit is the process of reviewing the delivery of healthcare to identify deficiencies so that they may be remedied.

Clinical audit is an essential tool within a clinical governance regime and over a period should cover all aspects of clinical practice. Clinical audit requires the collection and interpretation of data in a manner that can be repeated, to show that any changes resultant from the audit have been effective when re-audit takes place. Establishing an *audit cycle* in this manner provides a tool to demonstrate effectiveness.

Clinical audit is a cyclical process (Figure 3.1). It is conducted as follows: • look critically at a particular aspect of practice • think about how what is being done compares to a defined standard • measure what is being done against the standard • implement change • monitor progress by measuring again after change has been implemented.

Clinical audit is a practice-based procedure that should be owned and participated in by all members of the dental team. Clinical audit assumes much greater importance and relevance when it can be seen to address and reduce or remove existing problems or difficulties within the practice. However, to be effective it must also be anonymous so that individuals do not feel threatened by results that demonstrate a need for change of their particular practice.

In the absence of awareness of evident problems that require attention, patient questionnaires can provide useful ideas as to where to start a clinical audit. It is imperative to ensure that everyone within the practice is involved with the design of such questionnaires as they may receive criticism. Questionnaires must also be constructed in such a way that the collected data can readily be interpreted and the collection repeated in the future. It is also

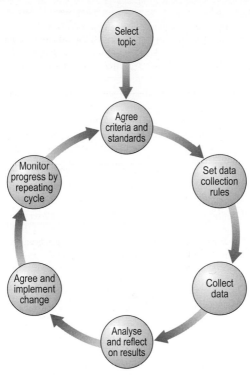

Figure 3.1 The clinical audit cycle.

essential to ensure that patients are given the opportunity to give positive as well as negative feedback concerning the practice.

Audits must be specific and not too wide ranging; results should be shared with all concerned and contained within a readily accessible clinical audit file. They should not be shared with third parties as a management or disciplinary tool; they must primarily be educative for those taking part.

Audit and research

It is important to understand the difference between research and audit. • Healthcare research is about extending the body of knowledge of best practice. • Audit is about measuring whether best practice is being adopted.

Peer review

Operates alongside clinical audit in general practice. Groups of dentists, usually four to eight, meet in an atmosphere of complete confidentiality to review aspects of practice. Not focused like audit, but standards emerge as part of the discussion. Less formal than audit.

Peer review provides an effective mechanism for reviewing clinical practice and procedures amongst colleagues; however, it requires a high degree of trust to be established and a mutual respect of participants one for the other. Over a period of time all aspects of practice can be reviewed. Although a culture can be established by participants within the same practice, peer review is most effective when more than one practice participates in the process. Peer review must of necessity be non-threatening. It must be educational and should remain the property of the participants. Although individual participants or practices should be able to identify their own results within the collected, analysed data, the results should be anonymous to all others, particularly regarding the identity of individual patients or practitioners.

EVIDENCE-BASED DENTISTRY

> Evidence-based dentistry implies the use of techniques and procedures that have been shown by both research and audit to be clinically effective.

The practice of evidence-based dentistry means integrating individual clinical expertise with the best available external clinical evidence from systematic research. Evidence comes from clinical trials, of which the randomized controlled trial (RCT) is viewed as the gold standard.

Systematic reviews collate evidence (both published and unpublished) from different studies (of one or more experimental designs), summarize and grade the evidence available.

Evidence is disseminated in the form of *clinical guidelines*.

CLINICAL EFFECTIVENESS

Treatment which is ineffective or unnecessary is unlikely to be regarded by peers as satisfactory. Practitioners therefore should carry out audits and hold records to demonstrate effectiveness: covering, for example, items such as longevity of particular treatments. If a practitioner perceives that a particular treatment fails or has short longevity in their hands, yet allegedly gives good results for others, the reasons for this disparity should be ascertained and if possible addressed. Records of such review are frequently an effective rebuttal to any allegation of failure of a practitioner's duty of care.

Improving clinical performance

Risk management and reporting of critical incidents are seen as important aspects of delivering quality care. Dental practitioners would be well advised to have in place, and to be able to demonstrate, procedures and protocols for dealing with risk, handling patient complaints, etc.

Protocols

The clinical record must be full, contemporaneous and accurate. However, if written protocols are developed within a practice and rigidly adhered to, the amount of detail in an individual patient record can be reduced. For example, if a dental examination always follows a standard protocol that defines all that is carried out, plus additionally the records confirm the necessary chartings, notes, etc., confirming compliance, the minutiae of the examination will not be required to be recorded each time.

It is part of clinical governance that patients receive care of consistent quality. This requires the establishment of guidelines which are developed into written protocols. The protocols must also be regularly audited and if necessary reviewed and updated.

A simple, but invaluable protocol should for example, cover how a dental practice receives and deals with telephone calls. Many practitioners fail to realize the potential pitfalls resulting from a failure in communication when a patient contacts the surgery – these are easily prevented with a robust protocol that is rigidly followed.

Patient and user involvement

Taking into account the views of patients and their carers is seen as an important aspect of quality healthcare.

CONTINUING PROFESSIONAL DEVELOPMENT AND LIFELONG LEARNING

Continuing Professional Development (CPD) is a requirement for all members of the practice team. The UK's General Dental Council lays down requirements for CPD to ensure that all members of the team keep up to date with current practice. Prescribed numbers of hours are required to maintain registration with the GDC.

This is divided into: • verifiable CPD (activities for which some form of confirmation of participation is available, e.g. formal courses) 15 hours per year • general CPD (e.g. self-directed learning, journal reading) 35 hours per year.

SIGNIFICANT EVENT ANALYSIS

Sometimes referred to as critical incident analysis. It should become an established part of the practice procedure for all members of the dental team to analyse what went well, not just what went badly and then subsequently establish how successes may be repeated and how any mistakes or shortcomings may be prevented. A good record of such events should be retained.

COMPLAINTS

It is imperative that complaints are dealt with appropriately, expeditiously and sympathetically, ensuring that all matters relevant and the patient's viewpoint are taken into account. Practices must have a written complaints policy which should be strictly followed; a rapid acknowledgement is essential. In the UK acknowledgement of receipt of the complaint should be made within 2 days, if possible, with a full response made within 10 days (general practice) or 20 days (hospital and community practice).

How a complaint is dealt with is obviously a matter of personal preference dependent on the circumstances. However, it is important that if the complaint is not dealt with entirely in writing, that prior to any meeting there is a note made of all the items of concern and that the meeting has a structured agenda. After such a meeting the issues raised and their resolution should be recorded as a minute and distributed and verified as accurate by all parties. An apology does not need to be an admission of liability; those complained about should never be afraid therefore to apologize if the facts deem this appropriate.

Complaints should be recorded anonymously so that they can be used as an educative tool as part of the practice clinical governance programme. Effective dental care requires the confidence of the patient and the dental care team members one for the other. If such confidence has never been apparent or has been lost and is incapable of restoration, it should be suggested to the complainant that it is in their own best interests to seek their dental care elsewhere; such an action should be regarded as a pragmatic, appropriate remedy rather than a failure.

UNDERPERFORMANCE

Practices must have a written underperformance policy that all members of the team endorse and follow. The causes of underperformance or inappropriate performance are myriad but it is important to separate dishonesty from underperformance and deal with each differently.

Honesty is an ethical requirement of dentists and DCPs. They are in a position of trust and any attempt to address dishonesty or resolve it must ensure that a position of trust can be restored.

Underperformance not associated with dishonesty should be dealt with sympathetically, ensuring that any danger to patients is immediately removed; it is also essential that the cause is identified and addressed.

Dealing with underperformance is difficult and harrowing for all involved but is an ethical obligation. The Dentist Help Support Trust, which can be contacted via the British Dental Association in London, does sterling work to assist dentists with alcohol, drug and health problems. Underperformance due to lack of ability or knowledge will require structured CPD or even retraining in some other discipline.

Data collection and retention

Governance in whatever sphere requires the collection and retention of accurate, relevant data in a usable format. Data must never be collected or computed in a fashion to give a specific desired result. Wherever possible, data should be anonymized, non-threatening and capable of being collected again in the future in a similar format.

The data itself should be used as an educational tool to verify performance and address performance issues; its collection, interpretation and retention should not be regarded as a chore by team members but as an essential clinical tool and a robust authentification to counteract allegations regarding inappropriate performance.

CONCLUSION

Research has shown that most patients have high levels of confidence in those providing them with dental care The dental profession can be proud of this but such good reputations are harder to achieve than to lose. In this litigious society we must strive to ensure than we have hard fact rather than anecdotal evidence to demonstrate that our patients' faith in the dental profession and the care it provides for patients is justified.

REFERENCE

1. General Dental Council 2005 Guidance for Dental Professionals. General Dental Council, London. www.gdc-uk.org

CHAPTER 4

DENTAL RADIOLOGY

The nature of X-rays, their production and interaction   34

Radiation dose measurement and radiation protection   36

Ionizing radiation regulations   42

Radiographic technique   43

Guidelines for the prescription of radiographs   50

Interpretation of radiographs   56

Differential diagnosis of radiographic lesions   56

References   58

THE NATURE OF X-RAYS, THEIR PRODUCTION AND INTERACTION

X-rays form part of the electromagnetic spectrum together with radiation such as radio waves and light. Radio waves, which lie at one end of this spectrum, have a long wavelength but are of low energy; X-rays on the other hand have a short wavelength but are of high energy.

X-rays were discovered in 1895 by Conrad Roentgen and were so-called because at that time the nature of the radiation was unknown. Later it was realized that X-rays were the same as gamma radiation. However, the beam generated by an X-ray tube (Figure 4.1) consists of X-ray photons with a range of different energies, whereas gamma rays that are produced by a radioactive source are of a single energy characteristic of that particular isotope. X-rays are produced in the X-ray tube by bombarding a tungsten target with a stream of electrons, accelerated by a high voltage (typically of 60–70 kV for a dental unit). The process is very inefficient, with only approximately 1% of the energy from the electron stream going into X-rays, 99% being lost as heat.

The larger the voltage, the greater will be the maximum energy of the X-ray photons within the beam, increasing its penetrative power (Figure 4.2). There will still be a range of energies, and this is of fundamental importance to the creation of a radiographic image, as it enhances the differential absorption of the beam by the different tissues of the body. Very-low-energy photons, however,

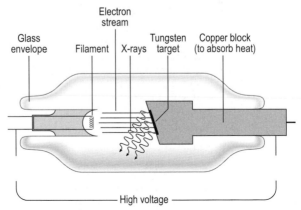

Figure 4.1 X-ray tube.

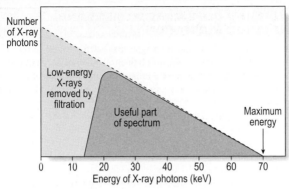

Figure 4.2 X-ray spectrum produced at 70 kV.

would not contribute to the radiographic image, being immediately absorbed by the skin. These are removed using an aluminium filter. The current flowing though the X-ray tube (typically 8–10 mA) will determine the quantity of X-rays produced. The higher the current the less time will be required for the exposure. However, many dental radiography sets have a fixed current, leaving the operator only to adjust the time.

When X-ray photons enter the body, two main interactions occur: *photoelectric absorption* and *Compton scatter*.

PHOTOELECTRIC ABSORPTION

The photoelectric effect predominates with lower-energy photons, the likelihood of this interaction occurring varying with the atomic number (Z) of the tissue. The probability is proportional to Z^3; consequently there is a big difference between the absorption by bone ($Z^3 = 1728$) and soft tissues ($Z^3 = 343$), which is why there is good contrast between these structures on a radiograph, particularly where a relatively low voltage (usually referred to as kV) is used.

COMPTON SCATTER

Compton scatter is the predominant interaction produced by high-energy photons and is not dependent on the atomic number. This accounts for the fact that as the voltage is raised there is less contrast between different tissues.

RADIATION DOSE MEASUREMENT AND RADIATION PROTECTION

The measurement of radiation dose is quite complex. Of particular interest is the assessment of the detrimental effect of a given procedure. To express this several factors must be taken into account.

> Absorbed dose = The amount of energy absorbed from a radiation exposure
> Unit: Gray (Gy) =1 joule absorbed/kg

This measurement can be made for different types of radiation (alpha, beta, gamma/X-rays, etc.) that vary in the degree of ionization that they cause. To assess their detrimental effect on biological tissues, it is necessary to adjust the *absorbed dose by a quality factor (Q)* specific to the type of radiation.

> Equivalent dose = the absorbed dose multiplied by Q
> Unit: Sievert (Sv)
> Q value: X-rays = 1
> Alpha particles = 20
> (therefore for X-rays the equivalent dose is equal to the absorbed dose)

To compare the potential harm caused by different radiographic examinations, it is necessary to make a further adjustment that takes account of the radiosensitivity of the tissues being irradiated. A list of weighting factors has been calculated for different organs of the body. For a particular examination the equivalent dose reaching each of these organs can be measured experimentally and this value is multiplied by the weighting factor for that organ. Adding up the resulting figures for all the tissues involved gives a value that represents the risk of causing biological harm from that procedure. It allows the risk from different examinations in different parts of the body to be compared.

> Effective dose = the equivalent dose multiplied by the tissue weighting factor
> Unit: Sievert (Sv)

When referring to the dose for a particular procedure it is usually the effective dose that is quoted.

DOSES FOR COMMON RADIOGRAPHIC EXAMINATIONS AND THEIR COMPARATIVE RISK

The effective doses of some common radiographic examinations are listed in Table 4.1, together with the amount of background radiation which would give the same risk of biological harm.

The risks from dental radiography can also be compared with those of other activities in everyday life. For instance, the additional radiation received by a patient having two bitewings puts them at the same risk as that from the additional cosmic radiation received in an aeroplane by flying from the UK to Spain and back. However, another factor which must be taken into account is the age of the patient. The figures in Table 4.1 are average figures for the population, but the risk to younger patients is higher for the same amount of radiation received and for older patients it is lower. Table 4.2 lists the multiplication factors to adjust the risk for different age groups.

THE BIOLOGICAL EFFECTS OF RADIATION

Radiation can have two effects on the body: *deterministic* and *stochastic*.

Deterministic effects

Deterministic effects are *certain* to happen if a high enough dose is given. Their severity is dose dependent and it is believed that there is a dose threshold below which no effect will occur. Following high radiation doses, such as in nuclear accidents, deterministic effects include reddening of the skin and the development of cataracts. However, if modern radiation safety rules are followed, none of these effects will result from dental radiography.

Deterministic effects: severity ∝ dose

Stochastic effects

Stochastic effects are those that *may* happen, the chance of their occurrence being proportional to the dose. Stochastic effects include the induction of malignant tumours and, if there is

TABLE 4.1 Dose levels and risks for various radiographic examinations

X-ray examination	Effective dose (mSv)	Risk of cancer (per million examinations)	Equivalent natural background radiation
Two bitewings (70 kV, rectangular collimation and F speed film)	0.0016	0.08	6.4 hours
Two bitewings (70 kV, rectangular collimation and E speed film)	0.002	0.1	8 hours
Two bitewings (70 kV, round collimation and D speed film)	0.008	0.4	32 hours
Two oblique laterals (70 kV and rare earth screens)	0.015	0.75	60 hours
Panoramic (rare earth screens)	0.007	0.35	28 hours
Panoramic (calcium tungstate screens)	0.014	0.8	56 hours
Skull view	0.1	0.5	16.5 days
CT head	2	120	331 days

TABLE 4.2 Risk in relation to age

Age group (years)	Multiplication factor for risk
<10	×3
10–20	×2
20–30	×1.5
30–50	×0.5
50–80	×0.3
80+	negligible risk

Multiplication factor at 30 years = 1.

irradiation of the reproductive organs, the induction of mutations, which may lead to congenital abnormalities. The induction of neoplastic disease is the main risk of radiography.

Stochastic effects: probability $\propto$ dose

DOSE LIMITATION IN DENTAL RADIOGRAPHY

The principles of patient dose limitation can be summarized by two terms: • justification • optimization.

Justification
The prescription of radiographs must, in every case, be of some positive benefit to the patient and influence their treatment. The clinician should be sure that the information required is not already available on any existing films, e.g. root morphology prior to an extraction.

Optimization
Where the decision has been made to request a radiograph, the dose must be kept *as low as reasonably practicable* (ALARP). This can be achieved by using appropriate equipment, good technique and by having a quality control programme in place to ensure that films are consistently of diagnostic quality.

Equipment
X-ray generator • Preferably constant potential rather than AC.
Voltage • 65–70 kV.

FSD • Minimum focus to skin distance of 200 mm for intraoral radiography.

Film holders • For bitewing and periapical radiography.

Collimation • Rectangular collimation for intraoral films. • For panoramic radiography the use of sectional views, where possible, limited to the area of interest and a reduced field of view for children.

Film/screens • Fast film: E or F speed for intraoral views. • Rare earth intensifying screens for extraoral views.

Technique

Radiography should only be undertaken by staff who have been appropriately trained.

The effect on patient dose of different equipment factors is summarized in Table 4.3.

Quality assurance (QA)

Inspection of X-ray equipment • *Critical examination* and *acceptance test* after installation • *Routine tests* at regular intervals, not exceeding 3 years and following relocation, repair or modification • Servicing as directed by the manufacturer.

Checks on darkroom, films and processing • Processing conditions and changing of chemicals • Light-tightness of darkroom • Performance of safe lights • Film storage and expiry dates.

Programme of staff training • Rigorous and ongoing.

TABLE 4.3 Equipment factors and dose

Equipment factors	Multiplication factor for estimating the effective dose
Digital system (phosphor plate)	×0.25–0.75
Digital system (CCD)	×0.5
Rectangular collimation	×0.5
F-speed film	×0.8
'DC' constant potential	×0.8
'Short cone' (10 cm fsd)	×1.5
50 kV set	×2
D-speed film	×2

Image quality • Subjective assessment of each film against a reference film kept on the viewing box. National Radiological Protection Board/Royal College of Radiologists[1] recommend a three-point quality rating (Table 4.4) and quality targets (Table 4.5) • Analysis of reject film on a regular basis to identify faults and to allow changes to be implemented to prevent their recurrence.

Audit • Records should be kept of the QA procedures and an audit of them carried out at least every 12 months.

LEAD APRONS AND RADIOGRAPHY IN PREGNANCY

There is no justification for the routine use of lead aprons for patients in dental radiography, and for panoramic radiography their use is positively discouraged as the apron may interfere with the movement of the machine. A thyroid collar is of value if the gland is in the primary beam, as occurs in an upper standard occlusal, but otherwise, if rectangular collimation and the paralleling technique are used, thyroid shielding is unnecessary.

TABLE 4.4 Subjective quality rating of radiographs[1]

Rating	Quality	Basis
1	Excellent	No errors of patient preparation, exposure, positioning, processing or film handling
2	Diagnostically acceptable	Some errors of patient preparation, exposure, positioning, processing or film handling, but do not detract from the diagnostic utility of the radiograph
3	Unacceptable	Errors of patient preparation, exposure, positioning, processing or film handling which render the radiograph diagnostically unacceptable

TABLE 4.5 Minimum targets for radiographic quality[1]

Rating	Percentage of radiographs taken
1	Not less than 70%
2	Not greater than 20%
3	Not greater than 10%

The Ionizing Radiation (Medical Exposure) Regulations 2000 prohibit the carrying out of a medical exposure on a female of child-bearing age without enquiry as to whether she is pregnant, if this is relevant. In dentistry this enquiry should not normally be necessary as the only view where the primary beam is directed towards the pelvic area is the vertex occlusal. This projection is rarely used now and is difficult to justify for a pregnant woman. Although some practitioners avoid radiography in patients known to be pregnant, essentially for psychological reasons, a more pragmatic approach is to explain to the patient that for the majority of dental projections, the pelvic area is not irradiated directly and that the dose received by the fetus from scattered radiation is so small that the associated risk can be regarded as negligible. Radiography should be limited to those films necessary for assessing an acute problem; any non-urgent radiography should be delayed until after the birth.

If these guidelines are followed it is unnecessary to use a lead apron even during pregnancy, although its use may be of some psychological benefit.

IONIZING RADIATION REGULATIONS

Dentists who use X-ray equipment in the UK must now comply with the Ionizing Radiations 1999 and the Ionizing Radiation (Medical Exposure) Regulations 2000. Guidance on the implementation of these regulations are contained in the Guidance Notes.[2]

The important points are as follows:

Notification The employer (practice principal) must notify the Health and Safety Executive before work with ionizing radiation is carried out for the first time.

Risk assessment This must be carried out by the employer to assess the risk to any employee from the use of radiographic equipment and to identify precautionary measures that may be required.

Radiation Protection Adviser (RPA) Dentists must now formally appoint an RPA, a physicist, who will advise on compliance with the regulations.

A controlled area This must be designated around an X-ray unit in consultation with the RPA. The standard approach is: • within the primary beam until sufficiently attenuated by distance or shielding • within 1.5 m of the X-ray tube or the patient's head.

Local rules These must be provided for any controlled area and a Radiation Protection Supervisor (RPS) must be appointed to ensure compliance with the regulations and the local rules. The RPS will usually be a dentist or a suitably trained person.

Personnel Three categories of staff are designated: the referrer (requests the radiograph), the practitioner (justifies the exposure – a radiologist in a hospital) and the operator (operates the machine). In a dental practice all three jobs will probably be carried out by the dentist unless there is a dental nurse with radiographic training who may act as the operator.

Training The practitioner and operator must have received adequate training and must undertake continuing education.

Justification and optimization No person shall carry out an exposure unless it has been justified by the practitioner as being of net benefit to the patient. Once the decision has been made to take a radiograph, the dose must be kept ALARP. To aid optimization each practice should set diagnostic reference levels (DRLs) for each type of projection. These are doses based on published guidelines,[3] which should not be exceeded.

Quality assurance (QA) Dental practices must have a QA programme for all procedures and this must be audited. X-ray equipment must be serviced regularly and radiation safety tests carried out at least every 3 years.

RADIOGRAPHIC TECHNIQUE

INTRAORAL VIEWS
Periapical radiography

Paralleling technique A film holder is used that aligns the film parallel to the tooth and also has a guide (beam aiming device) to position the beam at 90° to the film. This projection gives the most accurate and reproducible image of the tooth and periapical tissues.

Bisecting angle technique The film is placed against the back of the tooth and the X-ray tube is aligned at 90° to the plane halfway between the tooth and the film. The patient used to be asked to hold the film in place with their finger, but it is now advisable to use a film holder to avoid irradiating the hand. The advantage of the bisecting angle technique is that where there is a limited amount of space, such as in patients with a shallow palate, this technique can be easier to perform than the paralleling technique. The disadvantage is that the technique is prone to inaccuracy due to misjudgement of the vertical angulation of the tube. This leads to elongation or foreshortening of the image.

Bitewing

This projection is used to image the crowns of the teeth in both arches and usually allows the alveolar bone levels to be assessed.

The technique originally involved the patient biting down on a paper tab stuck on to the film packet (from which the name derives), but it is now advisable to use a film holder to facilitate more accurate positioning. The X-ray tube is positioned at 90° to the dental arch in the horizontal plane so that the beam passes between the contact points. In the vertical plane the beam is aimed down at 5–7° to the horizontal to avoid overlapping the cusp tips, which are inclined because of the curve of Monson.

Occlusal radiographs

Upper standard occlusal The film is placed centrally between the two dental arches with the beam aligned through the bridge of the nose with a 60° downward angulation. This view is used to detect pathology and buried or supernumerary teeth in the palate. Information about the position of a buried tooth relative to the dental arch can be gained using the principle of parallax by combining this view with another taken at different horizontal or vertical angle.

Upper true (vertex) occlusal The film is placed centrally between the two dental arches with the X-ray tube positioned at the vertex of the skull pointing down the long axis of the upper teeth. This view clearly shows the position of a buried or supernumerary tooth relative to the dental arch, but the projection results in a relatively high dose of radiation to the lens of the eye and consequently is no longer recommended.

Upper oblique occlusal The film packet is placed between the dental arches, positioned over to the side under investigation with the X-ray beam angled down at 65–70°. This view shows the posterior teeth, the surrounding bone and the antral floor. It is useful for imaging pathology, dentoalveolar fractures and roots displaced into the antrum.

Lower standard occlusal The film is placed centrally between the two dental arches with the beam aligned with a 45° upward angulation through the chin. This view shows the lower incisor teeth and surrounding bone and is useful for demonstrating pathology that extends beyond the limits of a periapical film.

Lower true occlusal The film is placed centrally between the two dental arches with the beam aligned at 90° to it. This film is used to assess mandibular fractures of the anterior mandible and the buccolingual expansion of lesions such as cysts and tumours. It is also used to identify calculi in the submandibular ducts.

Lower oblique occlusal The film packet is placed between the dental arches, positioned over to the side under investigation with the X-ray beam angled up from below and behind the angle of the mandible. This view is usually used in conjunction with the lower true occlusal for the detection of salivary calculi. It will identify stones in the posterior part of the submandibular duct and in the gland. It can also be used to assess the buccolingual expansion of lesions in the posterior part of the body of the mandible.

EXTRAORAL PROJECTIONS

Panoramic

Also referred to as a dental panoramic tomogram (DPT) or by a trade name, orthopantomogram (OPT/OPG). An image of the dental arches is produced by the technique of tomography that involves rotating the X-ray tube and film producing blurring of the structures on either side of the centre of rotation. In dental panoramic tomography a horseshoe-shaped in-focus plane (focal trough) is produced by moving the centre of rotation during the exposure. Care must be taken in patient positioning to ensure that the teeth lie within the trough. A panoramic image is magnified by 1.2–1.3 times. Failure to position the patient correctly results in changes in the horizontal magnification.

- Patient too far into the machine → narrow anterior teeth.
- Patient too far out of the machine → wide anterior teeth.
- Patient rotated posterior → teeth and rami are wider on one side and narrower on the other.

The anatomical features observable on a panoramic radiograph are illustrated in Figure 4.3.

Oblique lateral

Used to image the posterior maxilla and mandible but largely superseded by the panoramic. The patient is positioned with head tilted against the film. The beam is then aligned at 90° to it from under the angle of the mandible on the contralateral side.

Posteroanterior (PA) jaw

Used to assess fractures and pathology in the posterior mandible and condyles. The patient is positioned with nose and forehead against film. The beam is aimed horizontally from behind the head.

Reverse Towne's projection

Used to assess the condyles. The patient is positioned in a similar way to a PA but with the mouth open to bring the condyles out of

Bony anatomy:
1. Nasal septum
2. Nasal cavity
3. Inferior concha
4. Anterior nasal spine
5. Infra-orbital rim
6. Infra-orbital canal
7. Floor of nose/hard palate
8. Zygomatic buttress
9. Zygomatic arch
10. Pterygo-maxillary fissure
11. Lateral pterygoid plate
12. Articular eminence
13. External auditory meatus
14. Styloid process
15. Mandibular condyle
16. Sigmoid notch
17. Cervical vertebrae
18. Foramen transversarium
19. External oblique ridge
20. Internal oblique ridge
21. Mandibular foramen
22. Inferior alveolar canal
23. Mental foramen
24. Bony cortex of inferior border of mandible
25. Antegonial notch
26. Hyoid bone
27. Coronoid process

Soft tissue anatomy and air shadows:
A. Outline of adenoids
B. Outline of soft palate
C. Outline of ear lobe
D. Air in nasopharynx
E. Outline of dorsum of tongue
F. Outline of epiglottis
G. Outline of anterior wall of pharynx
H. Outline of posterior wall of pharynx
I. Air in nasal cavity

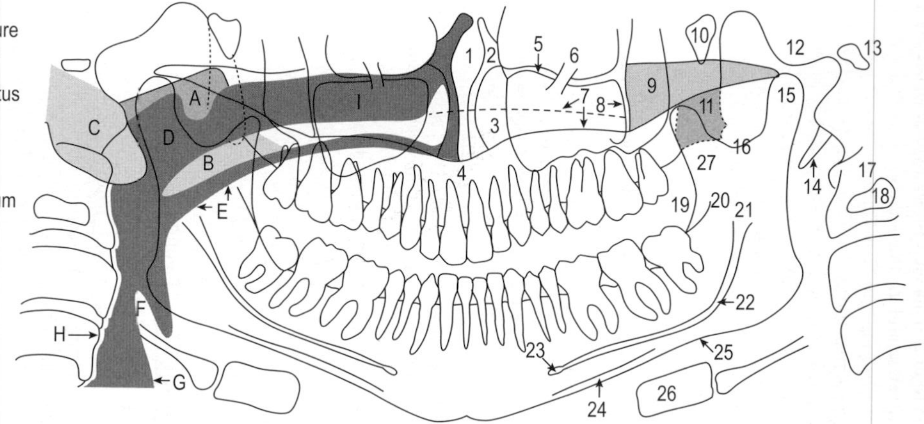

Figure 4.3 Anatomical features on a panoramic radiograph.

the fossae. The beam is then aimed upwards from behind the head from 30° below the horizontal.

Occipitomental
Used to assess the sinuses and fractures of the maxilla, zygomatic complex, orbits and coronoid process. The patient is positioned facing the film with head tilted back at 45° in the 'nose–chin' position, the X-ray tube aligned behind the head and angled down at 0–45° to the horizontal.

Submentovertex (SMV)
Used to assess fractures of the zygomatic arches and pathology in the palate and skull base. The patient is positioned with the head tilted back as far as possible against the film. The beam is then aimed upwards from under the chin. Contraindicated if there is any possibility of a fracture of the cervical spine.

Lateral cephalometric view
Taken for orthodontic purposes using a cephalostat to hold the patient in a standardized and reproducible position. The patient is positioned with their teeth in occlusion and with a natural head position or with the Frankfurt plane horizontal. The film is positioned parallel to the sagittal plane and the beam is aligned at 90° to it. For the majority of cephalometric analyses the cephalometric view can be coned down to show just the facial skeleton, auditory canal and the anterior cranial base.

ADVANCED IMAGING TECHNIQUES
Digital imaging
Uses conventional X-ray machine, but the film is replaced by either a sensor containing a charge-coupled device (CCD) or a photostimulable phosphor plate. In both cases the image receptors convert the information received into digital data. The digital data are stored on a computer and converted into a grey-scale image, which is displayed on a monitor.

Advantages • Lower radiation dose. • No need for conventional processing. • Software allows image manipulation and enhancement. • Very efficient image storage and retrieval.

Disadvantages • Expensive. • Sensors can be bulky, making placement difficult. • Some loss of image resolution compared to film. • Image manipulation can be misleading and can be misused. • A large amount of disk space is required for storage.

Conventional tomography (e.g. Scanora™)

Cross-sectional slices of the maxilla and mandible are produced using conventional tomography. The machines look similar to panoramic units but have a greater range of movement, allowing slices to be made through the jaws in almost any position. Used for implant planning and for assessing the buccolingual extension of pathology and the position of impacted teeth.

Computed tomography (CT)

An X-ray tube passes in a circle around the body and a series of detectors measure the attenuation (blocking) of the beam at each point. A computer then gives a value (Hounsfield number) to each unit of tissue within that slice and from this it constructs a picture of what structures must lie within that section of the body. CT shows both soft tissue and bone but does not demonstrate soft-tissue lesions as well as magnetic resonance imaging. It is particularly useful for assessing serious mid-facial trauma or disease involving bone.

Magnetic resonance imaging (MRI)

This involves placing the patient into a strong magnetic field and then applying a pulse of radio waves. The frequency of these waves is chosen specifically so that the abundant hydrogen protons in body fluid take up energy from the signal. The protons then emit a radio signal, which is picked up and processed by a computer. Several different images of each slice through the patient are produced. The main ones are T1, T2 and proton-density weighted images, each reflecting different characteristics of the tissue. T1 shows the anatomy well, whereas pathology is usually demonstrated better on T2. MRI gives good soft-tissue detail and is excellent for tumour staging and for the assessment of intracranial disease. It can also be used to image the TMJ as it allows direct imaging of the disc. MRI is not good for imaging bone as this tends to appear as a signal void due to the absence of fluid there. The advantage of MRI is that it does not involve ionizing radiation; however, it is contraindicated in patients with ferromagnetic surgical clips, pacemakers, cochlear implants and in the first 3 months of pregnancy.

Ultrasonography

This technique involves scanning the patient with a transducer that emits high-frequency sound waves (1–10 MHz) and then detects the waves reflected from various interfaces within the tissue. The time taken for the waves to be reflected back allows the machine to calculate the depth of the structures that reflected them and from this a picture is created. Ultrasound is excellent for the assessment of superficial soft-tissue structures such as salivary glands, lymph nodes and the thyroid. Fine-needle aspiration under ultrasound guidance can be used to provide further diagnostic information and Doppler imaging can be used to assess vascularity.

Contrast techniques in the head and neck

Radiographic contrast agents are radio-opaque substances containing iodine that when introduced into the body artificially alter the contrast. Adverse reactions to these agents are rare, but patients should always be asked if they have ever had an allergic reaction to iodine.

Sialography This involves the introduction of radiographic contrast into the ductal system of the parotid or submandibular glands.

Indications • Symptoms suggestive of ductal obstruction • suspected Sjögren's syndrome.

Contraindications • Acute salivary gland infection • suspected mass lesions – sialography can be misleading; other techniques are more appropriate.

Angiography This involves the injection of radiographic contrast into the vascular system, usually via a catheter introduced into the femoral artery. Under fluoroscopic control (real-time imaging) the catheter can be passed into a specific artery such as the external carotid to allow selective catheterization of its branches. This technique maybe used to investigate haemangiomas, arteriovenous malformations and suspected intracranial bleeds.

TMJ arthrography This involves the introduction of radiographic contrast into the joint space, usually the inferior compartment, to determine the disc position and to detect disc perforations and adhesions. This technique can give a truly dynamic assessment of disc position but it is uncomfortable for the patient and has largely been replaced by MRI.

Radionuclide imaging This involves the injection of a radioactive agent into the bloodstream that emits gamma rays, which can be detected by a gamma camera. Technetium-99m is the most commonly used isotope, but other substances can be attached to it so that the isotope is concentrated in a particular tissue – e.g methylene diphosphonate (MDP) for bone scans. Radionuclide imaging is useful for assessing the function or activity of a tissue, but the disadvantages are the relatively high dose, poor resolution and limited disease specificity.

Indications • Detection of bony metastases and bony invasion by tumours • Assessment of bone grafts • Assessment of growth in condylar hyperplasia • Investigation of salivary gland function • Assessment of thyroid function.

GUIDELINES FOR THE PRESCRIPTION OF RADIOGRAPHS

Radiographs should be requested only after taking the patient's medical history and completing a full clinical examination; in this way they are likely to contribute to a clinical diagnosis and management (Chapter 2). The use of panoramic radiographs to routinely screen new patients cannot be justified in view of the low diagnostic yield and the minimal impact it has on the management of the vast majority of patients. A panoramic radiograph may be of value for a patient with a very heavily restored or neglected dentition, but for most patients bitewings (which more accurately record early caries and periodontal bone loss) are more appropriate.

When requesting a radiograph, the operator should always ask the question 'Will this radiograph affect this patient's management or prognosis?'

PATIENTS IN PAIN (TABLE 4.6)

In a recent publication by the Faculty of General Dental Practitioners (FGDP)[4] evidence-based guidelines were produced. Guidelines based on this work are listed here, but for more detail the reader is advised to refer to the original text.

DIAGNOSIS OF CARIES

The FGDP recommend that the taking of 'routine' radiographs based solely on time elapsed since last examination is not

TABLE 4.6 Radiographs in the investigation of pain	
Symptom	*Appropriate imaging*
Dental pain with hot and/or cold, but not tender to pressure	Periapical of tooth (or teeth) under suspicion or a bitewing of affected side if pain difficult to localize

TABLE 4.6 (cont'd)

Symptom	Appropriate imaging
Tooth tender to percussion	Periapical radiograph
Dental abscess and/or facial swelling	Periapical view or sectional panoramic radiograph
Pericoronitis	See third molar assessment
TMJ pain	Specific TMJ radiography for these patients rarely reveals anything that affects the management of the condition. A panoramic film is sometimes helpful to exclude concurrent dental disease should there be any confusion following the clinical examination. A good view of the condyles can be obtained by asking for a panoramic radiograph with the mouth open and the jaw protruded
	If the patient fails to respond to conservative treatment, the most helpful investigation is MRI
	If the clinical examination suggests the possibility of condylar hyperplasia, then a panoramic radiograph is indicated together with a bone scan
Atypical facial pain	Suggest a panoramic radiograph of the affected side. An MRI scan may be indicated if there is no response to medical treatment
Trigeminal neuralgia	An MRI scan is indicated to check for a neoplasm along the course of the nerve or for evidence of multiple sclerosis (demyelination) in younger patients (under 40)
Sinusitis	Exclude dental disease using appropriate views Commence medical treatment and if no response a limited CT investigation may be requested if thought appropriate by an ENT specialist
	Occipitomental (OM) views are not routinely indicated as a normal OM view does not exclude the presence of potentially significant pathology particularly in the frontal, ethmoidal and sphenoidal sinuses

supportable. A patient should be exposed to ionizing radiation *only* after a thorough clinical examination, which should include an assessment of caries risk as high, medium or low (Table 4.7). The frequency of radiographic examinations should be based on this assessment, but must be kept under review as individuals move in and out of caries risk categories with time.

PERIODONTAL ASSESSMENT

The FGDP found no clear evidence in the literature regarding the frequency of radiographs for periodontal assessment. It was concluded, however, that bitewing radiographs should be used where possible as they offer the optimal geometry and fine detail of intraoral radiography and, when they are already indicated for

TABLE 4.7 Radiographs in the diagnosis of dental caries

Caries risk	Frequency of radiograph
High	Posterior bitewings at 6-month intervals until no new or active lesions are apparent and the individual has entered another risk category
Moderate	Annual posterior bitewings at intervals unless risk status alters
Low	Primary dentition: intervals of 12–18 months
	Permanent dentition: 2-year intervals, but more extended recall intervals may be employed if there is explicit evidence of continuing low caries risk

TABLE 4.8 Radiographs in the assessment of periodontal disease

Lesion	Radiograph
Uniform pocketing <6 mm and little or no recession	Horizontal bitewings
Pocketing of 6 mm or more	Vertical bitewings supplemented if necessary by intraoral periapical views, using the paralleling technique
Irregular pocketing	Bitewing radiographs (horizontal or vertical depending on pocket depth), supplemented if necessary by periapical radiographs taken using the paralleling technique

caries assessment, they provide information about bone levels without any additional radiation dose. Early loss of bone height can be captured on horizontal bitewings but in more severe cases vertical bitewings can be used (see Table 4.8).

ORAL SURGERY
Radiography before routine extractions

Opinion is divided as to whether a radiograph is required routinely before an extraction. However, from a radiation protection point of view each exposure must be justified on an individual basis and may be indicated where it is felt that there is some risk that the extraction may be complicated. If a film already exists that shows the root pattern, further radiography is probably unnecessary (see Table 4.9).

TABLE 4.8 (cont'd)

Lesion	Radiograph
Where there are concurrent problems for which radiography is indicated (e.g. symptomatic third molars, multiple existing crowns/heavily restored teeth and/or multiple endodontically treated teeth in a patient new to the practice)	A panoramic radiograph may offer a dose advantage over a large number of intraoral radiographs. However, in view of the limitations in fine detail on panoramic radiographs, supplementary intraoral radiographs may be necessary for selected sites
Periodontal/endodontic lesion	A periapical radiograph taken using the paralleling technique

TABLE 4.9 Radiography prior to routine extractions

Extraction	Radiograph
A broken-down tooth which may require a surgical procedure	Periapical radiograph
When there is a history of difficult extractions	Periapical radiograph
When there is a history of bone disease	Periapical radiograph
When the tooth is a lone standing upper molar	Periapical radiograph
Multiple carious teeth in several quadrants to be extracted	Panoramic radiograph
Extractions under general anaesthesia	Panoramic radiograph

Surgical procedures

See Table 4.10.

TABLE 4.10 Radiography prior to minor surgery	
Procedure	*Radiograph*
Removal of root fragments	
Small cysts	Periapical radiograph
Apicectomies	
Oroantral fistula/root displaced into antrum	Sectional panoramic radiograph or upper oblique occlusal

Third molar assessment

See Table 4.11.

TABLE 4.11 Radiographs in third molar assessment	
Symptoms	*Radiograph*
Unilateral symptoms	Sectional panoramic radiograph of symptomatic side
	A full panoramic is justified to enable the asymptomatic contralateral side to be assessed if a general anaesthetic is required
Bilateral symptoms	Full panoramic
Radiography is only justified prior to planned surgical removal; routine radiography of unerupted or asymptomatic partially erupted third molars is not recommended.	

Trauma

See Table 4.12.

TABLE 4.12 Radiographs in the assessment of facial bone fractures

Injury	Views required
Suspected dentoalveolar fracture	A combination of periapical views at different angles (paralleling and bisecting angle) or a periapical and an upper oblique occlusal are most likely to reveal the presence of a root or alveolar bone fracture
Suspected mandibular fracture	Panoramic and posteroanterior jaw view taken with the mouth open to show the mandibular condyles more clearly
Suspected zygomatic fracture	Occipitomental 10° ± 30° views supplemented by a submentovertex view where the fracture is found to be limited to the zygomatic arch (this view is contraindicated if the patient cannot safely extend their neck, e.g. possible cervical spine fracture)
Suspected Le Fort fracture	Occipitomental 10° ± 30° and lateral skull views initially, followed by CT scanning

Salivary gland disease

See Table 4.13.

TABLE 4.13 Radiographs in the assessment of salivary gland disease

Problem	Examination modality
Symptoms of obstruction	Plain films may reveal radio-opaque calculi. Submandibular gland – lower true occlusal, lower oblique occlusal and half panoramic radiographs. Parotid – anteroposterior soft tissue view ± periapical film of duct orifice
	Sialography – after acute symptoms have settled. May reveal radiolucent calculi or strictures and it can also be therapeutic
Suspected autoimmune salivary gland disease – Sjögren's syndrome	Sialography ± an ultrasound scan
A palpable lump in a salivary gland	Ultrasound scan followed by MRI or CT

INTERPRETATION OF RADIOGRAPHS

The features to consider when describing the radiographic appearance of a lesion are listed in Table 4.14.

TABLE 4.14 Principles of describing a lesion

Characteristic	Details
Number	Single or multiple
Density	Radiolucent, mixed or radio-opaque
Site	Anatomical position and whether it appears to be related to a particular structure (e.g. a buried tooth or the ID canal)
	If you have only one radiograph be aware of the possibility of superimposition, particularly if describing a radio-opaque lesion. Another view at right angles may be required to describe accurately the position of a lesion
Size	Take account of any radiographic magnification, or describe extension relative to anatomical structures
Internal architecture	Unilocular/multilocular, calcifications, etc.
Borders	Well defined or poorly defined
Affect on surrounding structures	Resorption of roots, displacement of ID nerve or expansion of the bone
Changes with time	If previous films are available

DIFFERENTIAL DIAGNOSIS OF RADIOGRAPHIC LESIONS

The differential diagnosis of lesions observed on a radiograph are described in Table 4.15.

TABLE 4.15 Radiological differential diagnosis

Well-defined unilocular radiolucent lesions	Well-defined multilocular radiolucent lesions	Pericoronal radiolucent lesions	Radiolucent lesions with indistinct borders	Radio-opaque lesions (well defined)
Apical granuloma	Keratocyst	Normal follicular space	Periodontal disease	Roots or buried teeth
Radicular cyst	Ameloblastoma	Dentigerous cyst	Osteomyelitis	Odontomes
Residual cyst	Giant cell granuloma	Paradental cyst	Osteoradionecrosis	Osteoma
Giant cell granuloma	Myxoma	Ameloblastoma	Primary malignancy	Calcified lymph nodes or tonsils
Nasopalatine cyst	Cherubism	Keratocyst	Secondary malignancy	Salivary calculi
Stafne's idiopathic bone cavity	Aneurysmal bone cyst	Developing odontome	Eosinophilic granuloma	Vascular calcification
Keratocyst	Central haemangioma	Ameloblastic fibroma		Sclerosing osteitis or dense bone island
Ameloblastoma	Arteriovenous malformation	Adenomatoid odontogenic tumour*		Osteomyelitis
Lateral periodontal cyst	Neurofibroma	Calcifying epithelial odontogenic tumour*		Fibrous dysplasia
Solitary bone cyst		Calcifying odontogenic cyst*		Paget's disease
Neurilemmoma				Cemental dysplasia
Neurofibroma				Osteosarcoma or osteogenic metastases

*May develop internal calcification as they mature.

REFERENCES

1. National Radiological Protection Board 1994 Guidelines on Radiology Standards for Primary Dental Care. Doc. NRPB, 5, No 3
2. Department of Health 2001 Guidance Notes for Dental Practitioners on the Safe Use of X-ray Equipment. HMSO, London
3. Napier ID 1999 Reference doses for dental radiography. British Dental Journal 186(8):392–6
4. FGDP (UK)-RCS 1998 Selection Criteria for Dental Radiography

CHAPTER 5

DRUG PRESCRIBING AND THERAPEUTICS

Drug prescribing   60

Analgesics and non-steroidal anti-inflammatory drugs (NSAIDs) 62

Antibiotics   68

Antifungal and antiviral agents   77

Anxiolytics, hypnotics and antidepressants   80

Antihistamines   84

Topical agents   85

Drug interactions of dental relevance   89

Note on drug nomenclature   89

DRUG PRESCRIBING

GENERAL

The BNF (*British National Formulary*) is an essential source of information on drug actions, uses and dangers. Within the BNF there is now a list of drugs which may be prescribed by dentists under NHS regulations although this no longer occupies a separate section of the publication as once was the case. This list is still known as the Dental Practitioners' Formulary. Dentists, however, may prescribe drugs outwith this list on a private prescription provided this is for a dentally related condition. Doses quoted in the BNF are conventionally the normal or accepted adult dose. Guidance on suitable children's doses is included where appropriate.

Abbreviations are used in the BNF. Important among these are:

CD (Controlled Drug)
Subject to regulations laid down under the Misuse of Drugs Act.
CSM (Committee on Safety of Medicines)
This body should be informed of any serious reaction to a prescribed drug.
POM (Prescription-Only-Medicine)
i.e. cannot be bought over the counter at a pharmacy.

The BNF is available on-line at www.bnf.org

PRESCRIPTION WRITING

 The prescription is the responsibility of the prescriber, *not* the pharmacist.

Essential information to be written in ink or indelible form:

1. Name and address of patient
2. Age of patient (if under 12 years)
3. Total number of days of treatment
4. The *generic* name of the drug, its form and strength (e.g. metronidazole tablets 200 mg)
5. Instructions as to how and when drug is to be taken, written in English with no abbreviations (e.g. 'one tablet to be taken three times daily with food')

6. Delete any space remaining on the form
7. Date and prescriber's signature

Note

More than one drug may be prescribed for a patient on one form.

The box marked 'NP' must be deleted if the prescriber does not wish the name of the drug to appear on the label of the container. This action is not really applicable to prescribing in dentistry.

For controlled drugs, marked CD, the prescriber's own handwriting should be used in indelible ink throughout and the total quantity of the drug in both words and figures is required. The prescription should be endorsed with the words 'For dental treatment only'. The only controlled drugs of relevance to outpatient NHS dental practice are pethidine and temazepam.

WARNINGS TO PATIENTS

- Always take the drug at the recommended time and finish the prescribed course.
- If any untoward reaction occurs (e.g. skin rash or severe diarrhoea) *stop* drug and contact prescriber immediately.
- Patients should be informed of known side effects or interactions, e.g.:
  — reduced effect of oral contraceptives with antibiotics
  — interaction of metronidazole with alcohol.
- Medicines should be kept safely out of the reach of children and the use of 'child safe' containers is essential. When no longer needed, medicines should be disposed of by returning them to the local pharmacist, *not* discarded where children may find and swallow them.

PATIENTS AT PARTICULAR RISK

Children Doses should be appropriately reduced by age or body weight. Appropriate doses are listed in the BNF and a BNF for children is now available. Elixirs are preferable for oral ingestion. If under 12 years, the age must be included in the prescription. 'Sugar-free' preparations should be prescribed where available.

Elderly Elderly people may show exaggerated reactions to drugs, and doses may need to be modified. Gastrointestinal (GI) haemorrhage is more likely with non-steroidal anti-inflammatory drugs and these should be prescribed with caution.

Polypharmacy is common in the elderly; possible interactions should be identified. Elderly patients often get confused about which drugs are to be taken at which times, with the possibility of neglecting important medication. Try to avoid adding to their confusion.

Pregnancy Only prescribe when absolutely essential. Use the well-tried, safer preparations. Teratogenic effects are most likely in the first trimester. Second and third trimester effects are mainly on growth, development and drug toxicity to the fetus.

Breast feeding Some drugs pass into the milk and are thereby ingested by the baby. This is potentially dangerous.

Liver disease Many drugs are metabolized through the liver. Impaired liver function may affect the breakdown of drugs; certain drugs may further damage the organ. Check BNF listings.

Kidney disease As many drugs are excreted through the kidney, impaired function may lead to: • increased drug levels in the plasma • rising sensitivity to certain drugs • poor tolerance to side effects.

Certain drugs should be avoided, and some may require dose reduction.

 For all the above groups check BNF listings under 'Guidance on Prescribing' and appropriate appendices.

ANALGESICS AND NON-STEROIDAL ANTI-INFLAMMATORY DRUGS (NSAIDs)

GENERAL

Most dental pain is inflammatory in origin whether it be pulpal, periodontal or, less frequently, temporomandibular joint or muscular. Non-steroidal anti-inflammatory drugs (NSAIDs) with their associated analgesic properties are therefore frequently appropriate prescriptions for dentally related pain.

The way in which analgesics are prescribed may have a significant bearing on the success of their actions. 'Just take aspirin if you have any pain' is not likely to induce confidence in patients, whereas an explanation of the positive qualities of the drug in the particular patient's context may well result in more benefit. No response to standard analgesics may indicate atypical facial pain, often of psychogenic origin, or a more sinister cause.

> ⚠ Most analgesics will have no perceptible effect on acute
> pulpitis, periodontal or periapical abscess if physical
> measures are not taken by the dentist to actively relieve the pain.

NON-STEROIDAL ANTI-INFLAMMATORY DRUGS

Examples of such drugs are aspirin and ibuprofen. The main
actions of these drugs are: • analgesic • anti-inflammatory
• antipyretic.

Aspirin

Pain control Trauma, infection or any inflammatory reaction leads
to the production of arachidonic acid from cell phospholipid.
Arachidonic acid is acted on by a number of enzymes including the
cyclo-oxygenase system. This leads to the production of
prostaglandins which, although not themselves pain-producers,
enhance the pain-producing effects of several other chemicals such
as bradykinin and 5-hydroxytryptamine by sensitizing the pain
receptors. Most NSAIDs interfere with the production or
conversion of arachidonic acid to prostaglandins.

Anti-inflammatory action Prostaglandins are vasodilators and have
an effect on capillary permeability, leading to redness and swelling
of tissues. Prostaglandin inhibition by NSAIDs reduces these
manifestations.

Antipyretic In the hypothalamic region of the brain, levels of
prostaglandins become raised in response to leucocyte pyrogens.
These higher levels appear to 'raise' the temperature-setting
mechanism of the body but are responsive to NSAIDs and the
temperature setting is thus lowered. The excess heat is lost by
peripheral vasodilatation. Normal temperature is unaffected.

   In addition to these therapeutic activities, aspirin has various
other metabolic effects:

Antidiabetic action Reduction of blood sugar in diabetics by
increasing peripheral utilization of glucose.

Increases basal metabolic rate (BMR)

Reduction of platelet adhesiveness This action is now widely
employed in the prevention and treatment of thromboembolic
vascular disease, where low-dose long-term therapy has proven

benefits in preventing thrombus formation. There is no requirement to alter regime for extractions or routine minor surgery.

Increase in thyroid hormone levels (with long-term use of aspirin).

Patient groups at risk from aspirin

Peptic ulceration Prostaglandins exert a moderating influence on acid secretion and stimulate mucin production in the stomach with a resultant protective effect on the gastric mucosa. Aspirin and most other NSAIDs hence cause increase in acid production and reduction in mucin, which may lead to erosive and ulcerative effects on the stomach and duodenum. This can cause bleeding even in normal conditions but may have more serious outcomes such as perforation in patients with pre-existing peptic ulceration. NSAIDs are therefore largely contraindicated in these patients; paracetamol may be given safely.

Bleeding disorders In patients with known clotting defects such as haemophilia, an increased bleeding tendency generated by the above mechanism may have serious implications and NSAIDs are therefore potentially dangerous and should be avoided.

Anticoagulants Coumarin-type drugs (such as warfarin) are enhanced by aspirin with increased anticoagulant effect. This can increase blood loss from the GI tract in addition to other systems. Paracetamol is a suitable alternative to any of the peripherally acting NSAIDs.

Children under 16 years Aspirin has been implicated in the aetiology of Reye's syndrome – a fatty degeneration in liver and kidney with an associated encephalopathy. The morbidity is high and the mortality from this condition is reported at 50%.

 Aspirin is contraindicated in children under 16 years.

Elderly All the NSAIDs, but aspirin in particular, can cause more severe effects on the gastric mucosa. Additionally they may be hazardous in older patients with cardiac disease or renal problems. In general paracetamol is a safer prescription for analgesia in elderly patients.

Asthmatics Hypersensitivity may precipitate severe bronchospasm.

Pregnancy Use in the third trimester may cause prolongation of labour and bleeding at birth in both mother and baby.

Renal or hepatic disease Dose may require reduction in renal disease. Worsening of bleeding problems may result with liver disease.

Dose 300–900 mg orally 4–6 hourly. Maximum adult dose: 4 g daily.

Overdose Tinnitus and metabolic acidosis.

IBUPROFEN
Similar but not identical effect to aspirin. Less anti-inflammatory activity. Less and more transitory effect on platelets than aspirin. Irritant to GI tract but less so than aspirin. Bronchospasm, especially if patient allergic to other NSAIDs. Many drug interactions possible, notably angiotensin-converting enzyme inhibitors, other NSAIDs, oral antidiabetic drugs and lithium.

Side effects GI discomfort and possible hypersensitivity but also several others.

Dose 1.2–1.8 g orally daily in 3 to 4 divided doses. Maximum adult dose: 2.4 g daily.

Children Reduced dose in paediatric suspension. Not recommended for children under 7 kg or under 1 year of age.

Elderly See above note on aspirin. All NSAIDs should be prescribed with caution in this group of patients.

ANALGESICS
Paracetamol
Similar analgesic properties to aspirin. Antipyretic but little or no anti-inflammatory action. No significant GI irritation. Not implicated in Reye's syndrome. Side effects rare but include rash and blood dyscrasias. A safer analgesic alternative for groups of patients with peptic ulceration, taking anticoagulants or in the elderly.

Dose 500 mg–1 g orally 4–6 hourly. Maximum adult dose 4 g daily.

Children Reduced dose in paediatric suspension.

Overdose Causes severe but delayed hepatocellular necrosis. In adults 7–10 g may be sufficient and, in children, as little as 3 g. *Symptoms occur 24–48 hours after ingestion.* Early symptoms are anorexia, nausea, vomiting and abdominal pain. Maximal liver damage occurs in 3–4 days. Plasma levels are required if overdose suspected. Liver may be protected by treatment with acetylcysteine or methionine if administered within the first few hours of the overdose. If patient reports taking what appears to be an excessive quantity, then this warrants immediate referral to an Accident and Emergency unit to assess the plasma level of paracetamol. Urgent medical assessment is required.

OPIOIDS

Opioids should not be given to patients with a suspected head injury as the drug may mask pupillary evidence of increasing intracranial pressure by its effect on the pupilloconstrictor centre.

Recourse to narcotic analgesics is infrequent in dentistry other than in oral and maxillofacial surgery. In general, opioids have depressive and stimulatory effects on the central nervous system.

Depression of pain centre, higher centres, respiratory and vasomotor centres and cough centre.

Stimulation of vomiting, salivary and pupilloconstrictor actions. The positive response to pain appears to be brought about more by an alteration in the patient's perception of pain rather than a reduction in the pain itself.

Dependence Patients may become dependent on opioids, both physiologically and psychologically, with craving for the drug and physical illness on acute withdrawal.

Tolerance This is an increase in dose to achieve the same level of therapeutic effect. This effect is restricted to the depressant effects on the central nervous system (CNS). Smooth muscle stimulation leads to constipation even with mild opioids such as codeine.

Codeine
Normally not used alone but added to other non-opioid analgesics such as aspirin or paracetamol. It is an efficient cough suppressant but not a particularly advantageous analgesic and it usually causes constipation.

Dihydrocodeine tartrate

Has a similar potency to codeine. Although recommended for more severe dental pain, its advantage over NSAIDs is far from conclusive, particularly after oral surgery.

Side effects Include nausea, vomiting, constipation and drowsiness. Larger doses may cause hypotension and respiratory depression. Serious interactions may occur with antidepressants, especially monoamine oxidase inhibitors, and several other interactions are recorded (see BNF).

Should be avoided or used with caution in the elderly, children, asthmatics, concomitant antihypertensive therapy, pregnant or lactating women and those with liver or kidney disease.

Dose 30 mg orally 4–6 hourly. Can be given intramuscularly (i.m.) 30–60 mg 4–6 hourly.

Pethidine

Pethidine is more suitable for ambulatory patients than morphine. Its side effects are less marked than morphine but it is liable to induce dependence and is unsuitable for prolonged use.

Dose Adult 50–100 mg orally 4 hourly. Can also be given by i.m., subcutaneous or i.v. routes.

POSTOPERATIVE PAIN

Particularly after oral surgical procedures, *good* pain control should be considered essential.

Use of local anaesthesia has benefits for patients undergoing surgery under general anaesthesia in that it: • lowers the requirement for volatile gaseous agents • reduces afferent induced arrhythmias in the heart • reduces the pain immediately postoperatively and hence the need for more powerful (opioid) analgesics • will also reduce local haemorrhage, where vasoconstrictor also used.

Patients should be instructed to start taking the prescribed analgesic before the local anaesthetic wears off as continuity of measures appears to prevent the pain becoming less receptive to analgesia.

CARBAMAZEPINE

This drug is used widely in the treatment of epilepsy but is also the main therapeutic agent in the management of trigeminal neuralgia.

It is not an analgesic drug but best considered as a membrane-stabilizing agent.

Carbamazepine will, in the majority of cases, reduce the frequency and the severity of the attacks. When used diagnostically, a dose of 100–200 mg daily is normally enough to confirm its effect, and the dosage can thereafter be increased incrementally until total comfort is achieved. Often a dose of 400–600 mg will be adequate, although some patients may require considerably more – up to 1.6 g daily. Such high doses, however, may lead to disturbing side effects. Plasma concentrations can be assessed in the laboratory but normally only to assess compliance, since the side-effect profile rather than blood levels tends to govern the maximum dose.

Side effects Nausea, skin rashes, drowsiness, ataxia and confusion are among the more common side effects; elderly people are particularly susceptible. The possibility of neutropenia and other blood disorders means regular blood counts for patients on long-term therapy. Liver function tests are advised on a regular basis.

Contraindications A-V conduction abnormalities, previous bone marrow disease and porphyria. Pregnancy: increased risk of neural-tube defects in the fetus so, where therapy is essential, appropriate counselling is advised. Dental use is normally for trigeminal neuralgia, which affects the older age group, and this latter problem is seldom encountered.

ANTIBIOTICS

> An antibiotic is a substance which causes the death of or prevents successful replication of micro-organisms.

Many antimicrobials are themselves products of micro-organisms (e.g. penicillin from the mould *Penicillium chrysogenum*); others are chemical therapeutic agents (e.g. metronidazole, sulphonamides).

> A **bactericidal** drug kills sensitive organisms.
> A **bacteriostatic** drug prevents successful reproduction.

SYNERGISM AND ANTAGONISM

Whilst some antibiotics enhance one another's activity, others when used in combination lead to reduced effectiveness. In general:

Bactericidal + bactericidal → synergism
Bactericidal + bacteriostatic → antagonism.

Spectrum of activity

> **Narrow-spectrum antibiotics** have a limited range of effect, normally against Gram-positive bacteria.
> **Broad-spectrum antibiotics** normally have activity against Gram-positive and Gram-negative bacteria, and sometimes *Mycoplasma*.

Provided the bacteria are sensitive, the narrower the spectrum of agent used the better. This reduces the GI side effects by limiting the destruction of the normal flora, and will also minimize the chance of overgrowth of opportunistic pathogens such as *Candida albicans* in the alimentary or urogenital tract.

Bacterial resistance to antibiotics

> **!** An increasing problem world-wide is that some micro-organisms are acquiring multi-resistance. The best known example is meticillin-resistant *Staphylococcus aureus* (MRSA). Prescription of antibiotics for dental purposes should be carefully assessed. Shorter courses (for 2–3 days) should be considered where appropriate as this reduces the chances of resistant forms emerging.

Bacterial resistance may be natural or acquired.

Natural resistance The micro-organism may have morphological or biological factors which exclude the target area(s) of the organism to the effect of the drug, e.g.: • many (not all) Gram-negative bacteria are resistant to penicillin by protecting the target inner cell wall with an impermeable outer cell wall (lipopolysaccharide) • aerobic micro-organisms are totally resistant to metronidazole by virtue of their metabolism • some bacteria (e.g. *Staph. aureus*) may produce β-lactamase enzymes which nullify the β-lactam antibiotics such as penicillin before they can act.

Acquired resistance This is an adaptive reaction of a bacterial colony to continued exposure to a drug, and is effected by mutation.

Side effect of antibiotics

Certain side effects may accompany the use of these drugs. Among the more important are:

Blood dyscrasias Rare, but include leucopenia, thrombocytopenia and agranulocytosis.

Gastrointestinal upsets Nausea, vomiting and diarrhoea are very common. Diarrhoea as a manifestation of the more serious condition of antibiotic-associated colitis (AAC) must be differentiated.

Superinfection AAC may occur during, or up to several weeks after, a course of antibiotics. The broad-spectrum antibiotics seem to be more commonly implicated but penicillins and cephalosporins can also be responsible. The cause is a toxin of *Clostridium difficile*, a gut organism. Symptoms include abdominal pain, severe blood-stained diarrhoea and fever. Treatment requires hospitalization where fluids and electrolytes are replaced and often oral vancomycin proves helpful.

Less serious problems can occur with candidal infections of the alimentary system (including the oral cavity) or urogenital tract. Candidosis is more likely with broad-spectrum antibiotics.

Hypersensitivity reactions These may range from itchy skin rashes to angio-oedematous swelling and full-blown anaphylactic shock (p. 527).

USES OF ANTIBIOTICS IN DENTISTRY

Use of antibiotics in dentistry can be considered under two headings: • prophylactic use (i.e. the prevention of infection) • therapeutic treatment of existing infection.

Prophylactic antibiotics
Prophylactic antibiotics
Prophylaxis of endocarditis Any manipulation of the teeth or gingival tissues and endodontic procedures may cause a bacteraemia which could, in theory, lead to infective endocarditis in

...eptible individuals. Endocarditis still has an unacceptably high
...rtality. However, it is known that many activities, such as
...ewing and toothbrushing, also cause a bacteraemia and so recent
...uidance on the prevention of endocarditis has relaxed many of the
previous 'rules' for antibiotic use (Guidelines for the prevention of
endocarditis: report of the Working Party of the British Society for
Antimicrobial Chemotherapy. Gould, FK *et al. Journal of
Antimicrobial Chemotherapy* 2006; 57:1035–42). Antibiotic
prophylaxis given immediately prior to the dental procedure may
protect damaged or prosthetic heart valves. Chlorhexidine
gluconate mouthwash (0.2%) used preoperatively for 1 minute is
known to reduce the oral load of bacteria and so may reduce the
chances of a patient developing endocarditis.

Which patients are at risk?
• Patients with a previous history of infective endocarditis.
• Patients who have undergone cardiac valve replacement surgery,
whether with mechanical or biological prosthetic valves. • Patients
who have had placed a systemic or pulmonary shunt or conduit.

Suggested regimens for endocarditis prophylaxis
A single oral dose of antibiotic is thought to achieve adequate blood
levels of the drug and should be used regardless of whether the
patient is to have dental treatment carried out under local or general
anaesthesia (Table 5.1). It is recognized that some clinical situations
may make the administration of intravenous antibiotics easier.
Dosages for both oral and i.v. administration are given in Table 5.1.
Further information is available in the *British National Formulary*.

Surgical prophylaxis Controversy exists in this context, particularly
for routine surgery. Many oral surgeons consider use of an antibiotic
such as amoxicillin or metronidazole peri- or postoperatively to be
justified particularly where the surgical site has been previously
infected (e.g. pericoronal infection) or where significant amounts of
bone have been removed. Few would disagree with use of such
antibiotic prophylaxis in treating facial fractures or closing
oroantral fistulae. Short courses in this context may reduce chances
of resistance being acquired. Routine use of antiseptic mouthwashes
further reduces the chance of postoperative infection.

Medically compromised Oral surgery or even multiple extractions
in some patients (immunocompromised, unstable diabetics or
debilitated) may well be justified, but each patient should be
individually assessed on the perceived benefit. Those with certain
bone conditions (e.g. previous radiotherapy to area, Paget's disease)

TABLE 5.1 Antibiotic prophylaxis for dental procedures

Population	Age			Timing of dose before procedure
	>10 years	>5 to <10 years	<5 years	
General	Amoxicillin 3 g p.o.	Amoxicillin 1.5 g p.o.	Amoxicillin 750 mg p.o.	1 hour
Allergic to penicillin	Clindamycin 600 mg p.o.	Clindamycin 300 mg p.o.	Clindamycin 150 mg p.o.	1 hour
Allergic to penicillin and unable to swallow capsules	Azithromycin 500 mg p.o.	Azithromycin 300 mg p.o.	Azithromycin 200 mg p.o.	1 hour
Intravenous regimen expedient	Amoxicillin 1 g i.v.	Amoxicillin 500 mg i.v.	Amoxicillin 250 mg i.v.	Just before the procedure or at induction of anaesthesia
Intravenous regimen expedient and allergic to penicillin	Clindamycin 300 mg i.v.*	Clindamycin 150 mg i.v.*	Clindamycin 75 mg i.v.*	Just before the procedure or at induction of anaesthesia

*Given over at least 10 min.

Where a course of treatment involves several visits, the antibiotic regimen should alternate between amoxicillin and clindamycin.

Preoperative mouth rinse with chlorhexidine gluconate 0.2% (10 ml for 1 min).

From Gould FK, Elliott TS, Foweraker J et al. 2006 Guidelines for the prevention of endocarditis: report of the Working Party of the British Society for Antimicrobial Chemotherapy. Journal of Antimicrobial Chemotherapy 57(6):1035–42. (Reproduced with permission of Oxford University Press.)

nould have an appropriate antibiotic prescribed both peri- and postoperatively.

Joint prostheses No requirement for antibiotic cover for oral operative procedures although some patients carry a card requesting this. Decision may need discussion with orthopaedic surgeon in charge of the patient's care. Regardless, such patients should have a dental assessment as part of their orthopaedic 'work-up' preoperatively and excellent standards of oral hygiene encouraged thereafter.

Cardiac pacemakers or indwelling intraperitoneal catheters
Confusion exists over the requirement for cover in patients with these devices; protocols should be discussed locally.

Haemodialysis for renal failure Many nephrologists in charge of patients on regular haemodialysis for renal failure request the use of antibiotic prophylaxis to maintain the viability and freedom from infection of the arteriovenous shunts (used to gain access for haemodialysis) during oral and dental surgery. Such protocols should be discussed locally.

Treatment of infection

Dentists often have the necessary skills to provide drainage for any collection of pus, whether by incision, pulp extirpation or extraction. Provision of drainage remains fundamental in purulent infections.

Ideally antibiotics must only *supplement* drainage, where drainage is possible, but certain clinical features might influence the decision to prescribe: • toxaemia (raised temperature and malaise) • associated regional lymphadenitis • trismus • dysphagia • inadequate drainage obtained surgically • medical history • rapid spread to soft tissues.

Certain principles should be observed and can be listed under 'do's and don'ts'

Do

Check previous history of possible allergy.

Sample pus (by aspiration if possible as this reduces contamination and helps preserve anaerobic bacteria) for antibiotic sensitivity testing.

Choose least toxic and narrowest spectrum drug consistent with desired effect.

Prescribe early as bactericidal agents such as the penicillins and cephalosporins are more active when micro-organisms are rapidly dividing.

Warn patient of any known serious and common side effects.

Choose route and dose appropriate to severity of infection.
Remember to reduce dose appropriately for children
Review patient within 2–3 days to assess response.

Don't
Substitute antibiotics for adequate provision of drainage.
Continue treatment if no response Re-think diagnosis (is it infection?) or change drug.
Use two antibiotics if one will suffice.
Change antibiotic if antibiotic sensitivity test suggests resistance but clinical response is good.

In severe infections where rapid spread is apparent, use of two or more antibiotics may be indicated. These patients normally require hospitalization for monitoring, and administration by infusion. Metronidazole with amoxicillin or erythromycin are frequent choices.

 Use of combined antibiotic treatment should be reserved for severe infections.

Commonly used antibiotics (Table 5.2)
Most courses of antibiotics are prescribed for 5 days in dentistry but each patient should be assessed individually in the light of his/her requirement. Frequent monitoring of patient response may allow a shortened course which may help reduce side effects and emergence of resistant bacteria. Regular review of patients with severe infection is essential until resolution is apparent.

Penicillins The penicillin group of antibiotics act by interfering with the transpeptidase enzyme which is responsible for alignment of peptidoglycan strands giving the bacterial cell wall rigidity. Gram-positive organisms are normally sensitive but most Gram-negative bacteria are protected by an outer lipopolysaccharide layer. Broad-spectrum penicillins such as ampicillin and amoxicillin have been developed to widen the range of susceptible micro-organisms by their ability to penetrate this outer cell wall layer.

Benzylpenicillin (Pen G) is not stable in acid and is given by parenteral routes. It is therefore seldom used in dental practice but still has value for hospitalized patients.

Phenoxymethylpenicillin (Pen V) is more acid stable and is widely prescribed orally by dentists. Its use for pyogenic dental infection

TABLE 5.2 Antibiotics commonly used in dentistry

Drug	Spectrum	Normal dose	Severe infection	Route	Dental uses	Important side effects
Penicillin V	Narrow	250 mg four times daily	500 mg four times daily	Oral	Pyogenic infections, ANUG	Skin rash
Penicillin G	Narrow	300–600 mg	1–2 g	i.m. or i.v.	Surgical prophylaxis	Anaphylactic reactions possible
Amoxicillin	Broad	250 mg three times daily	500 mg three times daily; or 3 g stat, or 500 mg–1 g every 6 hours	Oral i.v. infusion	Pyogenic infections Surgical prophylaxis Endocarditis prophylaxis (see Table 5.1)	Skin rash Anaphylactic reactions possible Candidosis or AAC if used for longer period
Metronidazole	Anaerobes	200 mg three times daily	400 mg three times daily; 500 mg every 8 hours	Oral i.v. infusion	Anaerobic infections, including ANUG Dental & periodontal abscess; pericoronitis; dry socket prophylaxis	Alcohol interaction, nausea, vomiting
Doxycycline	Broad	200 mg initial dose, then 100 mg daily	200 mg daily	Oral	Sinusitis; oral–antral fistula; chronic osteomyelitis	Staining of teeth (avoid in pregnancy and children under 12 years); nausea, AAC, candidosis
Erythromycin	Relatively narrow	250 mg four times daily	500 mg four times daily	Oral	Pyogenic infections; penicillin allergy	Nausea, vomiting, diarrhoea; jaundice on prolonged use

remains valuable although there appears to be an increasing number of resistant bacteria.

Amoxicillin This has a wider spectrum of activity than Pen G or Pen V and is a popular prescription for dental infections. Most dentists have to prescribe empirically on the basis of previous clinical experience, since microbiological culture and antibiotic sensitivity testing is not readily available. This wider range of effectiveness makes amoxicillin a popular choice but it is more liable to cause GI side effects than the more selective Pen V. Amoxicillin has a wide use in endocarditis prophylaxis in the form of a 3 g sachet orally 1 hour before any risk procedure in patients with no history of penicillin allergy (Table 5.1).

Ampicillin Broad-spectrum penicillin largely superseded by amoxicillin, which is better absorbed in the gut and may have a more rapid action.

Flucloxacillin If skin organisms are implicated, this β-lactamase-resistant form of penicillin may be a rational choice.

Dose 250 mg orally four times daily.

Metronidazole is not a conventional antibiotic but is an antimicrobial chemotherapeutic agent. It is broken down in the bacterial cell to an agent which disrupts DNA synthesis and causes breakdown of existing DNA. **It is only effective against anaerobes**. Metronidazole is an effective agent against most dental infections since they are usually polymicrobial and predominantly anaerobic in nature. Dental abscesses, pericoronal infections, acute necrotizing ulcerative gingivitis and wound infections normally respond well.

Local applications to periodontal pockets are available, although whether this therapy has long-term benefits or is superior to systemic administration has not yet been fully evaluated.

Prophylactic use of metronidazole in patients with a consistent history of repeated dry socket following extraction is also contentious since many believe the problem is more vascular than infective initially.

Doxycycline This broad-spectrum antibiotic has limited use for pyogenic infection but has been used for maxillary antral infection and for the now rare osteomyelitis. It is chelated by calcium ions and can become incorporated into developing teeth, causing unsightly staining. It should therefore not be prescribed during the period of tooth development. Both doxycycline and minocycline can be used in local applications to periodontal pockets but, as with all local agents, their efficacy is still to be established.

Other antibiotics

Clindamycin Dental uses include endocarditis prophylaxis, pyogenic salivary gland infection and sensitive anaerobic infections when severe (e.g. *Bacteroides* infection). Difficulties with the drug include antibiotic-associated colitis (AAC), although this is not regarded as a problem for one-dose endocarditis cover, and the association with AAC has probably been overstated in the past.

Dose 150–300 mg orally three times daily.

Cephalosporins Similar action but wider spectrum than penicillins. Approximately 10% of patients allergic to penicillin will also be allergic to cephalosporins.

Dose e.g. Cefalexin, 250 mg orally four times daily.

ANTIFUNGAL AND ANTIVIRAL AGENTS

ANTIFUNGAL AGENTS

Most fungal infections in the oral cavity are due to *Candida* species, most commonly *Candida albicans*. For clinical presentations and important considerations in the management of patients with oral candidosis see page 442.

Where candidosis is related to dentures, denture hygiene instruction should be stressed. Non-metal dentures should be soaked regularly overnight in sodium hypochlorite 1% (Milton's solution) and metal-containing dentures similarly in chlorhexidine 0.2% solution.

Nystatin and amphotericin (polyenes)

These agents attach to the fungal cell membrane and disrupt fluid and electrolyte permeability. They are not absorbed from the GI tract and hence act locally (see Table 5.3).

Miconazole (an imidazole)

Similar action to the polyenes. Effective against some Gram-positive bacteria such as *Staph. aureus*. More effective than polyenes in angular cheilitis due to possible mixed fungal/bacterial infection.

Available as oral gel, cream and in combination with hydrocortisone.

TABLE 5.3 Dosage regimens for nystatin and amphotericin

	Form	Dose	Frequency	Period
Nystatin	Pastilles	100 000 units	Four times daily	At least 2 but preferably 4 weeks
	Oral suspension	100 000 units/ml		
	Ointment/cream	100 000 units/g		
Amphotericin	Lozenges	10 mg	Four times daily	At least 2 but preferably 4 weeks
	Oral suspension	100 mg/ml		

Treatment for longer periods may be necessary, especially in chronic hyperplastic candidosis or in immunocompromised patients.

Oral gel (25 mg/ml) 5–10 ml held over area affected (after food) or applied to fitting surface of upper denture for the treatment of denture stomatitis (chronic erythematous candidosis).

Cream (2%) Apply to angles of lips 2–3 times daily.

Cream or ointment (2%) with hydrocortisone (1%) Apply to angles of lips 2–3 times daily. May be useful for clearing long-standing angular cheilitis but should not be used for longer than 10 days.

Fluconazole (a triazole)

This *systemically* acting agent inhibits fungal enzymes concerned with ergosterol synthesis. It appears to have low systemic toxicity.

Form Capsules (50 mg) and oral suspension (50 mg/5 ml).

Dose 50 mg daily for 7–14 days. Higher doses will be required in immunocompromised patients.

Cautions Avoid in renal disease, pregnancy and lactation, children.

Side effects Nausea, diarrhoea and allergic manifestations are the most serious effects.

Interactions Consult BNF for *all* antifungal interactions. Main interactions are with antihistamines, oral hypoglycaemic agents and warfarin.

Itraconazole is another potent triazole antifungal agent.

 Beware of the potential interactions of the imidazole and triazole antifungal agents with other drugs.

ANTIVIRAL AGENTS

Viruses exist intracellularly and agents used to treat viral infection run the risk of inducing host cell damage.

Aciclovir

Action Aciclovir is an analogue of the nucleotide purine. It is acted on by viral and cellular enzymes to form guanosine triphosphate, which disrupts viral DNA synthesis. It is used particularly in treating herpes simplex virus (HSV) and herpes zoster infections (see Table 5.4).

Forms Tablets (200 mg and 800 mg), suspension (200 mg/5 ml) and cream (5%).

TABLE 5.4 Dental uses of aciclovir

	Dose	Frequency	Duration
Primary herpes simplex infection	200 mg (Children <2 years: half adult dose in suspension form)	5 times daily	5 days
Secondary herpes simplex infection (cold sore)	5% cream	5 times daily	Must start at prodromal stage of cold sore
Herpes zoster (shingles)	800 mg	5 times daily	7 days

In primary herpetic gingivostomatitis, adequate rehydration measures must be taken along with bed-rest and a systemic analgesic/antipyretic agent such as paracetamol elixir.

Aciclovir should be avoided, if possible, in pregnancy, lactation and in renal disease.

Be aware of the newer agents for the treatment of shingles – **valaciclovir** and **famciclovir**.

Given the recent evidence that Bell's (lower motor neurone) facial palsy may be caused by HSV, many clinicians are now using aciclovir or a similar agent in the management of Bell's palsy.

Penciclovir

Penciclovir cream (1%) is available as a treatment for cold sores.

ANXIOLYTICS, HYPNOTICS AND ANTIDEPRESSANTS

> **Anxiolytics** are drugs that reduce anxiety, tension or fear.
> **Hypnotics** are drugs that induce sleep.

Anxiolytics and hypnotics may be used in dentistry for their primary effects. The benzodiazepines are by far the most common group of drugs used in this context.

BENZODIAZEPINES

Mode of action

All this group bind to γ-aminobutyric acid (GABA) receptors, mainly in the cerebral cortex. They augment GABA activity and have the following pharmacological effects: • reduction of anxiety • sedation and sleep induction (hypnotic effect) • muscle relaxation (centrally mediated) • anticonvulsant.

They *do not* have any analgesic effects.

Dental uses

Premedication Benzodiazepines may be used to help anxious patients achieve sleep before their dental treatment and to relieve nervousness by prescription an hour or two before appointments. Temazepam or diazepam is often used for this purpose. Patients should be warned of the sedative effects, should be accompanied to and from the surgery and should not drive a car or use potentially dangerous domestic or industrial machinery or appliances. Alcohol enhancement is known to occur and therefore concurrent use should be avoided. Long-term prescription will lead to addiction and there is no *justification for long-term use in dentistry* (see Table 5.5).

Muscle relaxation Many patients with myofascial pain dysfunction syndrome exhibit marked overactivity of the muscles of mastication and experience muscle pain due to spasm and fatigue. Diazepam (2–5 mg), taken an hour before bed for about 1 week, may have a good response, especially where muscle overactivity is nocturnal. It may also be prescribed at a dose of 2 mg three times daily.

Intravenous sedation Midazolam has largely superseded diazepam and diazemuls as an intravenous sedation agent (p. 104).

Anticonvulsant Intravenous diazepam may effect termination of status epilepticus. It may also be administered rectally (p. 530).

Unwanted effects

Overdosage is considered less dangerous than with other sedative or hypnotic drugs. Respiration may be depressed and hypotension may occur. Flumazenil is a short-acting antagonist to the benzodiazepines and may be used in overdose, but its effects are relatively transitory and careful monitoring of patients is therefore necessary.

Sedative effects such as drowsiness and ataxia (particularly in elderly people) are well recognized. Patients must be counselled on these effects, which may still be apparent on the day following use.

TABLE 5.5 Uses of diazepam, temazepam and nitrazepam

Drug	Use	Dose (mg)	Route	Time of administration
Diazepam	Hypnotic	5	Oral	Night before
	Premedication	5	Oral	1 hour pre-appointment
	Muscle relaxation	5	Oral	Before retiring
	(myofascial pain			(for no more than 1 week)
	dysfunction syndrome)	2	Oral	Three times daily
	Status epilepticus	10	i.v.	
Temazepam	Hypnotic	10	Oral	Night before
	Premedication	10	Oral	1 hour pre-appointment
Nitrazepam	Hypnotic	5	Oral	Night before

Elderly or infirm patients should take half the normal adult dose.

Dependence Both physical and psychological dependence occur on prolonged use. Together these may cause severe anxiety, nervousness and tremor on withdrawal. *There is no dental indication for long-term prescription.*

Prolongation of effect Some benzodiazepines have longer half-lives than others. For example, diazepam and nitrazepam have half-lives of around 30 hours, whilst others are significantly shorter (temazepam has a half-life of 8 hours) and may therefore be preferred.

Additionally, however, some (notably diazepam) are metabolized to cerebrally active breakdown products (e.g. nordiazepam), which are slow to be excreted, and may further delay full and safe recovery.

Contraindications

• Patients with chronic obstructive pulmonary disease (COPD).
• Patients with psychotic illness or who exhibit abnormal behaviour such as obsession or phobia. • Alcohol or drug misusers. • In children the effect of intravenous benzodiazepines is unpredictable, often resulting in 'paradoxical' excitation. However, oral premedication and sedation may be helpful in selected children.
• Pregnancy and lactation.

ANTIDEPRESSANTS

There are several classes of antidepressant drugs in clinical use:
• tricyclic antidepressants (TCAs) • monoamine oxidase inhibitors (MAOIs) • selective serotonin re-uptake inhibitors (SSRIs)
• serotonin-noradrenaline re-uptake inhibitors (SNRIs).

As far as dentistry is concerned, it is important to know that a patient is under treatment for depression since the condition may alter the patient's behaviour. The symptoms and their treatment may have effects on patient management.

Both TCAs and MAOIs may cause postural hypotension. As much dentistry is carried out in the supine position, care must be taken to upright the patient slowly and ensure no ataxia when ambulant and before discharge.

Both TCAs and MAOIs have atropine-like action, which may cause xerostomia. This, in turn, can increase the risk of caries and periodontal disease and may adversely affect denture retention. It may also predispose to oral candidosis.

Both TCAs and MAOIs increase risk of arrhythmias and hypotension with general anaesthetic agents; the use of opioids either pre- or postsurgically may cause hypo- or hypertension (especially pethidine).

There is *no* clinical evidence of significant interaction with local anaesthetics containing epinephrine (adrenaline) leading to hypertension in either TCA or MAOI groups.

Therapeutic dental use It is not the professional responsibility of dental surgeons to diagnose depression or prescribe accordingly. However, even in patients not suffering from depressive illness, there is an analgesic effect which some antidepressant drugs exert (dosulepin and amitriptyline in particular) that may be of value in atypical or chronic facial pain syndromes and in some non-responsive patients with temporomandibular disorders (dysfunction). This property may be related to enhancing monoaminergic nerve transmission, which inhibits pain afferents or as a direct antidepressant effect. It may take several weeks to achieve relief of symptoms and treatment may extend over several months or longer according to the individual patient's need.

This group of drugs also cause some muscle relaxation which may be beneficial in chronic orofacial pain syndrome.

Dosulepin

Dose Initially 25–75 mg at bedtime, increasing gradually if required.

Contraindications Recent myocardial infarction, cardiac arrhythmias, mania and liver disease.

Side effects and interactions See BNF
Liaison with patient's general medical practitioner is essential in prescription.

Amitryptiline

Dose Initially 10–25 mg at bedtime, increasing to 75 mg if required.

This drug has a good evidence base for use in patients with chronic orofacial pain syndromes. However, higher doses may be required as opposed to the 10 mg dose recommended generally for chronic pain.

ANTIHISTAMINES

The use of antihistamines in dental practice is restricted to the management of allergic reactions, the emergency treatment of anaphylaxis and for premedication and sedation in children.

Chlorphenamine maleate

A sedating antihistamine.

Form Tablets 4 mg

Dose 4 mg every 4–6 hours, maximum 24 mg daily.

Promethazine hydrochloride

A sedating antihistamine.

Form Tablets 10 mg and 25 mg, oral suspension 5 mg/5 ml.

Dose 25–50 mg at night or 10–20 mg 2–3 times daily.

Both of these drugs require appropriate dose reduction for children (see BNF). Both drugs may cause drowsiness and affect performance of skilled tasks (e.g. driving). The effect of alcohol is enhanced. For other important interactions refer to BNF.

Other agents, particularly non-sedating ones (e.g. cetirizine and fexofenadine) may be prescribed by a physician or bought in a pharmacy.

TOPICAL AGENTS

Various agents are available for topical use in the mouth. Among the more commonly prescribed are: • chlorhexidine • povidone-iodine • choline salicylate • benzydamine hydrochloride • carmellose sodium • lidocaine (lignocaine) • topical steroids • saliva substitutes.

Chlorhexidine

A biguanide antiseptic. Adheres to tooth enamel, pellicle and plaque. Causes changes in bacterial cell wall permeability. Mainly effective against Gram-positive bacteria but also against oral fungi. Adherent property allows longer duration of action. As a mouthwash, can cause dramatic fall in bacterial count in saliva (up to 90% reported).

Dental uses

Dental mouthwash 0.2% chlorhexidine gluconate solution. Particularly useful in the following situations: • oral surgery – pre- and postoperatively • periodontology – (p. 215) • oral ulceration – to prevent secondary infection and promote healing • disabled patients – where oral hygiene (brushing) is compromised • immunocompromised patients • antiseptic overnight 'soak' for dentures in patients with candidosis.

Irrigant 0.05% chlorhexidine gluconate: • surgical wounds, e.g. dry socket • pericoronal infections • root canals (*Savlon*: chlorhexidine and cetrimide).

Toothpaste gel 1% chlorhexidine gluconate.

Oral spray 0.2% chlorhexidine gluconate. May be useful for disabled patients.

It has been suggested that the use of chlorhexidine mouthwash before dentoalveolar surgery in the endocarditis risk group may reduce the resultant bacteraemia quantitatively and increase the protection to the patient.

Periodontal pockets Chlorhexidine is available in gelatin as a local delivery antimicrobial for periodontal pockets.

Side effects
• Staining (exogenous and removable) of teeth and tongue. Probably mainly due to dietary pigments adhering to the antiseptic-treated pellicle or plaque. • Taste disturbance. • Mucosal desquamation – leading to surface discomfort. • Parotid swelling (aetiology unknown).

Povidone–iodine
This mouthwash (1% solution) is a useful and palatable alternative to chlorhexidine. However, it does not have the antiplaque property of chlorhexidine and has several contraindications and cautions associated.

Contraindications Thyroid disorders, patients on lithium therapy.

Cautions Should not be used for longer than 2 weeks due to possible iodine absorption. Pregnancy and lactation: due to possible fetal absorption of iodine, other mouthwashes should be prescribed. Renal disease.

PREPARATIONS FOR ULCERATION OF ORAL MUCOSA

It is important that the cause of ulceration is correctly diagnosed and treated – e.g. dentures causing trauma should be suitably relieved, biopsy of suspicious ulcer performed and underlying haematological deficiencies excluded. However, symptomatic relief may be obtained by use of these agents (Table 5.6).

TABLE 5.6 Drugs for topical use

Drug	Form	Frequency	Action	Common uses	Dangers
Hydrocortisone sodium succinate (cromucosal tablets)	Tablets (2.5 mg)	4 times daily	Anti-inflammatory	Recurrent oral ulceration Erosive lichen planus	Pregnancy and lactation Should not be used for infected lesions
Hydrocortisone	Cream (1%)	3 times daily	Anti-inflammatory	Non-infected angular cheilitis	Use should not exceed 1 week
Triamcinolone acetonide	Paste (0.1%)	Thin layer 3 times daily	Anti-inflammatory	Recurrent oral ulceration Erosive lichen planus	Pregnancy and lactation Should not be used for infected lesions
Betamethasone sodium phosphate	Tablets (0.5 mg)	Dissolve in water and use as a mouthwash for 1 minute 2–4 times daily	Anti-inflammatory	As above	As above
Beclometasone dipropionate	Aerosol (50 µg per actuation)	Apply 2 puffs 2–4 times daily directly onto mucosa	Anti-inflammatory	As above	As above

TABLE 5.6 (cont'd)

Drug	Form	Frequency	Action	Common uses	Dangers
Hydrocortisone and miconazole	Cream or ointment (1%) with miconazole (2%)	3 times daily	Anti-inflammatory Antifungal Antibacterial	Angular chelitis	As above
Benzydamine hydrochloride	Mouth-wash (0.15%) Spray (0.15%)	15 ml 2–3 hourly	Topical anaesthetic	Oral ulceration Post-radiation mucositis	Not normally used for >1 week Avoid in children
Lidocaine hydrochloride	Ointment (5%)	Apply thin layer before meals	Topical anaesthetic	Oral ulceration	Excessive use may cause toxicity Avoid in children Development of allergy
Choline salicylate	Gel (8.7%)	Not more than 3 hourly	Surface analgesic	Oral ulceration	May cause damage to mucosa and salicylate toxicity, especially in children
Carmellose sodium	Paste (16.5%)	As required	Protective surface agent	Oral ulceration	No significant dangers

SALIVA SUBSTITUTES

Dry mouth can be the result of irradiation, salivary gland disease, drug therapy and psychopathology. Artificial salivas are available generically via the DPF list and prescribable by physicians via the BNF. Examples are Glandosane®, Luborant® and Saliva Orthana®, which are available as sprays. Saliva Orthana® is also available as a lozenge and Salivix® as a pastille. Biotène Oralbalance® and BioXtra® are available as a saliva replacement gel, mouthwash and toothpaste. The aetiology of xerostomia should *always* be established.

DRUG INTERACTIONS OF DENTAL RELEVANCE

The BNF is essential reading each and every time you reach for the prescription pad. Remember that all drugs have potentially serious interactions and the professional responsibility of prescribing drugs is an onerous one.

It is important to avoid polypharmacy where possible. Update the patient's medical history sheet by *direct questioning* at each visit. Almost any medical condition affects drug prescribing but be particularly cautious in pregnancy, breast feeding, liver and kidney disease, and in patients taking anticoagulant therapy.

The freedom to prescribe drugs is a great responsibility afforded to very few professional groups. Never abuse the privilege and always liaise with the patient's medical practitioner if any doubt exists in your mind.

Be aware of the Committee on Safety of Medicines' 'Yellow Card' Scheme for reporting adverse drug reactions. These yellow cards are available at the back of each BNF.

NOTE ON DRUG NOMENCLATURE

In the UK, in light of EU directive (92/27/EEC), the British Approved Names (BANs) of some drugs have been amended to accord with the Recommended International Non-proprietary Names (rINNs). The substances affected by the change of most relevance to dentistry are given in Table 5.7.

TABLE 5.7 Drug nomenclature

BAN	rINN
adrenaline	epinephrine
amoxycillin	amoxicillin
cephalexin	cefalexin
cephradine	cefradine
chlorpheniramine	chlorphenamine
doxycycline hydrocholoride	doxycycline hyclate
dothiepin	dosulepin
lignocaine	lidocaine

CHAPTER 6

ANALGESIA, SEDATION AND GENERAL ANAESTHESIA

Local anaesthesia 92

Sedation 101

Intravenous (i.v.) sedation 104

General anaesthesia 107

Hypnotherapy 113

LOCAL ANAESTHESIA

Local anaesthesia is more properly referred to as local analgesia, but the term local anaesthesia is normally used in modern dental practice. To avoid confusion the term local anaesthesia will be used throughout this chapter.

Local anaesthetic (LA) agents block conduction of nerve impulses reversibly and may be administered:

- topically
- by infiltration
- by regional block
- by intraligamentous injection
- by intraosseous injection.

Most commonly used local anaesthetics such as lidocaine and prilocaine have an *amide* link between the aromatic head and the rest of the molecule (Figure 6.1), which means they are broken down in the *liver* by *amidase enzymes*.

LOCAL ANAESTHETIC SOLUTIONS

Consist mainly of LA, usually in the form of a strong acid salt, a vasoconstrictor and physiological saline. Sodium bisulphite may be added as an antioxidant to prevent deterioration of the vasoconstrictor. In the local anaesthetic solution, most of the LA is present as the hydrochloride salt.

$$R \equiv N + HCl \rightarrow R \equiv NH^+ + Cl^-$$

When injected into the tissues, the cation $R-NH^+$ dissociates and liberates a certain amount of free LA, although most remains in the cation form.

$$R \equiv NH^+ \rightleftharpoons R \equiv N + H^+$$

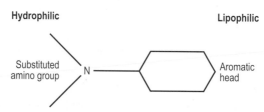

Hydrophilic   **Lipophilic**

Substituted
amino group   N   Aromatic
                            head

Figure 6.1 Basic structure of local anaesthetic.

Where the tissues are inflamed, even more cation is formed, leaving less free base. The free base liberated is important as it, being lipophilic and uncharged, passes through the axon wall; the cation, being positively charged is unable to do this. Within the cell (axon) the base LA again dissociates into the cation, and it is the cation which is believed to be mainly responsible for conduction block.

Mechanism

In general terms, local anaesthetics prevent nerve conduction by obstructing the depolarization, which is primarily effected by a massive influx of sodium ions. In the axon wall, there are numerous pores or sodium channels, which allow the ionic changes. LA cations block these channels and LA base may cause further distortion (membrane expansion).

Effect of LA on other systems

Cardiovascular
Myocardium: Reduces excitability. Reduces force of contraction.
Arterioles: Vasodilation.

Central nervous
Stimulation, e.g. restlessness, tremor. Increasing dose – respiratory depression especially dangerous.

Vasoconstrictors

Agents Usually epinephrine (adrenaline) or felypressin. These are included in most solutions for four main purposes: • to prolong length of action • to increase depth of action • to reduce toxicity of the LA (this is controversial as some consider the more significant danger to be related to the effect of epinephrine) • to obtain haemostatic effect (oral or periodontal surgery).

Epinephrine (adrenaline)

Systemic effects Mediated via α and β receptors (Table 6.1).
Possible dangers: excitatory effect on patients with heart disease • patients with uncontrolled thyrotoxicosis • pheochromocytoma (hypertension) • recent use of cocaine (hypertension).

There is *no* evidence of interactive clinical problems with tricyclic antidepressant or monoamine oxidase inhibitor drugs, but dosage should probably be limited to 5 ml of 1 : 80 000 concentration.

Felypressin

• Synthetic hormone similar to vasopressin • less vasoconstrictive than epinephrine • no cardiac effects • no known interactions • mild

TABLE 6.1 Systemic effects of epinephrine (adrenaline)		
Heart (β)	*Blood vessels (α and β₂)*	
Rate increases	Striated muscle	Dilates (β)
Force increases	Skin	Constricts (α)
Output increases	Coronary	Dilates (β)
Excitability increases	Blood pressure	Systolic rises Diastolic falls

In addition, bronchial muscle is relaxed.

oxytocic effect which, in theory, could impede placental circulation and therefore is probably better avoided in pregnancy.

Commonly used agents
- Lidocaine 2% with epinephrine 1 : 80 000
- Prilocaine 3% with felypressin 0.03 IU
- Prilocaine 4%
- Prilocaine 3% with epinephrine 1 : 300 000
- Articaine 4% with epinephrine 1 : 100 000

Other local anaesthetic agents less commonly used are mepivacaine, which is shorter acting, and bupivacaine, which is a long-acting anaesthetic and may act for 6–8 hours when given as a block injection.

Maximum safe doses
Calculated on the basis of possible effects of the local anaesthetic. The effects of the vasoconstrictor should not be ignored. For example, the addition of epinephrine to lidocaine raises the safe maximum dose by slowing its absorption into the circulation, but this 'slowing down' process may not be as significant as once thought.

- Lidocaine with epinephrine   4.4 mg/kg
- Prilocaine   6 mg/kg
- Articaine   7 mg/kg

These figures, when translated into volumes of the local anaesthetic solution for a fit, healthy patient of average weight, suggest the following:

2% Lidocaine with epinephrine   6–7 cartridges of 2.2 ml
3% Prilocaine with felypressin   5–6 cartridges of 2.2 ml
4% Prilocaine   4 cartridges of 2.2 ml
4% Articaine (with epinephrine)   4 cartridges of 2.2 ml

These maximum doses should be suitably reduced for: • elderly people • children • debilitated • cardiac disease.

Toxicity can be reduced for all patients by the following measures: • use of an efficient aspirating technique • slow deposition of the solution.

Controversy exists whether epinephrine-containing local anaesthetics should be used for patients with known heart disease. Epinephrine has powerful effects on the cardiovascular system and may also reduce potassium levels in the bloodstream – potentially of importance in patients on diuretic therapy who may be potassium depleted. Use of epinephrine-free solutions will avoid these problems. However, some clinicians consider lidocaine with epinephrine achieves a more profound anaesthesia and is therefore less likely to cause the release of endogenous epinephrine, which is evident when pain is felt during the operative procedure.

Practical aspects

Local anaesthetics are the most commonly used drugs in dental practice. They provide a reversible interruption to the transmission of nerve impulses, particularly in response to pain but also to touch, pressure and thermal stimulation. They are generally very safe and allow most dental procedures to be carried out without recourse to general anaesthesia.

Uses can be listed as follows: • comfort during operative dental procedures • diagnosis, e.g. differentiation between pain arising from upper or lower tooth where symptoms of pulpitis can make it difficult to isolate the source • reduction of bleeding for periodontal or oral surgery (due to the vasoconstrictor component) • reduction of arrhythmias during surgical manipulation under general anaesthesia • reduction of the depth of general anaesthesia during oral surgery due to decrease in afferent stimulation of the CNS, which in turn leads to less risk of arrhythmia • immediate postoperative analgesia after oral or maxillofacial procedures (reduces need for postoperative opiates) • pain control in acute 'flare-ups' of pain in certain chronic pain syndromes (e.g. trigeminal neuralgia). Long-acting locals may have a role in certain cases.

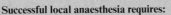

Successful local anaesthesia requires:
- **knowledge of the innervation of the oral cavity**
- **knowledge of the content and pharmacological nature of local anaesthetic agents.**

Administration

Local anaesthetic agents may be administered: • by surface application (topical agents) • by injection.

Infiltration

Here the solution is deposited at or near the apex of the tooth and diffuses through the bone to affect the periapical nerves and those nerves serving the periodontal ligament, adjacent bone and soft tissues. Bone porosity is needed to allow such diffusion; this precludes this form of local anaesthesia in the mandibular molar and premolar regions. Normally the needle is inserted in the buccal sulcus only 2–3 mm, such that the solution is introduced to the periapical region; usually 1–2 ml (roughly half to one 2.2 ml cartridge) is sufficient.

Technique

There are two distinct stages in the procedure:
1. Insertion of needle
   This requires firm stretching (with the finger or thumb) of the sulcus such that the mucosa becomes taut, and hence allows less discomfort on needle penetration. Only 2–3 mm of needle is generally inserted and the angulation of the syringe is approximately parallel to the long axis of the tooth.
2. Deposition of the solution
   Before depressing the syringe plunger, it is prudent, even with infiltration, to aspirate. The solution should be introduced *slowly* to avoid tissue damage, which may be considerable given the very narrow gauge of dental needles.

Regional block

Here, the solution is deposited around a nerve trunk and will cause anaesthesia to tissues within the distribution of the nerve peripheral to the point of block administration. In dentistry there are several nerve blocks which can be useful.

Inferior dental (ID) block All lower teeth.

Mental nerve block Lower first premolar to central incisor.

Infraorbital nerve block Upper central to second premolar.

Nasopalatine block Mucoperiosteum palatal to upper canines and incisors.

Greater palatine block Mucoperiosteum palatal to upper premolars and molars.

Posterior superior dental block Upper molars – seldom of any additional value to simple infiltration.

The most commonly given by far is the *inferior dental block injection*. Tissues anaesthetized will include tissues served by the lingual nerve in addition to tissues supplied by the inferior dental nerve.

ID nerve block
Tissues anaesthetized

ID nerve: • mandibular teeth – pulps and periodontium • bone of mandible in toothbearing area • buccal gingivae from premolars to midline • lower lip and chin • cheek variably adjacent to premolars/canine.

Lingual nerve: • anterior two-thirds tongue • floor of mouth • lingual gingivae.

Not anaesthetized fully: buccal gingivae and sulcus in molar region. These tissues are supplied by the (long) buccal nerve and require separate infiltration for surgery but not restorative work.

Technique

1. Patient seated comfortably – neck supported and slightly extended such that when the mouth is fully open, the lower occlusal plane will be approximately horizontal.
2. Index finger or thumb of the non-syringe-holding hand is passed posteriorly in the buccal sulcus until it lies in the retromolar triangle (formed by meeting of external oblique line and mylohyoid line).
3. Visualize the almost vertically running pterygomandibular raphe (runs from pterygoid hamulus to medial aspect of mandible in third molar region).
4. Introduce needle from premolars of opposite side such that:
   a. It is parallel to lower occlusal plane.

  b. It is halfway up the finger lying in the retromolar triangle.
  c. It passes *lateral* to the raphe.
5. The needle is advanced, usually 2.5 cm, until bone is felt – then withdrawn 1–2 mm.
   Never advance needle to hub as this will make retrieval impossible should the needle fracture.
6. Aspirate – if blood noted in cartridge, then move needle a millimetre or so and aspirate again.
7. Inject *slowly* – using most of 2.2 ml cartridge and keep injecting on withdrawal to deposit solution around the lingual nerve.
8. Mouth rinse (taste of LA is very unpleasant).

Assessment of block

This is accomplished by asking the patient to describe subjective feelings, most easily felt on lower lip and chin. Early anaesthesia is often described as a tingling sensation or 'pins and needles'. Later description may be of a puffy, swollen, rubbery or thick feeling. Objective assessment may be accomplished by using a sharp probe (sparingly!) on the gingivae. When testing anaesthesia, don't ask the patient simply to report if he/she feels *anything* (many will be aware of touch or pressure) – ask if *pain* or *discomfort* is felt.

Remember to supplement the ID nerve block with a long buccal nerve block for periodontal and oral surgical procedures in the mandible.

Mental nerve block

Tissues anaesthetized: • Pulp and periodontium of mandibular first premolar to central incisor with supporting bone. Variably, second premolar. • Lip, chin and adjacent sulcus and cheek to the above teeth. • For extractions or surgery, a lingual infiltration must also be given.

Technique

Essentially an infiltration technique around the mental foramen but aspiration prior to depositing solution is necessary. The mental foramen lies halfway between the gingival margin of the premolars and the lower border of mandible in the dentate mouth.

Infraorbital nerve block

Tissues anaesthetized • upper lip, cheek, side of nose and lower eyelid
• buccal gingivae and sulcus from midline to premolar region •
incisors, canine and premolars (anterior and middle superior alveolar
nerves arise from the infraorbital nerve in the infraorbital canal).

Technique

Similar to infiltration but:
- The needle should be aligned parallel to the long axis
  of the premolars.
- The needle enters the tissues about 1.5 cm lateral to
  the buccal alveolar bone surface where an infiltration
  would be given.
- The needle should be advanced about 1.5 cm vertically
  to the region of the infraorbital foramen before
  aspirating and injecting slowly.

Greater palatine nerve block

Tissues anaesthetized: Palatal mucoperiosteum up to the canine
region. Anterior to this, the innervation is derived from the
nasopalatine nerve.

Technique

A more compressible area can be found on palpation of
the hard palate between the midline and the palatal
gingival margin of the teeth. This is less bound down to
underlying bone and therefore less painful on injection.
The nerve can be blocked at any point along its
anatomical path depending on the surgical site.
   This injection is painful. Application of surface
anaesthetic and firm finger pressure for 10–20 seconds by
the non-syringe-holding hand before sliding the needle
in close to this finger can minimize the pain. Thereafter,
only a few drops need be introduced *slowly*. For upper
wisdom teeth, it may be less uncomfortable to inject a
few drops close to the palatal cervical margin of the
tooth on the attached gingiva.

Nasopalatine nerve block

Tissues anaesthetized: Palatal mucoperiosteum of anterior hard
palate related to canines and incisors.

Technique

This is a very sensitive region and injections in this area are unpleasant. Firm finger pressure over the nasopalatine papilla (after application of topical anaesthetic) and introduction of needle from one side of the papilla may reduce the pain. It is also worthwhile putting a drop of anaesthetic solution just under the epithelium before proceeding to inject deeper into the foramen region. Very small amount needed and delivered *slowly*. Immediate blanching of the area is often noted.

COMPLICATIONS OF LOCAL ANAESTHESIA
Systemic
Fainting This is the commonest systemic complication. Psychological aetiology most likely; patients may give a previous history. Can be minimized by administering LA with patient supine. (For management, see p. 523.)

Interaction See previous notes. Very uncommon problem.

Allergy Very uncommon but possible. Should not be confused with fainting. Collapse with rapid drop in blood pressure may be a feature of allergy. For management of collapse, see page 527. Requires confirmation by specialized allergy clinic, which may identify the particular allergen.

Cardiovascular collapse This may be related to stress in a susceptible patient. Excessive amounts of LA, lack of aspiration and excessive speed of delivery may be contributory. Epinephrine in the LA can have direct effects on the heart, which, if previously diseased, may lead to arrhythmia or even fibrillation.

Local
Failure to achieve anaesthesia Often related to a 'hot' pulp or apical abscess. Aids to gaining sufficient anaesthesia include:
• intraligamentous injection or intrapulpal • supplementing block with infiltration • supplementing infiltration with block • use of higher concentration of LA, e.g. 4% prilocaine • sedative dressing such as *Ledermix* and try again in 48 hours • ask a colleague to give LA (especially if block).

Haematoma Small haematomas (e.g. in sulcus) are of no consequence but aspiration during block injections will reduce chance in deeper tissues.

Trismus This may occur after ID block and is attributed to damage with haematoma formation in the medial pterygoid muscle. Injection given too low and excessive rate of deposition are possible factors. Management is difficult and generally involves reassurance, prescription of an antibiotic if diagnosed within the first few days, and encouragement to open mouth using progressive numbers of wooden spatulas.

Facial paralysis A complication of the ID block and due to the needle passing through the investing deep cervical fascia around the parotid gland, through which the facial nerve passes and separates into its five branches. Paralysis is normally short in duration (1 hour) and affects all branches (i.e. lower motor neurone distribution). Reassure patient. A protective eye covering is necessary until the blink reflex returns.

Needle fracture Very unlikely due to 'use once' policy. Needles should not be bent or inserted to the hub – both of which increase likelihood of fracture. Spencer Wells or 'mosquito' forceps should be near at hand to effect immediate retrieval.

Needle-stick injury Administration of LA is the most common cause of needle-stick injury. Risk can be minimized by a safe sheathing policy or use of 'safety' syringes now available. For management, see page 543.

Very uncommonly • An unusual blanching of skin in the cheek may be observed following ID block. This is short lived, not fully understood and of no consequence. • Visual disturbance including loss of vision. Very rare and may reflect intra-arterial injection in patients with anatomical variants of blood supply. Normally transient but persistence would demand immediate referral to an ophthalmic specialist.

SEDATION

CONSCIOUS SEDATION

Many patients have understandable anxiety when undergoing dental treatment. The sympathetic and reassuring practitioner has a major role in the successful management of such patients. There remains, however, a number of patients who need additional help, which can be achieved in a number of ways: • oral premedication – normally a benzodiazepine (p. 81) • inhalation sedation • intravenous sedation • hypnotherapy • oral or transmucosal (usually intranasal) sedation.

A patient who is sedated satisfactorily is one who accepts treatment with or without local anaesthesia and who previously tolerated such treatment only with difficulty, if at all.

> The General Dental Council defines sedation as follows:
>
> A technique in which the use of a drug or drugs produces a state of depression of the central nervous system enabling treatment to be carried out, but during which communication can be maintained and the modification of the patient's state of mind is such that the patient will respond to command throughout the period of sedation. Techniques used should carry a margin of safety wide enough to render unintended loss of consciousness unlikely.

Assessment

Ideally all patients for conscious sedation should be formally assessed. Questions relevant to each specific technique should include: • drug history • drug allergy • previous sedation/anaesthetic • dental anxiety history.

This visit also allows for informed written consent to be obtained and baseline vital signs (blood pressure and heart rate) to be measured.

There are a number of routes available for sedation in dentistry: • oral (p. 80) • inhalation • intravenous • transmucosal.

INHALATION SEDATION

Equipment The technique most used is that of nitrous oxide (N_2O) inhalation administered with oxygen. To deliver the correct mixture of these gases, specific equipment is required. The most common delivery system is the *Quantiflex* system.

 Written, informed consent is required for inhalation sedation.

Technique for inhalation sedation

1. The patient should be informed of the objectives of the technique and of the equipment to be used. He/she should be instructed to speak during the procedure only if distressed.
2. The subject should be seated comfortably.
3. After demonstrating the position of the nosepiece, the patient should settle the mask over the nose.
4. The flow control should then be adjusted to keep the reservoir bag full while 100% O_2 is breathed.
5. N_2O should be increased reasonably quickly at first, i.e. 10% to 15% to 20% at 1 minute intervals, thereafter at smaller increments.
6. The operator should talk quietly and encouragingly, asking only for nodding responses to avoid the patient speaking and therefore breathing air and losing (rapidly) the sedative effect.
7. When sensory disturbance is noted (see below), the N_2O concentration should be reduced by 2.5–5%.
8. The dental procedure should commence. NB: Local anaesthesia is still required.
9. When nearing completion of treatment, the N_2O concentration should be reduced.
10. The patient should breath 'pure' air for at least 5 minutes before discharge. (Some operators prefer to administer 100% O_2 for 2–3 minutes at completion of treatment.)
11. Recovery from N_2O sedation is rapid but it is wise to keep the patient for 15–20 minutes to ensure total elimination of the agent.

Subjective sensory disturbances

Although mainly subjective, some of the following features may be felt by the patient: • tingling sensations (pins and needles) in fingers, toes, lips and tongue • tinnitus (ringing noise in ears); or observed by the operator: • lethargy – delay or slowing of reaction to requests • mild intoxication.

The technique of inhalational sedation relies heavily on behavioural management skills.

The operator should continually reassure the patient by stressing the feelings of warmth and comfort. Patients should be able to understand and respond to requests by the operator at all times.

For medico-legal reasons, there should *at all times* be a trained third party present. This should normally be a female dental nurse, particularly if the operator is male and the patient female.

Contraindications

Local Nasal obstruction, e.g. polyps, heavy cold, intolerance of mask, lack of seal to mask (e.g. moustache), operative procedures to upper anterior teeth (obstructed by mask).

Systemic Severe respiratory disease, active neurological disease such as multiple sclerosis (MS), deafness, severe mental or physical impairment.

Problems

Surgery contamination with N_2O This is a recognized problem particularly in small, poorly ventilated surgeries. Frequency of use of the technique and the difficulty and high cost of effective scavenging systems may make this a limiting factor on provision of this form of sedation. Opening windows and doors to the surgery will reduce the contamination but not eliminate it. Active scavenging is best practice.

Cost In addition to the capital cost of equipment and maintenance, cylinders of oxygen and nitrous oxide are relatively expensive if the technique is used frequently.

INTRAVENOUS (i.v.) SEDATION

Various intravenous sedation agents have been used in the past. These included a mixture of pentobarbitone, pethidine and hyoscine (Jorgensen technique), methohexitone and, more recently, the benzodiazepine group of anxiolytic drugs. These latter drugs started to find favour for sedative purposes in the 1960s and were popular with practitioners as they: • induced reliable sedation without loss of consciousness • allowed good patient cooperation with verbal contact maintained • produced marked anterograde amnesia of 20–30 minutes' duration • could induce a convenient duration of sedation of around 30–60 minutes.

PHARMACOKINETICS OF BENZODIAZEPINES

As discussed in Chapter 5, benzodiazepine receptors are distributed widely in the CNS. The effect of the drug enhances the action of γ-aminobutyric acid (GABA), which is a major inhibitory neurotransmitter in brain synapses. GABA controls the synaptic flow of chloride ions, and activation of the benzodiazepine receptors enhances the flow of these ions. The overall effect of these drugs is therefore *inhibitory* and causes reduction in anxiety, sedative effects and muscle relaxation.

Early use of *diazepam* highlighted some disadvantages of this particular drug. Being insoluble in water, it had to be mixed with aspirated blood to reduce local irritation to the veins as thrombophlebitis was a problem. Furthermore, it was apparent that diazepam formed active metabolites (e.g. nordiazepam), which could cause prolongation of effects. Some improvement in the local discomfort of injection was achieved with the introduction of *Diazemuls*, which was an intralipid emulsion of diazepam. However, both these drugs have largely been superseded by *midazolam* which has several advantages over the earlier drugs. These are: • water solubility – less pain at injection and less chance of thrombophlebitis • faster recovery – short half-life and probably little activity from metabolites • less hangover – shorter half-life • lower dosage – about 2.5 times more potent than diazepam.

i.v. SEDATION WITH MIDAZOLAM

Preparation

- The patient should eat only a light snack up to 2 hours preoperatively.
- An escort *must* be available to accompany the patient after treatment.
- Written informed consent must be obtained.
- A trained assistant must be present at all times during treatment and recovery.
- Monitoring – pulse oximetry is mandatory.
- Means of i.v. access – ideally an indwelling cannula (e.g. Venflon®).

Technique

Midazolam is commercially available in two preparations: 10 mg/2 ml and 10 mg/5 ml. The latter is preferred in dentistry, giving a concentration of 2 mg per ml. The normal final dose will be in the range of 3–8 mg, and 10 mg should be considered the safe maximum in most patients.

Using the 2 mg/ml solution the technique is as follows:
1. Give 2 mg (1 ml) i.v. and wait for 1 minute.
2. Give 1 mg (0.5 ml) increments every 60 seconds.
3. The patient should be engaged in conversation during this period.
4. Watch for evidence of the patient showing less interest in the conversation.
5. Watch for evidence of the patient's gaze being directed forwards and blinking slowly.
6. Watch for yawning or drooping of eyelids; if the upper eyelid covers half the pupil (Verrill's sign), this should be considered slight overdosage.
7. Administer local anaesthesia as required.

Intravenous sedation produces no analgesia; therefore, careful local anaesthetic technique is important.

Safety

The technique is normally safe but a small number of patients may exhibit hypotension and/or respiratory depression. It is therefore important that this is recognized and treated promptly. The use of a pulse oximeter is a reliable early warning of such occurrences and most practitioners set the warning level of falling oxygen saturation at no less than 90%. Most patients have a saturation of 97–99%. The haemoglobin oxygen-carrying capacity drops rapidly after the 90% saturation level and effective measures to deal with this should be immediately available. These may include:

● Stop any further introduction of midazolam. Try to rouse patient with mild physical stimulation, reassess.
● Administer 100% oxygen and support ventilation if necessary (Ambu bag). Remember to extend neck, lift mandible and insert airway adjunct (nasopharyngeal tube) if respiratory obstruction is still present, reassess.
● Administer flumazenil, the competitive benzodiazepine antagonist and the antidote to midazolam. An i.v. injection of 200 μg is given over 15 seconds with a further 100 μg every 60 seconds until the patient shows evidence of recovery (maximum dose of 1000 μg).

Flumazenil has a much shorter half-life than midazolam and careful monitoring of patients is essential as relapse may occur. This drug should not be used to hasten normal recovery but be reserved for emergency use.

Recovery
This is normally uneventful but should be supervised, allowing discharge of the patient 60–90 minutes after first administration. The i.v. access should be left until recovery is complete. Patients should be escorted home, should not drive a motor vehicle, use complicated domestic appliances or make important decisions (e.g. signing legal documents) until the following day.

Other points to remember
• The technique is unsuitable for young children, especially under 10 years. • The patient should be in verbal contact throughout. • A trained assistant should be present at all times for medico-legal reasons. Such an assistant not only renders active help to the operator but, since some patients may hallucinate under sedation, may provide crucial testimony in any subsequent dispute.
• Procedures should not normally last for more than 1 hour.
• Patients who are currently taking oral benzodiazepines are more difficult to sedate. • Previously controlled emotions may be released with the technique and may require sensitive management, e.g. recently bereaved.

Future developments
Propofol is a commonly used intravenous general anaesthetic (GA) induction agent. It is presently being evaluated for use as a sedation agent in dentistry. The perceived advantages may be: • smoother, rapid onset • patient control of sedation level • quick recovery.

However, there are a number of important disadvantages:
• profound respiratory depression in overdose • no reversal drug • cost.

There has been recent interest in the use of midazolam both orally and intranasally, particularly for children or adults with learning difficulties. These techniques show promise but use bolus doses and should therefore not be preferred to the incremental use of i.v. midazolam, particularly in unexperienced hands.

GENERAL ANAESTHESIA

Dental patients will from time to time require GA to allow necessary treatment to be carried out.

> General anaesthetic agents cause a reversible disorganization
> of the functioning brain such that a state of unconsciousness
> is produced.

This allows dental or oral surgical procedures to be performed:
• without pain • without awareness • without movement • without
excessive bleeding • without detriment to central nervous system
function on recovery.

GENERAL DENTAL COUNCIL (GDC) GUIDANCE

The GDC has laid down strict guidelines for the use of general
anaesthesia in dentistry. Important among these are:

The referring dentist must:

● Discuss alternative treatment options for control of pain and
  anxiety.
● Give a clear explanation of the risk of a general anaesthetic.

The treating dentist must:

● Reiterate alternative treatment options and risk of a general
  anaesthetic.
● Obtain written consent.
● Give clear pre- and postoperative written instructions.
● Keep contemporaneous records.
● Ensure they have appropriately trained dental assisting staff.
● Ensure that the credentials of the anaesthetist meet GDC
  criteria.
● Ensure there is a written protocol for advanced life support and
  for immediate patient transfer to critical care if required.

Team training for emergencies is essential.

Certain categories of patient can be identified for general
anaesthesia.

Inpatient • Major oral and maxillofacial surgery, e.g. osteotomy.
• facial trauma often involving fracture(s).

Inpatient or day stay • Dentoalveolar surgery, e.g. difficult
impacted wisdom teeth.

Outpatient • Children with multiple carious teeth or too young to
allow local anaesthesia or local anaesthetic with sedation to be
used. • Adults with conditions not amenable to local anaesthesia

but otherwise requiring short procedures and who are medically fit, e.g. acute abscesses for incision and/or extraction of tooth.
• Children and adults with learning difficulties for restorative procedures and/or simple extractions. • Dental phobics may require restorative work if measures to control their fear have been unsuccessful.

INPATIENT GENERAL ANAESTHESIA

The advantages of having patients in a hospital ward are that nurses can ensure that the preanaesthetic checks are performed in an orderly fashion, and the anaesthetist has the opportunity to discuss the procedure with the patient and organize any particular tests thought appropriate to that case. Also postoperative recovery can be carefully monitored and analgesia controlled.

The following should be carried out before the patient is brought to theatre: • medical history taken, including any previous GA problems • routine medical assessment, mainly on cardiovascular and respiratory systems • special tests *where appropriate*, e.g. chest radiographs, ECG, full blood count • written informed consent with signature (covering both anaesthetic and proposed surgery) • patient starved for at least 4 hours preanaesthetic • premedication given at time indicated by anaesthetist • removal of dentures, make-up, jewellery.

Premedication primarily reduces anxiety and fear with its consequent epinephrine release, thereby facilitating anaesthetic induction. Various agents are used such as opiates or benzodiazepines. If an opiate is used there will be an increase in salivation, which, with bronchial secretion increase related to intubation and certain inhalation anaesthetics, is unwanted and is therefore countered by administering atropine or hyoscine. These latter drugs also counteract the bradycardia and hypotension caused by some anaesthetic agents, e.g. propofol, sevoflurane.

Anaesthetic procedure
When the patient arrives at the anaesthetic room, the following procedures are normally followed.

1. Nursing assistant ensures that the preoperative checks have been completed.
2. ECG leads are attached.

3. Intravenous access is gained.
4. Anaesthesia is induced, normally with a short-acting intravenous agent, e.g. propofol, but can be achieved more slowly by inhalation.
5. A muscle relaxant is given intravenously to relax the vocal cords (allowing easier endotracheal intubation), e.g. suxamethonium if the patient is to be allowed to breathe spontaneously, or vecuronium for longer procedures or with less fit patients. Breathing must be supported using intermittent positive pressure ventilation (IPPV). Atracurium is the drug of choice in renal or hepatic impairment.
6. A nasoendotracheal tube is passed using a laryngoscope to visualize the vocal cords, and the maintenance of the anaesthetic continues with oxygen, nitrous oxide (N_2O) and a volatile anaesthetic agent.
7. The cuff around the endotracheal tube is inflated.
8. A nasopharyngeal pack is inserted around the tube to absorb blood, saline irrigations or fragments not aspirated by the suction system.
9. The nasal part of the tube is stabilized with tape and the eyes protected with surgical tape.

Monitoring of anaesthetic
Vital signs are monitored using:

ECG Which shows the heart's electrical activity.
Pulse oximeter For pulse rate and oxygen saturation.
Capnograph Measures expired carbon dioxide (CO_2) concentration.
Airway pressure monitor (cm of water) Which indicates any obstruction to the airway or disconnections.

On recovery, pulse oximetry is usually continued until the patient is fully conscious and responsive.
On completion of the procedure:

1. The anaesthetic gases are diminished and subsequently stopped.
2. The dental operator normally dries the mouth thoroughly using a large-bore, high-volume aspirator,

and carefully inspects areas that may harbour fragments, e.g. under tongue, in sulci, and around the oropharyngeal aspect of the pack.
3. The pack is then slowly withdrawn with careful suction continuing and tongue depression to increase vision.
4. The anaesthetist extubates the patient (this requires skill and timing). The integrity of the airway is checked with a laryngoscope and appropriate suction.
5. Oxygen is administered (normally 4–5 litres/min) using a flexible disposable face mask held round the head with elastic fixation; a Guedel airway is also possible.
6. The patient may be turned on to his/her side in the 'recovery position'. This reduces the chance of obstruction by either tongue or secretions.

NB Most anaesthetists insert the pack and most oral surgeons or dentists remove them. Removal of the pack should be loudly communicated to all staff and many theatre sisters use a whiteboard 'pack-in-pack-out' display system.

OUTPATIENT GENERAL ANAESTHESIA

The vast majority of patients in this category are young children requiring extractions. The GDC places heavy ethical obligations on dentists referring patients for GA. All other treatment options should be discussed with the parent and discounted before GA is considered. The patient (or in the case of young children, parents) should be made fully aware of the implications of a GA. Furthermore, outpatient GA should only be performed in a hospital setting where intensive therapy unit facilities are immediately available.

The main concern is maintaining a good airway. The airway is particularly threatened by the following factors: • the relative shortness and narrowness of the respiratory tree in children • the presence of enlarged tonsils, adenoids or both • nasal stuffiness through excessive secretions • obstruction through inappropriate packing of the oropharyngeal region • obstruction by inappropriate dental manipulation, e.g. applying pressure to the mandible, as in molar extractions without adequate countersupport, may lead to the tongue being forced back on to the posterior pharyngeal wall • enlarged tongue, which may be a feature of Down syndrome • dental haemorrhage packs which can obstruct the airway during recovery • no artificial airway tube – although this may be used where problems are predicted or, less easily, when encountered. Either nasopharyngeal or endotracheal tubes may be appropriate.

Additionally, patients do not normally receive premedication and this, allied to their fear and apprehension, can lead to difficulties in delivering a smooth induction. Most inductions are by inhalation and, of necessity, take time.

Contraindications to outpatient general anaesthesia

- Medically unfit, particularly:
  - cardiovascular or respiratory problems
  - recent exposure to infectious fevers
  - medication which may interact, e.g. monoamine oxidase inhibitors, antihypertensives
- Not starved (at least 4 hours without food or drink is essential)
- Unaccompanied
- No valid consent
- Severe alcohol or drug abuse problems
- Pregnancy
- Trismus (would require inpatient facilities with fibreoptic technique for intubation).

Outpatient anaesthetic procedure

These patients should, as previously stated, be medically fit as far as can be assessed by accurate history taking (see Chapter 2) and this may be in written questionnaire format and signed by the patient. Parents or legal guardians should sign the medical history questionnaire for children. Full written consent to the proposed procedure is also required.

Despite the outpatient nature of the anaesthetic, the same monitoring equipment as for inpatients should be used and trained staff are essential. The Poswillo Report on dental anaesthesia also lists necessary drugs that may be needed for any complications. A parent is often asked to accompany the child into the surgery and some anaesthetists are happy to induce anaesthesia with the child on the parent's knee. This reduces the fear in the unpremedicated child and aids a smooth induction. Normally a mixture of nitrous oxide (N_2O), sevoflurane (or other volatile agents such as enflurane) and oxygen (O_2) is used.

The major preoccupation of the anaesthetist is the airway; the child's jaw is held forward with the neck slightly extended, to maintain the patency. Oral packs are inserted, and the mouth is kept open with a gag (Ferguson's gag) or prop (McKesson's prop). Many dental operators now infiltrate some local anaesthetic around the surgical site (mainly to achieve postoperative comfort) before extracting *but this should never be done without the full approval of the anaesthetist*. The prop or gag may be switched to the opposite side following initial extraction(s) if bilateral surgery is needed, and fresh packs (with trailing strings to ensure safe removal) inserted as haemostatic aids. The child is then transferred to a trolley and placed in the recovery position. Pulse oximetry is continued until the patient recovers, at which time any haemostatic packs are finally removed.

Modifications for restorative procedures

Restorative procedures under outpatient GA may be justifiable in the following groups (p. 193): • physical disability, e.g. cerebral palsy • learning difficulty, e.g. Down syndrome • needle or dental phobics.

For relatively short procedures, a laryngeal mask may be used to protect the airway, but excessive secretions or large volumes of irrigant or coolant may limit its use. Often the patients are fully intubated and the airway protected with nasopharyngeal packs. Limitation of space within the mouth may cause difficulties and experienced operators are generally required. Careful debridement is essential as fragments of old restorations, dental rolls and restorative materials are not always easy to clear before extubation.

HYPNOTHERAPY

Many consider that hypnotherapy has an important part to play in the longer-term management of dental and needle phobics. Relaxation induced by hypnotherapy may also be useful in the management of muscle tension and bruxism associated with myofascial pain dysfunction syndrome. Local and national courses are organized by regulated bodies for practitioners interested in developing skills in this field.

CHAPTER 7

DENTAL MATERIALS

Properties of materials   116

Dental amalgam   119

Resin composites   121

Glass ionomers   123

Cermets, resin-modified
glass ionomers and similar
materials   125

Adhesion and bonding
agents   126

Luting cements, linings and
bases   128

Temporary cements and
restorations   130

Impression materials   131

Porcelain and ceramics   136

Casting and wrought
alloys   139

Denture base
materials   141

Endodontic materials   143

Implant materials   144

Miscellaneous   145

Current 'growth areas' in
dental materials   147

PROPERTIES OF MATERIALS

The properties of dental materials can be classified as:

- mechanical, e.g. strength
- physical, e.g. thermal expansion
- chemical, e.g. corrosion
- biocompatibility, e.g. toxicity.

Dental materials can also be defined by their molecular form:

Metals Crystalline held by primary forces.

Polymers Large chain molecules held by physical entanglement and secondary forces.

Ceramics Ionic crystalline materials which can exist as an amorphous glass.

Composites A combination of two or more material types, displaying properties of both.

Mechanical properties

Stress Measure of the force per unit of cross-sectional area.

Strain The amount of deformation when a force is exerted.

Elastic modulus **(E)** Ratio of stress to strain; this is a measure of the rigidity of a material.

Elastic deformation The reversible deformation of a material under load.

Plastic deformation The irreversible deformation of a material under load.

Brittleness The fracturing of a material with little or no plastic deformation, e.g. glass ionomer cement.

Ductility A material that undergoes plastic deformation is ductile, e.g. gold alloy.

Hardness Material hardness is a measure of abrasion resistance and indentation resistance.

Strength This is the stress required to produce either plastic deformation or fracture.

Fatigue Plastic deformation or fracture of a material below the normal fracture strength due to repeated cyclic stresses.

Physical properties

Electrical conductivity Materials with free electrons (e.g. metals) conduct electricity; materials without them (e.g. ceramics) do not.

Thermal conductivity The transfer of thermal energy from one area of a material to another.

Thermal expansion Materials expand as temperature rises and contract as it decreases, due to atomic vibration.

Radio-opacity The amount of X-ray energy absorbed by a material depends on the composition and thickness of the material. Metals absorb X-rays well, polymers absorb X-rays poorly.

Optical properties Materials may absorb, reflect, refract and transmit light (Figure 7.1).

Chemical properties

Corrosion This is an electrochemical process which involves movement of ions in an aqueous environment, e.g. saliva.

Solubility This is how much a material will dissolve in a fluid, e.g. saliva.

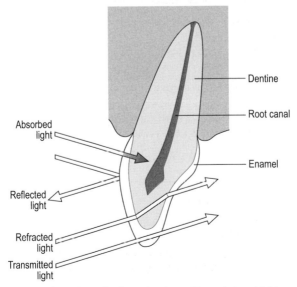

Figure 7.1 Absorption, reflection, refraction and transmission of light.

Formation of oxide layer All metals (except noble metals, e.g. gold) form an oxide layer on the metal surface; this can be either uneven and porous or uniform, tightly bound and non-porous.

Biocompatibility properties

> **Ideally, dental materials should produce no adverse effects on the oral tissues.**

Basic principles are that dental materials should: • not be carcinogenic • not readily induce hypersensitivity reactions • not produce systemic toxic effects.

Degradation products of materials should not produce the above effects.

Equally importantly, the dentist should be aware for each material in use (and their components, e.g. mercury in amalgam) of:

● relevant safe handling procedures
● safe disposal procedures
● what to do in the event of accident or spillage
● Health and Safety Law, e.g. COSHH regulations.

TESTING MATERIALS

In most countries, materials are subjected to in-vitro testing to determine their properties. Dentists should be aware of the limitations of in-vitro tests and when using new materials should, where possible, examine controlled, long-term clinical trials to determine a particular material's clinical efficacy. Systematic reviews and meta-analyses which combine the results of several trials provide evidence of clinical effectiveness.

Problems with testing

Materials testing should be to standard specifications and involve both laboratory tests and controlled clinical trials. British (BSI) and International (ISO) Standards are produced to help standardize laboratory testing. This is often difficult to achieve and sometimes materials are released for use before their long-term clinical efficacy has been established. It is important that materials are evaluated not only for their final properties but also for: • storage properties (e.g. shelf life, need for refrigeration) • mixing properties (e.g. ease of mix, time) • setting properties (e.g. time, method of set, dimensional and temperature changes).

> ⚠ **When selecting a material for use in the mouth, it is the dentist's responsibility to ensure the properties of the material are appropriate to the particular clinical situation.**

DENTAL AMALGAM

An alloy of mercury with silver and tin.

Basic properties

• Very strong restorative material • composite nature • corrodes • no adhesion to enamel or dentine • dimensional changes on setting • cheap • simple to use • some concerns about biocompatibility and toxicity • creep • much higher thermal conductivity than tooth tissue • similar proportional limit to enamel • double the thermal expansion of tooth.

Components and metallurgy

Dental amalgam is a polycrystalline solid solution and is therefore composite in nature.

Silver Gives corrosion resistance, strength, setting expansion. Rapid reaction with mercury (67–74%).

Tin Setting contraction, weakens material. Slows down the silver/mercury reaction (25–27%).

Copper Prevents formation of weak and corrosion-prone gamma 2 phase (0–6%).

Mercury Liquid metal, toxic.
   Need Ag:Sn ratio of 3:1 for gamma phase, which is strong, brittle and has a small setting expansion.

Setting reaction

$$Hg + Ag:Sn \rightarrow Ag_2Hg_3 (\& Ag_5Hg_8) + Sn_{6\text{-}8}Hg$$
   Gamma   Gamma 1   Gamma 2

Mercury reacts with outer layer of alloy particles and sets. New mercury/tin and mercury/silver alloys surround cores of original particles.

Gamma	Strongest phase
Gamma 1	Intermediate
Gamma 2	Weakest and corrodes

Copper is added to decrease gamma 2 phase by making Cu_3Sn or Cu_6Sn_5.

Need minimum mercury for optimum mechanical properties; 50 : 50 by weight is ideal. Mechanical mixing using minimum mercury and proper condensation into the cavity results in controlled expansion.

Alloy formation

Lathe cut Ingots of solid alloy are turned on a lathe and homogenized. Traditional method.

Spherical Spray cooled and atomized in an inert environment. Better packing and easier to mix. Low setting expansion. Greater strength but no 'squeaky' sound on condensation.

Dispersion Mixture of lathe cut and spherical. Maximizes properties of spherical but with 'squeaky' sound on condensation.

Uses
- Cavities in posterior teeth taking high occlusal loads.
- Cores (with or without pins) for crowns.

Practical tips

- Mix mechanically to manufacturer's recommendations.
- Condense quickly and correctly.
- Ensure no unsupported enamel in cavity preparation.
- Use matrices and wedges for marginal control.
- Use rubber dam for moisture control.
- Do not polish for at least 24 hours.

Safety and biocompatibility

Dental amalgam has been widely used for many years. Nevertheless, in several countries its use is declining due to concerns over its safety and environmental pollution. A patient receiving an amalgam restoration is exposed to fairly high doses of mercury during restoration placement, polishing and replacement. Over the years a small continuous dose occurs due to amalgam corrosion products being released.

Safety concerns, because of mercury release: • fetus • pregnant women • multiple sclerosis • prolonged exposure CNS problems.

Environment: • mercury from crematoria emissions • mercury in the water supply.

Dentists should bear in mind that there will be an increasing amount of concern in the future from patients and they should be prepared to answer difficult questions and provide alternative treatments. A very small percentage of patients exist, however, who seem to selectively absorb mercury and exhibit signs of mercury toxicity; in these rare cases amalgam restorations should be removed by a controlled procedure. It is good practice to remove and place amalgam restorations under rubber dam and in a well-ventilated room.

Amalgam allergy

(To mercury, ammoniated mercury or amalgam.) Rare; lichenoid reactions, often adjacent to amalgams, can be confirmed by patch testing.

Disposal

Amalgam separators within dental suction apparatus will minimize amalgam entering the water supply and food chains – these have recently been made mandatory in the UK. Waste amalgam should be stored in solution and sent to a recognized waste disposal company for recycling.

RESIN COMPOSITES

Based on BIS-GMA resin and glass fillers.

Basic properties

• No inherent adhesion to enamel or dentine • tensile and compressive strength comparable to tooth • lower elastic modulus than tooth • higher thermal expansion and contraction than tooth • polymerization shrinkage.

Components

Filler Strong, hard, brittle filler, e.g. quartz, borosilicate glass, silica. Filler decreases curing shrinkage and decreases thermal expansion. Glass surface undergoes *silinization* to ensure chemical bond to resin. Barium glasses used for radio-opacity. Filler loading of >60% by volume for posterior use and <60% for anterior use.

Resin Based on *bis*-phenol A and glycidyl methacrylate (BIS-GMA or 'Bowen' resin). *Bis*-phenol A has aromatic groups which increase stiffness of polymerized chain and decrease shrinkage. Other resins (e.g. urethane dimethacrylate) sometimes used. Acrylate diluent present, e.g. TEGDMA tri-ethylene glycol dimethacrylate, as BIS-GMA is very viscous. These diluents increase curing shrinkage a little.

Resin/filler composition affects refractive index and hence aesthetics.

Setting

By formation of polymer chains. Reaction can be initiated by:

Two paste (base and catalyst system) Reaction between tertiary amine and peroxide; superseded by visible light curing; used occasionally for core materials.

Visible light cure Uses light reacting with 1,2-diketone (e.g. camphoroquinone) and a tertiary amine; widely used. Works best at 470 nm wavelength.

Composite types

Based on size of filler particles.

Coarse Large filler particles; good wear resistance; poor aesthetics; difficult to polish

Microfill Small filler particles (less than 1 μm) enhances aesthetics; poor wear resistance; easier to polish

Hybrid Combines coarse and microfill particles to improve aesthetics without compromising wear.

Flowable composites

Uses
Direct composites

Microfine; Class III and V cavities, small Class I cavities
Hybrid; Class IV and larger Class I and Class II cavities, core build up
Flowable; repair of marginal defects, liner, initial increment at
   bottom of approximal box (improves adaptation)

Indirect composites Class I and II cavities, composite veneers (hybrid resin)

Practical tips

- Choose correct composite for given situation (e.g. anterior teeth – aesthetics of prime importance; posterior teeth – mechanical properties more important).
- Essential to use rubber dam for moisture control.
- Use retraction cord for arrest of gingival haemorrhage.
- Build deep cavities incrementally to achieve full depth cure.
- Acid etch enamel.
- Use dentine bonding agent where appropriate.

Problems with direct composites • reduced longevity compared with amalgam • shrinkage • microleakage • caution in patients with high caries rate • surface finish • wear resistance • radio-opacity • light-cured materials have a limited depth of cure • lights should be checked by a radiometer regularly to ensure correct intensity • placement time doubled versus amalgam.

Improving mechanical properties of direct composites Strength and wear resistance can be improved by addition of mega filler such as silane coupled beta-quartz inserts within small cavities.

Indirect composites
Require two clinical visits. Need to use a dual-cured luting cement. Inlay cured by photocure; then oven or hydropneumatic heat polymerization (120°C, 6 bar pressure for 6 minutes). Improved aesthetics as have time to mix shades.

Problems with indirect composites • microleakage • flash from luting cement • two visits required • wear resistance still a problem with high occlusal loads, e.g. bruxists • more expensive • ditch around inlay due to differential wear of softer luting cement.

GLASS IONOMERS

Alternative name is glass polyalkenoate cement. Developed in the 1960s at the Laboratory of the Government Chemist.

Typical constituents
Fused ion-leachable aluminosilicate glass. Glass is mainly SiO_2, Al_2O_3 and CaF_2 and is presented in a powder. Vacuum-dried

polyacrylic/itaconic (polyalkenoic) acid co-monomer, tartaric acid (to improve handling and snap set), water.

Setting reaction

Acid–base reaction between glass and polyalkenoic acid. This is complicated because of the presence of glass cations (calcium and aluminium). Thus three stages of set:

Dissolution phase; protons displace calcium ions from glass surface, these ions cause initial cross linking of polyacid chains

Gelation phase; protons displace aluminium ions and these further cross link polyacid chains. The gelation phase takes about 24 hours, during which physical properties improve.

Maturation phase; takes place over weeks and months and involves further cross linking of polyacid chains by calcium and aluminium ions.

Set cement is a composite structure with particles of unreacted glass surrounded by 'siliceous' hydrogel embedded in a matrix of cross-linked polyalkenoic acid.

Tooth surface pretreatment

Many substances have been evaluated as dentine pretreatment agents, e.g. 50% citric acid. In general, pretreatment does not result in worthwhile improvement in bond strengths.

Properties

• Hard and brittle • chemical adhesion to tooth (adversely affected by salivary contamination) • susceptible to erosion in first few minutes • increase in surface roughness in mouth over time • low translucency (aesthetics not as good as composite) • low abrasion wear resistance • release fluoride ions (some anticariogenic effect) • biocompatible.

Critical factors which can alter properties: Optimum powder:liquid ratio is 7 : 1. Reducing glass powder size improves cement properties.

Uses

• Cervical abrasion and erosion cavities • deciduous tooth restoration • fissure sealing • root surface caries • small Class III cavities • luting cement • Class I cavities in permanent molars/premolars (early carious lesions with minimal occlusal stress) • 'sandwich restorations' with composite • structural lining.

Clinical tips

- Difficult to mix, and powder : liquid ratio critical – consider use of encapsulated forms.
- Use a matrix where possible.
- Protect freshly set cement with unfilled resin.
- If need to polish, avoid desiccation.

CERMETS, RESIN-MODIFIED GLASS IONOMERS AND SIMILAR MATERIALS

CERMETS

A cermet is a *Cera*mic *Met*al glass.

Cermets were developed to combat the wear resistance problems of glass ionomers by reinforcing them with metal.

Components

Fused aluminosilicate glass with sintered silver or gold (3.5 mm). Glass ionomer type setting reaction. Sintered silver usually used, as gold has prohibitive cost.

Properties

• Better wear resistance than glass ionomer • very little marginal leakage • hydrolytically stable • poor aesthetically • metal gives radio-opacity • less fluoride release than glass ionomer.

Uses

• Class V cavities • restoration of primary molars • crown cores (but need substantial amount of supporting dentine) • intermediate restorations for teeth undergoing endodontics.

RESIN-MODIFIED GLASS IONOMERS AND SIMILAR MATERIALS

These materials have components of both a resin composite and a glass ionomer.

Often setting is light cured, chemically cured and has a glass ionomer type set. The light curing is faster than the chemical cure.

Types of materials

Modified composites Where filler has been replaced by an ion leachable aluminosilicate glass with no acid–base chemical reaction.

Compomer (acid-modified composite) Where resin has acidic components to generate acid–base chemical reaction but still is mainly set by resin polymerization. May release more fluoride.

Resin-modified glass ionomers Powder–liquid materials consisting of a methacrylate resin, a poly acid, an ion leachable glass, water and HEMA (hydroxyethylmethacrylate). This hybrid material has acid–base, light-cured and chemically cured setting.

Properties
• Long-term clinical trials remain sparse; early results encouraging • improved wear resistance over glass ionomer • improved aesthetics over glass ionomer • compomers and resin-modified glass ionomers adhere to tooth substance • fracture toughness greater than glass cermet • less fluoride release than glass ionomers.

Uses
• Class V cavities • restoration of primary molars • currently popular for crown cores.

ADHESION AND BONDING AGENTS

> Adhesion occurs when two surfaces are held together by interfacial forces – can be molecular attraction or mechanical forces.

Micromechanical adhesion
Due to surface irregularities and dimensional changes. Can get a strong bond in the absence of molecular attraction, especially under shear forces. Close adaptation of adhesive and surface increases molecular attraction. Ultimate bond strength depends on cohesive strength of the adhesive.

Molecular attraction
So-called chemical adhesion occurs due to ionic, covalent and metallic bonds or van der Waals' forces.

How to achieve adhesion
Material *must* 'wet' the other surface. Wetting is the ability of a material to cover a surface. Material must convert from liquid to

solid with negligible dimensional change. This can be achieved by evaporation, cooling or polymerization.

Factors promoting adhesion

Surface roughness Improves adhesion by exposing greater surface area.

Low viscosity or free flow Enhances adhesion.

ENAMEL BONDING

Based upon acid etching.

Types of etchants

Strong acids e.g. 37% phosphoric acid used for 15 seconds. Must clean to remove unwanted phosphates.

Weak acids e.g. 2.5% nitric acid or 17% maleic acid. These are universal or total etch (6th generation) bonding systems for enamel and dentine and need longer application, usually 30–60 seconds.

Three types of etching • intraprismatic • interprismatic • general roughening.

DENTINE BONDING

Usually contain three components:

● Etchant/conditioner – phosphoric acid/weak organic acid
● Primer, e.g. HEMA
● Bonding resin – usually BIS-GMA based or similar

Usually referred to as different generations of dentine bonding agents:

4th generation – three stages; etchant/primer/bonding resin (current gold standard)
5th generation – two stages; etchant/ combined primer and bonding resin (usually require two applications)
6th generation – combine all three components

 Always follow manufacturer's instructions fully.

METAL BONDING

Use *solvent-based* adhesives.

Stages in adhesion

1. *Metal conditioning* A rough surface for micromechanical adhesion is needed. This is achieved by sandblasting, chemical etching, electrolytic etching or tin plating.
2. *Metal priming* Acid-methacrylate resins, which adhere to metal oxide layer.
3. *Wet surface* Unfilled resin.

PORCELAIN BONDING

Use *solvent-based* adhesives.

Stages in adhesion

1. *Porcelain conditioning* Etching by either hydrofluoric acid or acidulated monofluorophosphate. Usually done in laboratory as hydrofluoric acid very corrosive.
2. *Silane coupling* Surface active coupling agents that react with methacrylate in the bonding resin and silica in the porcelain. Enhanced bonding if apply at chairside before cementation. May also be used to enhance retention of fibre posts.
3. *Wet surface* Unfilled resin.

Porcelain bonding can be very useful for repair of porcelain with composite. In addition, porcelain bonding is useful for ceramic veneers, inlays and onlays, ceramic orthodontic brackets and dentine-bonded porcelain crowns.

LUTING CEMENTS, LININGS AND BASES

Luting cements are setting pastes that retain indirect restorations in tooth.
Linings provide a bland thermal barrier.
Bases provide a strong barrier, structural lining.
Used to give a thermal, mechanical and chemical barrier to dentine and be biocompatible.

BASIC PRINCIPLES

• All involve acid–base reactions – powder is base • composite when set • no ideal material • different types for different clinical situations.

Calcium hydroxide

Properties • can be used as setting or non-setting in different clinical situations • lining sets with salicylic acid or light-cure set • alkaline, pH 9–10 • weak material – often requires structural lining • possible antibacterial action • calcific bridge formation.

Uses • dentine desensitizing • indirect pulp cap • direct pulp cap • endodontic intracanal dressing (non-setting) • root fractures, perforation, resorption (non-setting) • apexification (non-setting) • root canal sealer.

Zinc oxide-eugenol

Composition Zinc oxide and magnesium oxide, fillers in powder. Eugenol, olive oil and acetic acid in liquid.

Properties • bland material • weak • no adhesion to tooth • set accelerated by moisture • can be strengthened by, e.g., polystyrene or acrylic • possible pulpal irritation.

Uses • temporary luting cement • lining • temporary dressing • impression material (edentulous patients).

EBA cements

Composition • based on zinc oxide–eugenol • ortho-ethoxy benzoic acid added • resin added for strength, e.g. polystyrene.

Uses • intermediate restoration • retrograde seal in endodontic surgery (also consider MTA)

Zinc phosphate

Composition • zinc oxide with about 10% magnesium oxide • phosphoric acid • a crystalline set occurs so set material is fairly opaque.

Properties • no adhesion to tooth • slight setting contraction • some pulpal effects, so in vital teeth requires lining • exothermic set.

Uses • structural lining • luting cement (especially post cores) • temporary restorations.

Zinc polycarboxylate

Composition • mainly zinc oxide with freeze-dried polyacrylic acid and trace of fluoride • on setting, zinc ion cross-links polymer chains • some adhesion to tooth via a chelate, possibly calcium polyacrylate.

Properties • some adhesion to tooth • non-irritant to pulp • opaque • more soluble than zinc phosphate.

Uses • luting cement • structural lining • temporary restorations.

Glass ionomers

Widely used as luting cements, structural linings (p. 123).

Miscellaneous

Occasionally *cavity varnishes* are used, particularly with amalgam restorations. These consist of *natural resin* (e.g. copal, rosin) and a solvent (usually ether).

Many clinicians now use dentine bonding agents in place of cavity varnish as they seal freshly cut dentinal tubules and help minimize postoperative sensitivity.

Light curing units

Need around 400 mW/cm^2 to cure efficiently.

Output reduced by debris, bulb ageing, damage to internal filters; therefore need to check regularly.

Various lights are available:

● *Halogen* most commonly available
● *Ramped/soft start* halogen based but power output begins at 100 mW/cm^2 and increases up to 800 mW/cm^2 over 40 s. Thought to counteract clinical effects of polymerization shrinkage (marginal leakage, staining and secondary caries)
● *Plasma curing lights* much more intense with higher energy rating giving quicker polymerization times. No significant benefit over conventional curing apart from reduced placement time.
● *Light-emitting diodes (LEDs)* recently introduced, quieter (no fan), cordless, lighter, greater depth of cure, lower heat output, longer bulb life.

TEMPORARY CEMENTS AND RESTORATIONS

TEMPORARY CEMENTS

Must be strong enough for short-term retention of a restoration but weak enough for easy removal by the dentist.

Usually use zinc oxide–eugenol or non-eugenol-containing cements. Occasionally may need stronger temporary luting cement, e.g. if high occlusal load. Often choose zinc polycarboxylate with lower powder : liquid ratio. Can use temporary cements to 'try in' definitive restorations by making them non-setting, e.g. proprietary brands or zinc oxide with petroleum jelly.

TEMPORARY RESTORATIONS

Must be bland, withstand occlusal forces for several weeks, easy to remove and have low thermal conductivity. Usually use zinc oxide–eugenol. Can be strengthened with polystyrene. For more intermediate restoration can use ortho-ethoxy benzoic acid containing material which has better wear resistance than zinc oxide–eugenol.

Other temporary restorations
Gutta-percha

Natural rubber contorted polymer chain based on *cis*-polyisoprene.

Properties Include easy distortion, poor adaptation to cavity margins, needs pressure for insertion. Used occasionally as temporary restoration but much more commonly for root canal obturation.

Temporary putties

EBA or eugenol based single pastes which harden on contact with moisture.

Usually used as access cavity temporary restorations in teeth undergoing root canal treatment. Some use in patient-applied commercial 'dental emergency kits'.

IMPRESSION MATERIALS
Properties of ideal material
Should be: • accurate • dimensionally stable • biocompatible • easy to mix • short working and setting times.

Classification
Rigid
1. Plaster of Paris (impression plaster)
2. Impression compound
3. Zinc oxide–eugenol

Elastic
1. Hydrocolloids
   – Reversible (agar)
   – Irreversible (alginates)
2. Elastomers
   – Polysulphides (addition/condensation curing)
   – Silicones
   – Polyethers

RIGID IMPRESSION MATERIALS

• Cheap • relatively weak • used for edentulous impressions, i.e. where no undercuts present.

Impression plaster
Use decreasing, based on plaster of Paris.

Setting reaction:

$$CaSO_4.2H_2O \rightarrow CaSO_4.\tfrac{1}{2}H_2O \rightarrow CaSO_4.2H_2O$$

Gypsum   Plaster   Recrystallization

Also contains 4% potassium sulphate (accelerates set and anti-expansion agent) and 0.4% borax (retards set and anti-expansion).

Properties: dimensionally accurate and stores well, but difficult to disinfect without altering surface.

Impression compound
Type I low fusing, used for primary edentulous impressions.

Type II high fusing, used for peripheral adaptation of edentulous and dentulous individual trays.

Composition: • thermoplastic resins and waxes • lubricants, e.g. stearic acid • fillers, e.g. pumice.

Properties: • thermoplastic • poor accuracy • distortion and memory effects • cheap.

Clinical tips

> Heat in warm water. If too hot will stick to teeth. If too
> cool will not distort sufficiently.

Zinc oxide–eugenol

Zinc oxide-eugenol based. Adheres to denture acrylic, so is useful
for relining/rebasing impressions.

Properties: • setting accelerated by moisture • accurate • use with
close-fitting individual tray • irritant to oral mucosa.

Occasionally impression waxes can be used to correct minor
faults in impressions made with impression paste. Such waxes
require a high flow at body temperature.

ELASTIC IMPRESSION MATERIALS –
HYDROCOLLOIDS

> **Hydrocolloid is so-called as 'hydro' (water) is used as a
> plasticizer and 'colloid' (initial polymer is colloidal in
> size – approximately 0.2 mm diameter).**

Two types of hydrocolloids: *reversible* (agar) and *irreversible*
(alginate).

Setting reactions Goes from a *sol* to a *gel* by particles forming
fibrils which cross-link. If cross-linking and fibril formation
involves van der Waals' forces alone, is *reversible*; if in addition
involves ionic forces, is *irreversible*. Set *gel* is weak so need fillers to
strengthen gel.

Properties Hydrocolloids exhibit poor dimensional stability caused
by:

Syneresis Continued cross-link formation after initial set so
impression shrinks and water is forced out; happens almost
immediately.

Imbibition Impression swells as water is imbibed by osmosis due to
presence of electrolytes between polymer chains.

Evaporation Water evaporates so impression shrinks and becomes
hard and brittle.

Clinical tips

- Place damp gauze over impression to decrease syneresis
- Pour impressions as soon as possible to decrease effects of imbibition and evaporation
- Disinfect impressions prior to sending to laboratory.

Reversible hydrocolloid

Agar Sulphated polysaccharide. Agar is accurate but has poor dimensional stability and, as a water bath is required, it has largely been superseded by elastomer impression materials.

Irreversible hydrocolloid

Alginate Carboxylated polysaccharide based on alginic acid. In widespread clinical use. *Gels* by cross-link formation with calcium ions.

Composition: • sodium alginate • calcium phosphate • sodium sulphate (retarder) • fillers, e.g. zinc carbonate • some contain pH indicators (chromatic alginates); change colour – pH drops as gel forms.

Setting reaction

Sodium alginate + calcium sulphate $\rightarrow$ calcium alginate + sodium sulphate

ELASTIC IMPRESSION MATERIALS – ELASTOMERS

Basic types

• polyethers • polysulphides • addition silicones • condensation silicones.

Amount of filler present determines heavy, regular and light bodied material.

Polyethers

A polyether is a polyimine and is self cross-linking.

Composition Has base and catalyst pastes both containing plasticizer and filler. Catalyst is usually an *aromatic sulphonate ester*.

Properties: • rigid when set (difficult to remove from large undercuts) • dimensionally stable (can absorb water) • strong; automated mixing machine simpler than manual mix.

Uses: • crown and bridge impressions • cobalt–chromium denture impressions • implant impressions.

Polysulphides

Contains a prepolymer which has a sulphur bridge, an ether link and an ethyl group (plasticiser). Sets by cross-linking when oxidized using lead peroxide catalyst.

Properties: • accurate • high tear strength • set accelerated by moisture • poor medium-term dimensional stability (cast in first 24 hours) • noxious odour (free mercaptan groups) • stains clothes.

Uses: • crown and bridge impressions • cobalt–chromium denture impressions • implant impressions • master edentulous impressions • particularly useful for multiple preparations.

Addition silicones

Based on dimethylsiloxane, which polymerizes by addition to an unsaturated end group via a complex platinum-based catalyst.

Properties: • accurate • dimensionally stable • not as strong as other elastomers • fairly quick setting time.

Uses: • crown and bridge impressions • cobalt–chromium denture impressions • implant impressions • master edentulous impressions • particularly useful for one or two units of crown and bridgework (setting time can be a problem for multiple preparations).

Addition silicones are the most commonly used elastomer-type impression materials.

Condensation silicones

> Based on dimethylsiloxane, which polymerizes to
> polydimethylsiloxane, which acts as an alcohol. This
> undergoes transesterification with tetraethylsilicate (acid),
> releasing ethanol (i.e. condensation). A fatty acid salt catalyses
> the reaction.

Properties: • shrinks on curing • loses ethanol on storage
• intermediate tear strength.

Uses: • crown and bridge impressions • maxillofacial prosthetics
• use declining as superseded by other elastomers.

 **Remember the relative advantages and disadvantages of
the different impression materials – important to select
the correct material for the clinical situation in question.**

PORCELAIN AND CERAMICS

> Porcelains are inorganic salts that fuse when heated.
> Porcelains have a composite-like structure – hard brittle
> particles between fused glass.

Composition: • hard particles, e.g. silica and alumina
• glass-forming particles, e.g. boron oxide • fluxes, e.g. feldspar and
fluorospar • opacifiers, e.g. tin oxide • binders, e.g. starch • tints, e.g.
iron oxide • fluorescers, e.g. rare earth oxides.

Firing of porcelain Porcelain must be fired for inorganic salts to
fuse.

Two types:
High fusing 1200–1400°C; used for porcelain denture teeth, kaolin
used as a binder.
Low fusing 850–1100°C; used for crowns; starch as a binder within
a fused fritted powder.

DENTAL PORCELAIN

Crowns and bridges are individually made in a laboratory. First, an opaque core and then progressively glassier layers of porcelain are applied to mimic dentine and enamel. Tints can be applied to mimic cracks, gingival staining, irregularities, etc.

Laboratory handling

Firing shrinkage Shrinks 30% on firing.

Compaction If vibrate and blot reduces shrinkage to 10%.

Firing Vacuum firing, pressure cooling and slow firing reduces porosity.

Finish Self-glaze by putting in furnace for a short time.

Cooling is important as surface layers go into compression so fewer microcracks. Microcracks will lead to *crack propagation* when material is put under tension and result in failure.

Properties of dental porcelain: • hard • biocompatible • good aesthetics • brittle • good compressive strength • good abrasion resistance (can be a problem as unpolished porcelain can abrade enamel).

Improving porcelain strength

Aluminous porcelain This is strong and hard but opaque so used mainly as core porcelain. Can double crown strength but still get microcracks.

Bulk alumina slabs Useful on palatal surfaces of crowns, where it can dramatically increase strength.

Sintered alumina cores Involves difficult slip cast core construction; high flexural strength and improved ceramic translucency.

Injection-moulded ceramics Superior strength, good aesthetics but poorer fitting accuracy and marginal openings.

CAD-CAM ceramics Optical impression taken and ceramic milled on milling machine; marginal fit problems; fewer inherent flaws and cracks as restoration milled from a homogeneous ceramic 'blank'

Leucite-reinforced porcelain Good strength and aesthetics.

METAL–CERAMIC CROWNS

Ductile metal core often based on nickel–chrome, high and low gold or silver–palladium alloys. Porcelain adhesion to metal achieved by ceramic melting and wetting metal surface in a vacuum. Requires a high melting metal with matching thermal properties to porcelain. Acts as a laminated composite so any cracks present cannot propagate. Poorer aesthetics as 'metal shines through'. Good for 'tight occlusions' as can have metal palatal surfaces to crowns which are thinner than porcelain.

Uses of dental porcelain: • crowns and bridges • veneers • adhesive crowns • inlays and onlays • inserts within direct composites • denture teeth.

Aesthetics

Crown aesthetics are very important as a crown must mimic how light is *reflected*, *refracted*, *transmitted* and *absorbed* through a natural tooth (see Figure 7.1).

The dentist must select shades for crown restorations. This is usually based on the three-dimensional *Munsell Colour System*:

Hue – family, e.g. red, green, blue.
Chroma – intensity, i.e. the amount of hue.
Value – brightness or dullness.

Problems in choosing shades

Metamerism Objects appear as different colours in different lights.
Colour washout An object stared at for too long a time appears lighter.
Observer errors Different people are 'better' than others at shade selection.
Technical problems Different technicians and laboratories produce 'different shades' for same operator choice.

Electronic shade guide systems are also slowly being introduced to reduce some of the subjectivity in shade taking.

Tips for choosing aesthetic shades

• Communicate clearly to technician, e.g. map different shades for one crown • choose shades under natural daylight (choose surgery lighting that uses tubes as close to this as possible) • stare only briefly at object then rest eyes by looking at a grey object • ensure you are not colour blind • involve dental nurse in shade selection for 'second opinion' • in difficult cases consider use of photography to communicate with technician • recent development includes use of colour-corrected digital imaging systems • take great care when choosing shades for individual central incisor crowns and crowns next to dentures • do *not* permanently cement a crown if the patient is dissatisfied with the shade.

CASTING AND WROUGHT ALLOYS

BASIC METAL MICROSTRUCTURE

A metallic bond is non-directional so as atoms cool from a melt, crystals form. Metals are *crystalline*. As many nuclei form during cooling, metals are *polycrystalline*. Crystals grow *inwards* in a melt and have various shapes. Crystals are called *grains* and meet other crystals at *grain boundaries*. Crystals grow from a nucleus *dendritically*. Pure metal atoms are *close packed* and form one of *three lattices*.

Metal lattices

Alloys are combinations of metals in solid solutions.
  • Body-centred cube • face-centred cube • hexagonal.
  An alloy is often harder due to *solution hardening*. Alloy metals can combine by precipitation, crystallization or immiscibility in solid solution, depending on the metals involved.

Two basic types of alloys

Interstitial solid solution Here a very small atom is in the basic lattice space and does not really alter the lattice but stops dislocation, e.g. steel (carbon and iron).

Substitutional solid solution An atom of one metal replaces a lattice atom of another metal, distorting the lattice and altering properties, e.g. dental gold (gold and copper).

Altering metal properties

Metal properties can be altered by mechanical, chemical or heat treatment processes.

Work hardening Metal crystals are imperfect and are *ductile* due to imperfections called *dislocations*. When a metal is worked, e.g. tightening a cast clasp, dislocations accumulate at grain boundaries and microcracks form, the cracks propagate and the metal becomes *brittle* and work hardened.

Annealing This can reverse work hardening by heating the metal to encourage stress relief, recrystallization and grain growth.

Cooling Slow cooling gives larger grains which have fewer boundaries and are softer. Fast cooling gives smaller grains, more boundaries and produces a harder metal.

Polishing During polishing, metal atoms are smeared over the surface in a random way, which looks amorphous under a microscope but is aesthetically pleasing.

Etching Surface etching causes crystals to be etched in different directions. Produces poor aesthetic appearance but improves area for bonding.

Oxide layer All metals have an oxide layer on their surface. This can be seen as a *tarnished surface*. Some metals have an oxide layer which is tightly bound to metal and is useful for adhesion to porcelain or resin cements. Appropriate metals are incorporated into dental alloys so that an optimum oxide layer for bonding is produced by controlled surface oxidation.

Dental gold alloys

Composition Basic gold and copper. Copper causes *order* hardening where a random face-centred cube becomes an ordered face-centred tetragonal superlattice. Achieved by slow cooling then reheating. Copper causes gold to be red in colour. Other metals are introduced in small quantities to lighten the material, e.g. platinum, palladium, silver.

Properties: • biocompatible • good corrosion resistance • easy to cast • aesthetically appealing • ductility and hardness dependent on type of gold alloy chosen.

Uses Use of cast gold alloys depends on type:

Type I Class III or V inlays.
Type II Most inlays.
Type III Crowns/bridges.
Type IV Posts and dentures.

White gold Contains silver and palladium. White or pale yellow in colour. Used in crown and bridgework and is harder but more difficult to cast.

Cobalt–chromium alloys

Composition: • cobalt 40–60% • chromium 25–35% • small amounts of nickel (improves ductility) • carbon (hardens) • iron (solution hardening) • molybdenum (refines metal grains).

Properties: • strong and hard • high corrosion resistance • little ductility • very work hardenable • less expensive than gold • ×2 casting shrinkage compared with gold • less flexible than gold • does not bond to porcelain.

 Due to low ductility and work hardening, bend a cobalt–chromium clasp and it may break (due to brittle grain boundary carbides).

Uses: partial denture bases and clasps.

Nickel–chromium alloys

Composition: • nickel 70–80% • chromium 15–20% • trace metals.

Properties: • bonds to porcelain • casting accuracy • ductile • not as strong as cobalt–chromium • nickel is a possible carcinogen and common allergen.

Uses: crown and bridgework.

Steel alloys

Composition Iron and carbon alloy system where carbon acts as a metal in an interstitial position in the iron lattice. Steel contains less than 2% carbon. Steel may be brittle or ductile depending on heating and quenching.

Types

Martensite Hard and brittle but not corrosion resistant; used for scalpel blades, some surgical tools and dental hand instruments.

Stainless steels Austenitic steel of 2 types: 18/8 (18% chromium/8% nickel) and 12/12 (12% chromium/12% nickel). These have good corrosion resistance and can be used intraorally as clasps in orthodontic appliances or dentures.

DENTURE BASE MATERIALS

Two types: • polymer based • metal based – cobalt–chromium (p. 140).

POLYMER DENTURE BASE MATERIALS

Composition Come in powder and liquid form.

Powder Polymethylmethacrylate granules, benzoyl peroxide.
Liquid Methylmethacrylate, ethylene glycol dimethacrylate.

Curing reaction Cure occurs in several stages:

1. *Granular*: particles are wetted.
2. *Stringy*: particles become tacky.
3. *Dough*: molecular entanglement begins.
4. *Rubber*: complete molecular entanglement.

Cure is exothermic. 20% shrinkage in volume. Can be *heat cured* (above peroxide decomposition temperature) or *cold cured* (addition of amine causes peroxide to decompose at room temperature). Because of curing shrinkage, mould is *overpacked* and *pressurized*. Typical heat cure prewarms to 60°C then 70°C and up to 100°C over time – reduces residual monomer and decreases porosity. Cold cure leads to increased porosity and yellowing due to amine.

Properties: • poor impact resistance • moderate strength • generally non-toxic • low density • cheap • easy to process • not radio-opaque • poor thermal conductivity • weak in thin section • poor wear resistance • easy to add to, permitting ease of repair, reline or addition.

Uses: • dentures • orthodontic appliances • individual impression trays.

Developments
High-impact acrylics Have comonomers and rubber fillers.
Radio-opacity Heavy metals or halogenated compounds but
    weaken material.
Bonding to cobalt–chromium Can be improved by mechanical mesh,
    silicoating or metal conditioning.
Methacrylate sensitivity Although rare, can be a problem in some
    individuals.

Alternative denture base materials
Polycarbonates Have to be injection moulded.
Vulcanite Poor aesthetics (now used rarely).
Nylon Absorbs water and distorts denture.

Used in conjunction with porcelain teeth.

SOFT LININGS
Temporary
Polyethylmethacrylate gelled with ethanol. Ethanol is leached and lining often hardens.

Uses: • functional impressions • temporary linings to immediate dentures • as a tissue conditioner following surgery (especially implant surgery).

Permanent

Silicone, modified acrylic or polyphosphazine based. Adhere to acrylic with difficulty, attract bacteria.

Uses: • obturator • denture support problems.

ENDODONTIC MATERIALS

Materials used in endodontics can be classified as: • root canal cleansers • preformed root canal fillings • root canal sealers • retrograde root filling materials • intracanal medicaments.

Root canal cleansers

Sodium hypochlorite 1–5%, antibacterial action in the canal by release of chlorine.
EDTA solution 17%, chelating agent that removes smear layer.
EDTA and urea peroxide Releases nascent oxygen, which leaves environment unsuitable for anaerobes and lifts debris from canal. Lubricates canal.
Chlorhexidine Antibacterial.

Preformed root canal fillings

Gutta-percha cones Isomer of natural rubber with an isoprene unit. At room temperature, gutta-percha is 60% crystalline (crystals of transpolyisoprene) and 40% amorphous. Contains inert zinc oxide filler and antioxidant, which reduces brittleness. Available in either *standardized* (sizes compatible with files) or *non-standardized cones*. Gutta-percha becomes soft at 65°C and melts at 100°C.

Heated gutta-percha Various techniques. Uses *alpha* gutta-percha, which is more tacky and flows easier than conventional beta gutta-percha.

Silver points 99.8% pure silver. Useful for fine curved canals but poor fit to canal shape and relies on sealer for obturation. Antibacterial. Corrosion is a problem. Rarely used.

Root canal sealers

Zinc oxide–eugenol based contain setting retarders to increase working time and barium sulphate for radio-opacity.
Calcium hydroxide based Hygroscopic, antibacterial.
Glass ionomer based Some bonding to dentine, smear layer removal.

Dentine bonding agents Epoxy-based resin sealer. Very slow setting.

Formaldehyde-containing sealers Fix tissue. Problem if it escapes into periapical tissues. Generally thought to have no place in modern endodontics.

Retrograde root filling materials

- Modified zinc oxide–eugenol-based cements
- Ethoxy benzoic acid
- Hydroxyapatite and similar materials
- Mineral trioxide aggregate (MTA)

Intracanal medicaments

Non-setting calcium hydroxide Commonly used as it is antibacterial and hygroscopic.

Camphorated monochlorophenol and betamethasone 35% solution, anti-inflammatory, antiseptic, may be carcinogenic.

Combination of antibacterial agent and a steroid Occasionally useful in painless death of an hyperaemic pulp.

IMPLANT MATERIALS

TYPES OF IMPLANTS

• Subperiosteal • transmandibular • osseointegrated.

Subperiosteal

Used rarely nowadays. For edentulous mandible only. Involves impression of bone, manufacture of a casting with parallel copings made from *castable titanium*, which sits under the periosteum.

Transmandibular

Used rarely for very atrophic edentulous mandibles only. Made from *gold* in a rigid box frame.

Osseointegrated

Most common implant in current use (p. 330).

Uses: • single tooth replacement • edentulism • partial edentulism.

> Osseointegration is a direct and functional connection between ordered, living bone and the surface of a load-carrying implant.

Commercially pure titanium Most commonly used material. In form of hollow cylinder. 'Fracture healing' between implant and bone. Capable of bearing load 3–6 months after insertion of implant depending on oral site. In some instances immediate loading is possible.

Properties: • titanium oxide is chemically inert • biocompatible • strong • high dielectric constant of titanium oxide.

Other materials used for osseointegration
Titanium alloys Less good results.
Plasma-sprayed surface to titanium Increases surface area.
Aluminium oxide Good for immediate tooth replacement but poor mechanical properties.

MISCELLANEOUS

WAXES

Waxes occur naturally from animal, mineral and plant sources. In addition, some distillation products of petroleum may exist as a wax (e.g. paraffin wax). Addition of natural gums and resins may give wax adhesive properties. Dental waxes are a combination of natural and synthetic waxes.

Types of wax in dentistry
Inlay wax 40–60% paraffin wax, maximum flow at 45°C.
Sheet casting wax Used for wax patterns in laboratory.
Sticky wax Hard, brittle and adhesive – used in laboratory for locating casts, etc.
Carding wax High flow at room temperature so can be hand moulded. Good for boxing impressions before casting.
Modelling wax 70–80% paraffin wax. Flows at 50–58°C. Used extensively in denture construction for record blocks, jaw registration, etc.
Shellac resin Thermoplastic; high in fillers; good as baseplate in denture construction as stable at mouth temperature.

FISSURE SEALANTS

Properties of ideal sealant: • adhesion between enamel and sealant • need flow of sealant into pits and fissures • sufficient strength and wear resistance to withstand occlusal forces.

Materials used for fissure sealing BIS-GMA resins (p. 121), glass ionomer cements (p. 123).

 It is absolutely critical when fissure sealing to ensure that caries is not present in the fissure.

PERIODONTAL MATERIALS

Periodontal pack or dressing Two-paste zinc oxide–eugenol system.

Uses: • post surgery when bone exposed, protects wound surface from mechanical trauma • prevents excessive granulation tissue formation • provides a physical barrier to bacterial contamination • used mainly after gingivectomy, apically repositioned flaps and free gingival grafts.

INVESTMENT MATERIALS

These are used in lost wax processes, e.g. metal casting, denture bases.

Properties: • withstand high temperature • set at room temperature • expand slightly to compensate for casting shrinkage • reproduce detail • porous to let gases escape • strong.

Types of dental investment
Low temperature – gypsum bonded. Used for gold casting.
High temperature – phosphate bonded : silica bonded. Used for cobalt–chromium casting.

Lost wax processes often involve addition of a *sprue* or *vent* to release gases from the mould. This is particularly important in silica-bonded investment, which is the least porous.

POLISHING

Polishing involves surface restructuring and surface loss or abrasion.

Abrasion polishing
Using successively finer abrasives reduces scratch width to below wavelength of light. In addition, it produces *surface restructuring*

by either transfer of high spots to low spots or, in metals, creation of finer crystal grains, so surface is virtually amorphous. Polishing abrasive *must* be harder than surface to be polished.

Relief polishing

Surfaces of varying hardness polish in relief, i.e. hard bits stick out of surface. This is undesirable and is why microfine composites with smaller particles polish better and have superior aesthetics than composites with coarse particles.

TEMPORARY CROWN MATERIALS

Properties: • cheap • moderate strength • reasonable aesthetics • set easily and quickly • non-adhesive to tooth • often use cartridge mixing systems.

Materials in use

Epimine polymers Based on *bis*-phenol A and polyether rubber; highly translucent, low shrinkage.

Polyethyl or polybutyl methacrylate Fairly high shrinkage on setting, good aesthetics.

Composite Good aesthetics often different shades available.

Preformed polycarbonate crowns Good aesthetics for anterior teeth.

Preformed stainless steel crowns Good for full veneer crown preparations on posterior teeth.

DENTURE TEETH

Types Acrylic or porcelain.

Acrylic Injection or dough moulded; acrylic is highly cross-linked for greater wear and surface characteristics, can lead to debonding problems from denture base; can surface stain teeth for better aesthetics.

Porcelain Mechanical attachment to denture base via diatoric hole or pin; use nowadays limited to acrylic allergy or highly demanding aesthetic problems; less abrasion than acrylic teeth.

CURRENT 'GROWTH AREAS' IN DENTAL MATERIALS

Although there is active research in all areas of dental materials, much attention surrounds the following:

Adhesion
Current trends in dental adhesion involve the development of multipurpose adhesives that can bond enamel, dentine, composites, amalgams and ceramics rather than individual kits for separate materials.

Casting
The 'lost wax' technique remains the main method of casting. There is currently some interest in spark erosion as an alternative method.

Posterior composites
Direct resin composites, which are 'packable' in a similar manner to amalgam, are showing some early signs of promise for use in posterior teeth. Long-term clinical evaluation is required.

Hydrophilic silicone impression materials
Hydrophilic silicone impression materials are being developed for use in situations where moisture control is a problem; although promising, they have a problem with poor tear strength.

Amalgam
There appears to be a slow progression to an 'amalgam-free mouth' due to patient pressure and environmental concerns regarding mercury. Satisfactory alternatives, e.g. gallium, are at an early stage of development.

CHAPTER 8

PREVENTIVE AND COMMUNITY DENTAL PRACTICE

The philosophy of prevention   150

Health promotion   150

Changing disease levels   151

Dental caries   152

Caries risk   155

Microbiology of dental caries   156

Diet and dental caries   156

Fluoride   159

Smoking and oral health   163

Frequency of dental attendance   164

Prevention in elderly patients   165

Dental care professionals   165

THE PHILOSOPHY OF PREVENTION

The major oral diseases – dental caries, periodontal disease and mouth cancer – are not inevitable, but are to a large extent influenced by environmental, social and lifestyle factors. The aetiology of these conditions is increasingly well understood and prevention is largely possible if people will adopt appropriate changes in behaviour.

Prevention has traditionally been defined in three stages:

Primary prevention – steps taken to ensure disease does not occur.
Secondary prevention – promoting early intervention in those already affected to halt progression at incipient stage of disease.
Tertiary prevention – treatment of well-established disease to restore function and avoid further episodes.

The prevention of oral disease can also be regarded as measures applied either on a *population (community) basis*, or at an *individual level*. Measures applied on a population basis include water fluoridation and health promotion campaigns. Preventive measures on an individual basis can be applied either by a dental professional (e.g. fissure sealants, diet counselling) or by the subject, e.g. toothbrushing.

In the developed world, dentistry has traditionally taken a 'treatment-oriented' approach, with the view that individuals were reliant on dental professionals for maintenance of oral health. However, recent decades have seen a change to a more 'preventive-oriented' approach. Factors influencing this transition include: • increased understanding of the nature of dental caries and periodontal disease • increased appreciation of the shortcomings of traditional restorative dentistry • advances in dental materials and restorative techniques • perhaps of greatest importance, changing aspirations of patients.

HEALTH PROMOTION

Health promotion describes activities and actions designed to enhance positive health and prevent ill-health by a combination of prevention, health education and health protection.

Prevention Described above.

Health education Involves the provision of information aimed at influencing beliefs, attitudes and behaviour relating to oral and dental health. In its widest sense includes provision of information about access to and appropriate use of health services.

The key messages are: • Reduce the intake of sugar-containing food and drink, particularly the frequency of sugar consumption. Avoid between-meal sugar snacks. • Brush teeth twice daily with a toothpaste containing fluoride. • Attend the dentist regularly • Do not smoke.

Health protection Comprises laws, regulations, policies and voluntary codes of practice aimed at preventing disease and enhancing health, e.g. legislation making use of car seat-belts compulsory, thereby reducing the prevalence of maxillofacial injuries due to road traffic accidents.

BARRIERS TO HEALTHY BEHAVIOURS

The principle of health promotion is that by provision of appropriate information and circumstances, beliefs and attitudes of individuals will be affected sufficiently to result in the adoption of behaviour likely to enhance health and diminish the chance of disease. However, dental disease is heavily influenced by socioeconomic and other constraints that may restrict the choices available (p. 2). Whilst parents may realize that fresh fruit is preferable to chocolate bars, non-availability or price may preclude its provision. Similarly, sugar-containing foodstuffs are given to children not only when they are hungry but also as a reward or a pacifier.

CHANGING DISEASE LEVELS

Dental disease levels in the UK population have reduced significantly in the last two decades; the 1998 Adult Dental Health Survey demonstrated that the proportion of edentulous adults fell from 30% in 1978 to 13% in 1998. The 2003 national survey of children's oral health showed the mean number of decayed, missing and filled teeth in 15 year olds fell from 93% in 1983 to 49% in 2003. Marked regional variations in the percentage of children affected by tooth decay were however apparent. The average number of decayed, missing and filled teeth (DMFT) at age 12 ranged from 1.0 in England to 1.4 in Wales and 2.7 in Northern Ireland. In contrast to the improvements shown in levels of decay in children's permanent teeth, the mean number of dmft in

5 year olds in the United Kingdom has seen little improvement in the past 20 years, being 1.8 in 1983 and 1.6 in 2003.

Caries still affects large numbers of children in lower socioeconomic groups and within some ethnic minorities. There is a threefold difference in levels of decay between the least and most deprived communities.

DENTAL CARIES

Dental caries is a dynamic process involving the exchange of calcium and phosphate ions between tooth structure and saliva (plaque fluid), in the presence of acids produced by the fermentation of carbohydrates by oral micro-organisms.

The factors involved in caries production are illustrated in Figure 8.1.

Enamel caries The earliest clinical appearance of caries is a 'white spot'. This is caused by loss of calcium and phosphate ions from the enamel prisms. Initially, loss is greater subsurface and the tooth surface remains intact. • Found in plaque stagnation areas such as: pits and fissures; just under contact points between adjacent teeth; at gingival margin. • May become discoloured – known as 'brown spot lesion'. • Is cone shaped with base on surface. • If lesion progresses, surface breaks down and a cavity is formed. • When surface breakdown occurs, requires restoration.

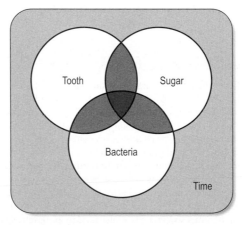

Figure 8.1 Factors involved in the aetiology of dental caries.

Fissure caries Describes caries occurring in the stagnation area at the base of pits and fissures. • Frequently the first site to be attacked.

Dentine caries Occurs when enamel caries extends to amelodentinal junction. • Spreads laterally and, as progresses, is cone shaped with base on amelodentinal junction. • As dentine is vital, can respond by laying down reactionary or secondary dentine at surface of the pulp chamber – depends on the rate of caries progression.

Occult caries Describes extensive dentine caries in the presence of minimal or no clinically apparent enamel breakdown. • Most commonly occurs under occlusal surfaces. • An increasing problem in older children/teenagers. • May be due to increased resistance to enamel breakdown as a result of exposure to fluoride.

Root caries Occurs following gingival recession. • Varies from light yellow to dark brown in colour. • Increasing problem in elderly patients.

Recurrent caries Continuation of caries after placement of restoration.

Secondary caries New caries occurring at restoration margins.
    Both secondary and recurrent caries indicate restoration failure, which accounts for a considerable component of operative dentistry.

Rampant caries Describes gross caries, frequently in deciduous dentition.

Early childhood caries Also known as 'nursing bottle caries'.
• Describes extensive caries in primary incisors due to prolonged exposure to sugar-containing drinks in a feeding bottle or cup.

Arrested caries Under favourable conditions, a lesion may become inactive – black or dark brown in colour – and has a hard or leathery consistency.

Caries diagnosis
Clinical diagnosis
Requires careful inspection of each tooth surface • good light is essential • drying the teeth enables easier visualization of white spot and early lesions • occult caries or caries at approximal surfaces appears as grey/black discoloration • don't use sharp probe – risk collapsing incipient lesions • probe should only be used to remove plaque/food debris.

Radiographic diagnosis
Bitewing radiographs are a crucial aid to the diagnosis of caries on approximal surfaces and for occult dentine caries under occlusal surfaces. They are also used to diagnose caries in restored teeth.

Bitewing radiographs are required for all new patients if the approximal surfaces of the teeth cannot be examined clinically. At recall visits, the frequency with which bitewings should be taken is dependent on the age of the patient and perceived caries risk. The interval ranges from 6 months for children at high risk to 2-yearly for adults at low risk (p. 52).

 Remember, caries can be difficult to diagnose by clinical examination alone. If in any doubt, bitewing radiographs should be taken.

Fibreoptic transillumination (FOTI)
In this technique, a bright light is conducted along a fibreoptic cable and can be directed interproximally. Approximal caries appears as a dark shadow. Whilst the technique is of benefit in epidemiological investigations, bitewings are superior for diagnosis in individual patients.

Electronic caries detector
Designed for detecting fissure caries – has been researched quite extensively but not in widespread clinical use.

Dyes
For use in cavity preparation. Claimed that dye is taken up by carious dentine to enable easier visualization.

Variability in caries diagnosis between individual clinicians is frequently a subject of debate. This reflects the difficulties encountered in caries diagnosis. Consistency in diagnosis is crucial in epidemiological studies and considerable effort must be made to train and calibrate the clinicians involved to achieve satisfactory reproducibility.

DMFT index
The decayed, missing and filled index is the most widely used method of recording caries experience.

D = decayed
M = missing
F = filled
T = teeth
DMFT applies to permanent teeth
DMFS applies to permanent tooth surfaces
dmft/dmfs applies to primary dentition

Components of DMF can be used to determine:

$$\frac{D}{DMF} = \text{Index of treatment need}$$

$$\frac{F}{DMF} = \text{Index of restorative provision (also known as Care Index)}$$

$$\frac{M}{DMF} = \text{Index of treatment failure}$$

CARIES RISK

The ability to determine susceptibility to dental caries on either a population or individual patient basis would offer a number of advantages.

Population basis permits targeting of resources, location of clinics, implementation of preventive programmes.

Individual basis determines the need for caries control measures, timing of recall appointments, decisions as to suitability for advanced restorations, suitability for orthodontic treatment.

Various tests have been devised for determining caries risk. Based on: • counts of salivary lactobacilli (*Dentocult LB*), mutans streptococci (*Dentocult SM*) • tests of salivary buffering capacity (*Dentobuff*) • tests based on socioeconomic factors • existing caries status • clinical judgement of dentist.

These have met with limited success as, due to the multifactorial aetiology of dental caries, variation precludes accuracy and consistent estimation of the caries susceptibility of an individual patient at the chairside. Of the above tests, the clinical judgement of the dentist and current caries experience have proven the most reliable indicators of future decay. Determination of disease risk is an important factor in determining how frequently patients should attend for dental care (p. 164).

MICROBIOLOGY OF DENTAL CARIES

It has been shown that caries does not develop in germ-free animals, even when fed a cariogenic diet. Caries results, not from the action of a single bacterial species, but from acid production by a range of organisms – the '*non-specific plaque hypothesis*'. The formation of *biofilms* and the complex interaction between bacteria and their extracellular products are important in creating an environment conducive to demineralization of tooth structure.

Most important organisms are:

- Mutans streptococci. A group of Gram-positive cocci, which includes *Streptococcus mutans* and *Streptococcus sobrinus*. Have the ability to metabolize sugars at low pH (acidogenic) and are important in the initiation of caries.
- *Lactobacillus* species. Gram-positive bacilli. Have the ability to survive at low pH (aciduric). Isolated in large numbers from carious dentine.

Whilst dental caries will not develop in the absence of dental plaque, and plaque removal is essential in maintaining periodontal health, dietary control and use of fluoride are more important in caries prevention than plaque removal per se.

The control of dental plaque is discussed on page 212.

DIET AND DENTAL CARIES

Carbohydrates in a form that can be metabolized by oral bacteria are a necessary prerequisite for caries development (Figure 8.1).

CLASSIFICATION OF SUGARS (TABLE 8.1)

TABLE 8.1 Classification of sugars

Intrinsic sugars – sugars forming an integral part of certain unprocessed foodstuffs. Called intrinsic because they are enclosed within a cell. Found in whole fruits and vegetables; mainly fructose, glucose, sucrose.

Extrinsic sugars – in food outwith cellular structure. Further classified as:
Milk sugars – in milk and milk-containing products; mainly lactose.
Non-milk extrinsic sugars – in confectionery, soft drinks, biscuits and cakes. Include sucrose, fructose and glucose. Constitute two-thirds of all sugar in the diet and have the greatest cariogenic potential.

EVIDENCE THAT SUGAR CAUSES CARIES

There is clear and extensive evidence of the correlation between the frequency and amount of sugar consumption and the prevalence and severity of dental caries: • epidemiological data show a correlation between sugar consumption and caries on a national basis • caries prevalence is higher in communities with high sugar intake, e.g. sugar cane and confectionery industry workers • caries prevalence increases following introduction of a sugar-containing diet in isolated communities, e.g. the Inuit, island communities such as Tristan da Cunha • caries decreases following restriction of sugar, e.g. wartime diets.

Recently a number of research papers have argued that the increased availability of fluoride has lessened the impact of sugar in the aetiology of dental caries. However, there can be little doubt that a diet rich in sugar, particularly if consumed at frequent intervals, will result in caries development.

FACTORS INFLUENCING CARIOGENICITY OF FOODS

Cariogenic potential is related to consistency: sticky retentive foods are more cariogenic than liquid non-retentive forms, e.g. toffee is more cariogenic than chocolate.

The frequency of consumption is crucial. Snacking or 'grazing' results in plaque pH being below the point where net outflow of calcium and phosphate ions from the tooth surface occurs for prolonged periods (Figure 8.2).

DIETARY ADVICE

The factors related to changing behaviour (p. 4) are particularly important in encouraging patients to adopt a less cariogenic diet. Effective dietary counselling requires knowledge of a patient's habits relating to non-milk extrinsic sugar consumption.

Diet diary

- Useful for those with high caries experience
- Must encourage patient to complete accurately
- Should cover a 3-day period including either Saturday or Sunday
- When completed, analyse with patient; highlight cariogenic foodstuffs, particularly hidden sugars

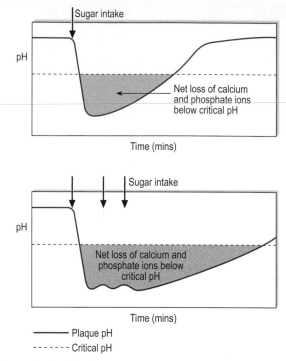

Figure 8.2 The effect of repeated sugar consumption on plaque pH.

- Allows formulation of personal advice for each individual
- Where possible, advise patient (and parent) in both written and verbal form.

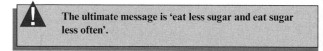

> ⚠ **The ultimate message is 'eat less sugar and eat sugar less often'.**

Non-sugar sweeteners Non-cariogenic and useful sugar substitutes.

Bulk sweeteners e.g. sorbitol and xylitol, provide calories and bulk; useful as sugar substitutes in confectionery, chewing gum and medicines.

ntense sweeteners e.g. saccharin and aspartame, are calorie free; popular in slimmers' foods.

From a dental point of view, whilst bulk and intense sweeteners are non-cariogenic and therefore useful sugar substitutes, use of artificial sweeteners perpetuates the craving for sweet foods.

'Tooth-friendly' sweets Identified by the 'tooth friendly' logo, these sweets contain non-sugar sweeteners. Their use should be restricted in small children due to possible side effects on the gastrointestinal system (e.g. diarrhoea).

Chewing-gum Sugar-free chewing-gum stimulates saliva and thus increases salivary buffers and enhances washout of sugar. May be of benefit in some patients, but should not be viewed as a prime caries preventive measure.

Carbonated beverages Carbonated drinks have a pH of 2–3 and can cause marked loss of tooth structure via erosion, an increasing problem in teenagers. Even 'diet' varieties can lead to erosion (p. 279).

Detersive foodstuffs Contrary to previous beliefs, detersive foods are of little or no benefit in removal of plaque. Effective plaque removal is dependent on toothbrushing. However, carrots, apples, etc., are preferable to high-sugar snacks.

FLUORIDE

Evidence for the efficacy of fluoride in the prevention of dental caries is incontrovertible. A series of systematic reviews published by the Cochrane Library have concluded that children who brush their teeth at least once a day with a toothpaste that contains fluoride will have less tooth decay. These reviews have also shown that fluoride has a caries preventive action when delivered in vehicles other than toothpaste.

MODES OF ACTION

Systemic (pre-eruptive) effect Fluoride ions are incorporated into enamel structure in the form of fluorapatite during the period of tooth formation. This decreases the mineral solubility.

Topical (posteruptive) effect Fluoride ions are associated with the tooth surface posteruption. The chemistry of fluoride interaction with hydroxyapatite is complex; fluoride interacts with the tooth structure either by incorporation into the crystal lattice or by binding to crystal surfaces. Calcium fluoride at the tooth surface not only reduces the solubility of the apatite but also encourages *remineralization*.

Whilst fluoride may cause decreased acid production by cariogenic bacteria, its effect on mineral solubility is of much greater clinical significance.

Historically it was thought that fluoride availability during tooth formation for incorporation into the hydroxyapatite was most important. It is now realized the topical effect at the tooth surface posteruption is very important. Thus, methods that apply fluoride on a regular (daily) basis are most effective.

EVIDENCE THAT FLUORIDE PREVENTS CARIES

- Caries prevalence is lower in areas where fluoride is present naturally in the water supply.
- Addition of fluoride to the water supply is effective in preventing caries.
- Fluoride-containing toothpastes are effective in preventing caries.

MECHANISMS FOR DELIVERING FLUORIDE

Water fluoridation Fluoridation of the public water supply at 1 ppm (part per million) has been shown in numerous studies to reduce caries incidence. It is more effective on smooth surfaces of teeth than in pits and fissures. However, in the UK, in spite of its proven benefits and safety, currently only 10% of the population receive fluoridated water.

Fluoride toothpaste The main mechanism whereby fluoride is delivered is via toothpaste (dentifrice). Most formulations contain sodium fluoride (NaF) or sodium monofluorophosphate (SMFP) or a combination of both, at a concentration of either 1000 or 1500 ppm. Used twice daily, this will reduce caries incidence by around 30%.

Restrict the amount of toothpaste used by children to a pea size/smear amount at each brushing.

Children's formulations containing either 125 or 550 ppm F^- are available, although there is little evidence that at this concentration they are truly effective in preventing caries, particularly in high-risk children. Available in mild minty taste or fruity flavours. Mint flavours are preferred to discourage children eating the paste.

Fluoride drops and tablets Given during the period of tooth formation, fluoride drops and tablets can exert both a systemic and topical effect. Dosage is related to age and the fluoride content of the local water supply. The regimen currently recommended in the *British National Formulary* is shown in Table 8.2.

Give fluoride tablets last thing at night and allow to dissolve slowly in the mouth.

If using fluoride toothpaste, additional supplementation is required only in those judged at high risk of developing caries. However, to be effective, supplements must be given over a prolonged period. Compliance is problematic. Those children who would benefit most (high caries risk/lower socioeconomic groups) are the least likely to be given supplements.

Fluoridated salt Fluoridated salt has been used successfully as a caries preventive measure in Switzerland and France. However, given the general health promotion message of *decreased* salt intake and the fact that most salt is added during the manufacturing process, this is unlikely to be a realistic mechanism for community fluoridation.

Fluoridated milk/fruit juices Whilst proven to be successful vehicles for fluoride delivery, they are difficult to implement as a public health measure and a recent systematic review has questioned the quality of evidence for the effectiveness of fluoridated milk. In addition, fruit juices are acidic.

Fluoride gels Topically applied in individual trays. Given current views on the importance of the frequency of fluoride application, if

TABLE 8.2 Recommended daily dosage of fluoride tablets and drops (mg F/day), related to age and concentration of fluoride in the drinking water

Age	Water F (ppm) <0.3	Water F (ppm) 0.3–0.7	Water F (ppm) >0.7
0–6 months	0	0	0
6 months–3 years	0.25	0	0
3–6 years	0.5	0.25	0
Over 6 years	1	0.5	0

fluoride therapy is required in addition to toothpaste, mouthwashes are preferred.

Fluoride mouthwashes Most contain NaF at 0.05% for daily use or 0.2% for weekly use. Daily use is preferred.
Indications Teenagers with high caries activity • patients prone to root caries, e.g. xerostomia • non-carious tooth surface loss (p. 279) • dentine hypersensitivity.

Fluoride varnishes Contain F⁻ in an alcoholic solution of natural varnishes at 2.26% F (Duraphat). Fluoride varnishes applied professionally two to four times a year have the ability to substantially reduce tooth decay in children.

Fluoride foams Used in a similar form to fluoride varnishes. Are professionally applied.
Indications To promote remineralization of early enamel caries • to encourage remineralization of exposed dentine.

Fluorosis

Fluorosis or mottled enamel occurs due to the excessive intake of fluoride during the period of tooth formation. This results in hypomineralization and affects mainly the permanent dentition. Ranges from 'white flecks', which are barely noticeable, to brown stains in more severe cases. Symmetrical in distribution.

Treatment Mild forms diminish with time. Can be markedly improved by etching and polishing. Most severe cases may require veneers. In the UK, fluorosis is most likely to occur due to excessive consumption of fluoridated toothpaste. For this reason, it is vital that the volume of toothpaste used by children should be restricted to a pea size/smear amount at each brushing and children discouraged from swallowing paste.

Safety of fluoride

The safety of fluoride at 1 ppm in the public water supply has been the subject of numerous studies and has been established. However, acute toxicity may occur above 5 mg F/kg body weight.

Antidote <5 mg F/kg body weight – drink large volumes of milk, seek medical advice; >5 mg F/kg body weight – refer to hospital for gastric lavage without delay.

  Fluoride tablets, toothpaste and mouthwashes should be stored out of the reach of children.

SMOKING AND ORAL HEALTH

The adverse impact of smoking on health is well recognized and it has been shown that about one-half of all smokers will die directly as a result of their smoking habit. This means that in the UK alone about 13 people die of a smoking-related illness every hour. Worldwide the toll is enormous and will increase in the future due to the high and increasing prevalence of smoking in the developing world.

Smoking has many effects on oral health (Table 8.3).

Stopping smoking has significant benefits both for general and oral health. It is now recognized that members of the dental team have a key role to play in helping smokers stop. The 'four As' smoking cessation routine, originally devised in the USA, has been suggested as a useful aide-memoire:

ASK – all patients about smoking
ADVISE – all smokers about the benefits of quitting

TABLE 8.3 The effects of smoking on oral health

- There is a dose–response relationship between tobacco and mouth cancer
- White patches occur on the oral mucosa six times more frequently in smokers than non-smokers
- Smoking causes cellular changes within the oral epithelium, which most commonly presents clinically as smokers' keratosis
- Smokers are 2.5 to 5 times more likely to develop periodontal disease than non-smokers. These odds may be even higher in younger people
- There is evidence of a direct correlation between the number of cigarettes smoked and the risk of developing periodontitis
- Reduced gingival redness and oedema in smokers (due to the vasoconstrictive effects of nicotine) may mask underlying attachment loss
- Acute necrotizing ulcerative gingivitis occurs predominantly in smokers
- Sinusitis occurs 75% more frequently in smokers than in non-smokers
- Taste and olfactory senses are dulled in smokers
- Tooth staining is more common in smokers
- Smokers are predisposed to halitosis
- Wound healing is delayed in smokers – dry sockets occur more commonly in smokers
- Osseointegrated implants are significantly more likely to fail in patients who smoke
- The outcome of most forms of periodontal therapy, including root planing, flap surgery, guided tissue regeneration and local antimicrobial therapy, is less favourable in smokers than in non-smokers

ASSIST – those patients who express an interest in stopping, either personally or by referring them to a formal smoking cessation programme

ARRANGE – follow-up visits.

Because of the cyclical nature of the process, follow-up of patients is important and the dental team is well placed to assist with this because of their ongoing and regular contact with patients (Figure 8.3).

There is good evidence that nicotine replacement therapy in the form of patches, chewing-gum and nasal sprays increases the quit success rates. Other drugs, such as bupropion, have also been used in helping smokers quit.

FREQUENCY OF DENTAL ATTENDANCE

An important consideration in prevention of oral disease is the frequency with which patients should attend for a routine oral examination, or 'check-up.' Traditionally patients were advised to visit the dentist on a 6-monthly basis. However, it is recognized that patients differ in their risk of oral disease, and as oral health improves, a 'one-size' fits all recall interval is no longer appropriate.

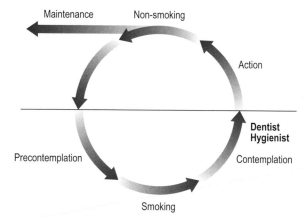

Figure 8.3 The potential contribution of members of the dental team in promoting smoking cessation (after Prochaska JO, DiClemente CC 1983 Stages and processes of self-change of smoking: toward an integrative model of change. Journal of Consulting and Clinical Psychology 51:390–5).

Recall intervals should therefore be tailored to individual patients needs or circumstances.

In the UK the National Institute for Health and Clinical Excellence (NICE) has issued guidance on the timing of dental recalls. This recommends that the interval between oral health reviews should be determined specifically for each patient and tailored to individual needs based on an assessment of disease levels and risk of or from dental disease. For patients younger than 18 years, recall intervals can vary between 3 and 12 months. For those over 18 years, intervals can range between 3 and 24 months.

A guiding principle in deciding on recall intervals is to start with a short interval and then gradually increase if the patient's oral health remains stable and risk factors remain constant or reduce.

PREVENTION IN ELDERLY PATIENTS

As oral health improves, an increasing number of elderly patients will retain their teeth for longer. Also, demographic changes have seen the total number of people of pensionable age in the UK increase by 4.2% between 1985 and 2001. By 2025 this will have increased by 31.1%. Thus, care of the elderly patient will become increasingly important to the dental profession.

Factors complicating prevention in elderly patients

Plaque control Gingival recession; migrated and tilted teeth increase the number of inaccessible surfaces • Partial dentures increase plaque retention. • Poor eyesight and reduced dexterity make toothbrushing difficult. • Polypharmacy is common in the elderly; some drugs reduce salivary flow.

Diet Increased tendency to snacking – cakes and biscuits – following retirement. Particularly prone to recurrent caries and root caries.

Denture care Encourage removal of dentures at night and good denture hygiene. • Emphasize the importance of annual dental examinations, even if edentulous, because this permits early detection of mucosal disease (e.g. mouth cancer).

DENTAL CARE PROFESSIONALS (DCPs)

Known variously as dental auxiliaries, professionals complementary to dentistry, a varied group of oral healthcare workers support dental surgeons. These include:

Dental nurses

Remit varies considerably depending on where they work and who employs them. Main role is assisting at the chairside but may also undertake receptionist and administrative duties. Require registration with the General Dental Council.

Dental hygienists

Role involves patient education, scaling (both sub- and supragingivally), polishing and application of prophylactic materials including fissure sealants. Can administer local anaesthesia by both infiltration and block. Can also replace crowns with a temporary cement in an emergency, remove excess cement using instruments which may include rotary instruments and treat patients under conscious sedation, provided that a registered dentist remains in the room throughout treatment. Currently must work to the written prescription of a dentist who has first examined the patient, though this may change in the future. Registered and regulated by the General Dental Council.

Dental therapists

Undertake the same work as hygienists, but can also do simple restorations, restore primary teeth by means of pulp therapy, place preformed crowns on primary teeth and extract primary teeth. Can be employed in all branches of dentistry, including general dental practice, working to the prescription of a supervising dentist.

Dental health educators

Frequently have a dental nursing, hygienist or therapist background. Specialize in the promotion of oral health.

Dental technicians

The second largest group of DCPs after dental nurses. Work mainly in commercial laboratories. Construct all forms of fixed and removable prostheses. Some specialize in maxillofacial prosthetics.

Orthodontic therapists

Assist orthodontics with the provision of orthodontic care.

A team approach to dental practice is viewed as a potential means of improving the delivery of care and of overcoming workforce shortages. In the UK, details of the current legislation applying to DCPs are available from the General Dental Council website (www.gdc-uk.org).

CHAPTER 9

PAEDIATRIC DENTISTRY

Organizing treatment for children   168

Managing behaviour in children   170

Development of the dentition   172

Maintenance of the operating field   174

Pit and fissure sealants   176

Restoration of carious primary teeth   177

Pulp therapy   180

Traumatic injuries   185

Oral pathology in children   190

Children with special needs   193

ORGANIZING TREATMENT FOR CHILDREN

The basic principles underlying history taking and examination described in Chapter 2 apply equally in paediatric dentistry. However, organization of treatment for children is made difficult by their lack of dental experience. Many adults ascribe lifelong dental anxiety and phobias to negative experiences of dentistry in childhood. A planned *atraumatic* introduction, using appropriate behaviour management techniques, is necessary to provide children with the appropriate skills to cope with dental treatment. This is complicated if the child first presents in pain.

Aims of treating children
- Provide a positive introduction to dentistry.
- Provide child with the skills necessary to accept dental treatment.
- Institute good preventive practice.
- Provide any necessary restorative care in a planned and organized fashion.

History
May rely on parent/carer for accurate history. Should include:
• when pain is present; features as described on page 232 • previous experience of dental treatment – e.g. has child had local anaesthetic before, or experience of rubber dam? • medical and social history • details of oral hygiene practices, including who brushes.

Examination
Extraoral Much information can be obtained from observing how the child enters the surgery, relationship with parent, behaviour.

Intraoral Young children (<3 years) may be best examined on a parent's lap. Note overall condition of the mouth, oral hygiene, caries experience, evidence of previous dental treatment, occlusion/development of the occlusion, soft tissue pathology. Radiographs should be taken when clinically indicated (Chapter 4).

Treatment planning
Obviously pain relief takes priority. In the absence of pain a sequential, gradual approach including prevention, restorative care and planned follow-up is required.

First visit Introduction to environs of surgery. Limit to history taking, examination and, possibly, radiographs, details of oral hygiene and dietary practices.

Second visit Preventive advice, acclimatization and simple treatment, e.g. dressing open carious lesions, application of fissure sealants, polishing.

Third and subsequent visits Commence restorative care, beginning with most easily restored cavity. Introduce local anaesthesia. Progress to more advanced procedures. Reinforce preventive messages. At the final visit the recall interval should be decided based on the individual's caries risk status (p. 164).

Preventive versus restorative care

The adoption of good dental behaviour is crucial in preventing further decay and avoiding the 'restoration cycle', i.e. repeated replacement of restorations. Preventive measures such as diet modification, oral hygiene instruction, prophylaxis, application of fluoride varnish, fissure sealants, etc., provide a good means of building confidence and cooperation but should not be used as an excuse to avoid dealing with decayed teeth.

Choice of preventive regimen

Preventive aspects of dental care are discussed in Chapter 8. While all preventive regimens have the common themes of reduction of non-milk extrinsic sugars, provision of fluoride and improved plaque control, the technique employed should be tailored to individual patient requirements. Thus, in a caries-free child, brushing with a fluoride toothpaste may suffice as a means of delivering fluoride, whilst a toddler presenting with rampant or nursing bottle caries would benefit from both systemic and topical fluorides as well as specific diet advice (p. 159).

Practical points

- For maximum benefit, children should spit, not rinse, after brushing.
- Under 7 years, children lack sufficient manual dexterity to brush their teeth effectively.
- Young children should be supervised when brushing to:
  — ensure effective brushing
  — limit amount of toothpaste consumed.
- Sugar-containing foods and drinks should be kept clear of bedtime.
- Keep preventive messages simple, build up gradually.

Role of parents or carers

Children are brought to the dentist; they do not choose to come. It is important to ensure that the adult accompanying the child is a parent, or a carer who is able to give consent. Parents can influence the organization of treatment in a number of ways. With a young child, the history must be obtained from a responsible adult. Additionally parents may:

- have to organize time off work or care for other siblings in order to attend; hence need to explain:
  — what treatment is required
  — likely number of visits
  — need to build child's confidence
- be responsible for implementing home strategies (e.g. brushing, diet control)
- wish their main concerns are dealt with promptly
- be guilty about the child's dental disease or behaviour
- adversely affect the child's behaviour because of their own anxiety about dental treatment
- be overly protective or demanding.

There are no hard and fast rules as to whether a parent should stay with the child during treatment or remain in the waiting room. Best judged on an individual basis, except for children under 4 years, who benefit from having a parent present.

Remember
- Attention span is short – plan treatment accordingly.
- Call child by his/her correct name.
- Children are very sensitive to environment and non-verbal communication – so smile!
- Child-friendly environment is important – posters, toys, etc.
- Skills of other members of team. A member of the surgery staff may be particularly adept at putting children at their ease.
- Ensure parents understand their role in the process.
- Consider referral to a colleague when failing to make progress.

MANAGING BEHAVIOUR IN CHILDREN

An important aspect of treating children is the ability to enable them to relax in the dental setting and learn how to cope with treatment. The child's attitude and behaviour will be influenced by many factors including:

- age, maturity, personality
- attitude of parents
- previous dental experience
- previous medical experience

- attitude of dental staff
- environs of surgery
- whether (s)he has a dental problem.

Various techniques for managing behaviour of children in the dental setting have been described. Whilst the terminology may be unfamiliar, most dentists routinely employ these methods when dealing with children as they are largely a matter of common sense. Remember some techniques require good verbal skills that some very young children and some children with specific disabilities may lack.

Behaviour management techniques

Remember non-verbal communication occurs continuously and may reinforce or contradict verbal signals. Where possible, treatment is organized as described on page 168, progressing from simple to more complex procedures.

Tell–show–do This technique is widely used to familiarize a patient with a new procedure. The *tell* phase involves an age-appropriate explanation of the procedure. The *show* phase is used to demonstrate the procedure, for example demonstrating with a slow handpiece on a finger. The *do* phase is initiated with a minimum delay, in this case a polish. It is important that the language used be appropriate to the child's age, and the whole dental team must adopt the same approach: specifically, emotive or negative words should be avoided.

Enhancing control Feeling out of control is a major cause of dental anxiety. The use of a 'stop signal' can give the child a degree of control over the dentist. The stop signal, usually raising an arm, should be rehearsed and the dentist should respond quickly when it is used. It is also possible to use a signal to proceed with treatment.

Modelling A child learns by watching others, e.g. siblings, other children. It is important that the patient can relate to and identify with the model and that the model exhibits appropriate behaviours. Videos or DVDs can be employed. Used for children with little or no dental experience.

Behaviour shaping and positive reinforcement Dental procedures require complex behaviours that need to be learned. For children, small clear steps leading to ideal behaviour are required. Rewarding good behaviour by paying compliments makes it possible to selectively reinforce positive behaviour, which is therefore more likely to be repeated. If possible, do not abandon treatment completely as a result of temper tantrums, etc. – this simply reinforces negative behaviour. In these circumstances attempt a compromise, e.g. dressing placed instead of final restoration, which finishes treatment session on a positive note. Stickers, badges and praise act as positive reinforcers, but the most powerful reinforcers are social stimuli such as facial expression, positive voice modulation and verbal praise. To be effective, praise must be continuous and specific.

Distraction This approach aims to shift the patient's attention from the dental setting to some other situation, or from a potentially unpleasant procedure to some other action. Short-term distractors such as diverting the attention by pulling the lip as a local anaesthetic is given or having patients raise their legs to stop them gagging during radiography may also be useful. Talking to patients or telling them stories while treating them uses the voice as a distractor.

Desensitization This technique helps individuals with specific fears or phobias overcome them by repeated contacts. A hierarchy of fear-producing stimuli is constructed, and the patient is exposed to them in an ordered manner, starting with the stimulus posing the lowest threat. In dental terms, fears are usually related to a specific procedure such as local anaesthetic. First, patients are taught to relax, and in this state exposed to each of the stimuli in the hierarchy in turn, only progressing to the next when they feel able. Friendly and caring attitude of dental staff is very important. The technique is useful for children who can clearly identify their fear and who can verbally communicate.

Behaviour management techniques may not always work with extremely anxious patients. May have to resort to pharmacological approach – sedation or general anaesthesia (Chapter 6).

DEVELOPMENT OF THE DENTITION

The timing of tooth formation and eruption is variable. The order of eruption is more important than precise age. Average dates of mineralization and eruption of the teeth are recorded in Appendix C. Development of the dentition can be divided into the following stages.

Pre-teeth
Usually there are no teeth until about 6 months. The upper gum pad is wider and longer than the lower. Palatal vault is almost flat, and the frenum of upper lip is attached to the crest of the gum pad and is continuous with the incisive papilla. Occasionally children

are born with teeth (natal teeth) or erupt them within a month (neonatal teeth). They are usually mandibular and mobile, having no root development. Left in situ, normal root development occurs, but if they are at risk of inhalation of interfering with feeding they should be extracted.

Development of primary dentition

Timing of tooth eruption is variable (about 6 months to 24/36 months). Lower incisors usually erupt first. Primary incisors are more upright than their successors and tend to be spaced. By age 5 attrition of primary teeth is common and incisors may be edge to edge. Varying degrees of space at this stage – if no space or crowded, then crowding in the permanent dentition is likely.

Mixed dentition to permanent dentition

Begins with eruption of first permanent molars or lower central incisors at about age 6 years. Upper central incisors and lower lateral incisors erupt around the age of 7 years with upper lateral incisors a year later. A variation of ±1 year is within normal limits but the eruption sequence should not vary. If the upper lateral incisor erupts ahead of the central incisor, pathology should be suspected (supernumerary or dilacerated central). Permanent incisors develop slightly behind the roots of the primary incisors, and are larger than them. The extra space is gained from:

- spacing of primary incisors
- permanent incisors are more proclined
- increases in inter-canine width at this time.

Lower incisors often erupt lingually and are moved forward by tongue pressure. Commonly an upper midline space is present when the upper incisors erupt and the crowns are distally inclined (it closes as lateral incisors and canines erupt). Canines move buccally and should be palpable high in the buccal sulcus from age 9 years onwards. Lower canine and first premolars begin to erupt at 10 years, followed by second premolars at age 10–12 and upper canines at 11–12. Normal pattern and symmetry of eruption is more important than chronological guidelines. A given pair of teeth normally erupt within 6 months of each other; if they fail to do so the non-eruption should be investigated. Most leeway space is taken up by the molars moving mesially. Whilst the sequence of eruption is also variable, in lower is usually canine, first premolar, second premolar, and in the upper is usually first premolar, second premolar, canine. Second molars erupt at about 12–14. Third molar eruption is quite variable.

Late changes

These include an increase in lower incisor crowding and an increase in the interincisal angle. May be a slight increase in mandibular prognathism.

MAINTENANCE OF THE OPERATING FIELD

Adequate isolation of the tooth during operative procedures is essential and can be achieved by retractors, saliva ejectors, cotton-wool rolls, absorbent pads, high- and low-volume aspirators and rubber dam.

Retractors Various forms are available. Care should be taken not to traumatize soft tissues, particularly when anaesthetized.

Saliva ejector Attached to low-volume aspirator this aids patient's comfort and reduces the need to swallow or spit out.

High-volume aspirator Essential when using high-speed handpieces (or ultrasonic scaler). Aids vision and reduces aerosol.

Cotton-wool rolls Place buccally and lingually. Of limited value in patients who produce copious saliva.

Absorbent pads Triangular in shape. Placed buccally, these are useful when fissure sealing upper molar teeth.

  Both cotton-wool rolls and absorbent pads should be moistened before removal to prevent adherence and damage to the oral mucosa.

RUBBER DAM

Provides the optimum means of isolation. (Although referred to traditionally as 'rubber dam', it may be better referred to as 'dental dam' as it is available in a latex-free formulation for patients with latex sensitivity.)

Advantages
- Moisture control. Prevents salivary contamination. Particularly important during pulp therapy and acid-etch procedures.
- Protects airway. Prevents inhalation or ingestion of foreign bodies.
- Prevents contamination of materials.
- Controls soft tissue and aids visualization.

- Protects patient from potentially irritating materials such as endodontic irrigants. Be very careful to ensure no leaks under the dam.
- Provides physical barrier from oral fluids and reduces bacterial load of aerosols.

In spite of the above advantages, rubber dam has not been routinely employed in the UK, with perhaps the exception of endodontic therapy. However, with practice, rubber dam can be applied easily in most situations and is generally well tolerated by patients.

 When operating under rubber dam, be sure to check angulation of burs, etc., as it is easy to become disorientated.

Technique

Several techniques for application of rubber dam are available depending on whether clamp is placed before, after or at the same time as the rubber dam sheet. The following describes clamp placement before rubber dam using a split dam technique which is most useful in the child patient.

1. Punch two holes in the dam about 1–2 cm apart and join the holes by cutting with scissors.
2. Select appropriate clamp.
3. Attach floss to the bow of the clamp. (Aids retrieval should the clamp become dislodged.)
4. Use forceps to place clamp on the most posterior tooth. Ensure it is firmly seated and not traumatizing the gingivae.
5. Stretch the slit anteriorly and place between anterior teeth (usually mesial of canine).
6. Stretch the periphery of the dam over a frame.
7. Rubber 'wedjets' may be used to anchor the dam anteriorly.

Rubber dam can be used to isolate a single tooth or a number of teeth depending on the procedure to be undertaken. In the anterior region as an alternative to clamps, floss ligatures, rubber 'wedjets' or orthodontic elastics can be used to hold a rubber dam.

PIT AND FISSURE SEALANTS

A resin (BIS-GMA) based material applied to pits and fissures of teeth that mechanically adheres to dental enamel, preventing bacteria and substrate from gaining further access.

Sealant
- Filled or unfilled.
- Light cured or self-polymerizing.

Selection of patients
It is not cost-effective to seal all occlusal surfaces. In selecting cases consider:

Children at high risk Indicated by extensive caries in primary dentition, socially disadvantaged background. Caries in a first permanent molar indicates a need to seal the remaining first molars and second molars as soon as erupt.

Children with special needs Medical, mental, behavioural or physical disability (p. 193).

Teeth at high risk Teeth with deep fissure or pits, e.g. lateral incisors.

Sealants should be applied as soon as whole occlusal surface has erupted and within 2 years of eruption. Only sound teeth should be sealed. Where there is any suspicion of caries, investigate with small bur and provide sealant restoration.

If cooperation is not good enough for sealants, fluoride varnish should be applied.

Technique for application of fissure sealant

1. Clean the tooth surface with rotary bristle brush and pumice to remove pellicle.
2. Wash, isolate and dry tooth.
3. Apply 30–50% phosphoric acid etchant for 30 seconds. Gel is easier to control than liquid.
4. Wash tooth for 15 seconds.
5. Dry tooth for 30 seconds.
6. Apply resin and cure.
7. Check resin – use probe to ensure covers entire fissure system and to remove flash. Add if deficient.
8. Check occlusion.

Moisture control is crucial. Salivary contamination will reduce the etch markedly and lead to poor retention and loss of sealant.

RESTORATION OF CARIOUS PRIMARY TEETH

The principles of cavity preparation and restoration placement described in detail on pages 242–250 apply equally to primary teeth. However the anatomy of primary teeth differs from permanent teeth and influences cavity design and restoration placement accordingly (Table 9.1).

The preparation of Class I (occlusal), II and III (proximal), IV (incisal) and V (cervical) cavities is described on pages 244–248. In primary teeth the following should be noted.

Class II (proximal) For amalgam the width of the isthmus (junction between box and occlusal part of restoration) should be restricted to about one-third distance between buccal and lingual cusps. For adhesive materials a box preparation alone is

TABLE 9.1 Influence of primary tooth anatomy on cavity design and restoration placement

Anatomy of primary teeth	Implications for cavity design and tooth restoration
Enamel thinner than in permanent teeth	Dentine involved more rapidly Pulp horns nearer the surface
Crowns more bulbous than permanent teeth, particularly in the cervical area	Influences placement of floor of interproximal box in Class II cavities Adaptation of matrices more difficult Help retain preformed metal crowns
Cervical constriction apical to the cervical bulge	Can make it difficult to establish the floor of box
Primary molars are narrower occlusally, especially Ds	Cusp strength is influenced by width of occlusal restoration
Broad contact points in molars	Implications for approximal caries diagnosis. Need bitewing radiographs to detect early lesions
Pulp chamber is larger, pulp horns are more pointed, pulpal outline follows dentinoenamel junction	Cavity size must be restricted. Limited space for sufficient bulk of restorative material to resist fracture

sufficient; supplemental grooves are not recommended. The box should be a third of the width of the tooth. Where caries results in a wide flared box with no retention, stainless steel crowns show greater durability.

Class III (proximal) A palatal lock should be incorporated to aid retention.

Class IV (incisal) Due to size, retention may be a problem. Consider composite build-up using a celluloid strip-crown form.

Class V (cervical) Adhesive materials should be used.

Miniature handpiece heads and small burs should be used,

Materials

A wide variety of restorative materials may be use to restore a primary tooth. The choice will depend on the type of cavity, the required durability, patient cooperation and operator preference.

Amalgam Remains the most durable intracoronal material for restoration of Class I and II cavities in primary molars but requires mechanical undercut. However, environmental and health concerns continue to be raised.

Composite materials Have the advantage of aesthetics and additional adhesion via acid-etching of enamel in anterior teeth. Are very sensitive to moisture contamination.

Glass ionomers Adhere to dentine and leach fluoride, decreasing the chance of recurrent caries. However they lack wear resistance. They are useful in cases where cooperation is less than optimal or where short duration is required.

Resin-modified glass ionomers Have the advantages of glass ionomers but are light cured. Recent studies show good durability in Class I and II cavities.

Compomers (poly-acid modified composites) Bond to enamel and dentine using a bonding agent. Show good durability in Class I and II cavities and, like glass ionomers, do not require undercut.

When caries involves the whole marginal ridge or 3+ surfaces, a preformed metal crown should be used.

Atraumatic restorative treatment (ART)

In this technique, caries is removed using hand instruments with no local anaesthesia and restored with glass ionomer. Designed for use in developing countries where facilities and staff are limited it can be useful as part of acclimatization with young children or in dental-phobic patients.

Chemomechanical caries removal

Chemomechanical removal has become more reliable with commercial kits now available (e.g. Carisolv™). Two gels are mixed to create the active agents (sodium hypochlorite and amino acids) which separate carious from sound dentine – the addition of dyes improves visibility. The mixed gel is placed on carious dentine for 20 seconds, then scraped gently with specifically designed hand instruments. The gel becomes cloudy and is removed by washing; the process is repeated until the gel remains clear. The tooth is restored as normal.

Preformed metal crowns (PMC)

Festooned and precontoured, they are designed to fit the anatomical (not clinical) crown margins and are thus placed subgingivally. They are the most durable restoration for primary molars.

Uses:

- extensive caries precluding cavity preparation
- following pulp therapy in primary molars
- recurrent caries
- as initial restoration in amelogenesis imperfecta, dentinogenesis imperfecta or severe enamel hypoplasia.

Technique

1. Administer local anaesthesia.
2. Remove caries.
3. Select crown of appropriate size. Dividers can be used to measure mesiodistal dimension of tooth.
4. Create space to accommodate crown:
   a. Reduce occlusal surface by 1–1.5 mm.
   b. Use tapered diamond to reduce axial surfaces. Extend to level of gingival margin, do not leave a ledge.
5. Crown should 'click' onto preparation; the gingivae will blanch.
6. Trimming using scissors is required with only very overextended margins.
7. Contour using crimping pliers and polish after trimming.
8. Check occlusion.
9. Cement using polycarboxylate cement or glass ionomer – adheres to tooth.
10. Remove excess cement and re-check occlusion.

PULP THERAPY

This section describes pulp therapy in primary teeth and in immature permanent teeth. Pulp therapy in mature permanent teeth is described on pages 287–295.

PULP THERAPY IN PRIMARY TEETH

When a child presents with pulp pathology the dentist must decide whether to extract the tooth or carry out pulp therapy.

Advantages of pulp therapy
- maintains an intact arch
- tooth acts as a space maintainer
- introduces child to operative dentistry
- avoids physical and psychological trauma of extraction
- avoids need for extraction in cases where surgery is contraindicated, e.g. patients with haemophilia.

Pulp therapy is contraindicated when
- pathological mobility of tooth is present
- caries involves root canals or bifurcation
- general condition of the mouth is poor – numerous carious teeth
- poor cooperation
- congenital or acquired heart condition where haematogenous spread of infection could be a problem
- tooth to be shed within 2 years.

Diagnosis of pulpal and choice of therapy
The diagnosis of pulpal pain is discussed in detail on page 232. In children, obtaining a pain history is complicated by the fact that patients may be unable to be accurate and information must be obtained from the parent/carer and from clinical examination. Marginal ridge cavitation greater than 4 mm is associated with pulp pathology in over 90% of cases. Positive pain history suggests pulp pathology. Nature of pain reflects type of pulp pathology and thus influences choice of therapy.

Transient pain Suggests vital pulp and pathology limited to coronal pulp. Can be due to:
- exposed dentine or leaking restoration – treated by *covering exposed dentine/replacing restoration*
- limited carious exposure – treated by *single-visit pulpotomy*.

Spontaneous pain Occurs in absence of direct stimulus, frequently at night. Indicates: • inflammation throughout pulp chamber and extending into canals • non-vital pulp and periapical infection. Single-visit pulpotomy is contraindicated. Treated by either *multivisit pulpotomy* or *pulpectomy*.

Pulp therapy techniques

Pulp capping (p. 251) Poor results in primary teeth; therefore, where pulp is compromised, pulpotomy is preferred.

Pulpotomy involves removal of the entire coronal pulp.
   Can be performed on either vital or non-vital teeth. A pretreatment radiograph is required. Formocresol is no longer recommended because of concerns over the carcinogenic effects of formaldehyde.

Ferric sulphate vital pulpotomy Vital pulps may be hyperaemic and bleed vigorously. Following amputation of the coronal pulp the bleeding should arrest; if this occurs, the tissue is presumed to have the capacity to recover. Under these conditions the medicament of choice is ferric sulphate. Rubber dam is recommended to avoid salivary contamination.

Technique

1. Having given LA and removed all caries, remove roof of pulp chamber.
2. Use sharp sterile excavator to remove coronal pulp.
3. Irrigate with saline, stop bleeding with light pressure. If bleeding stops...
4. Apply cotton-wool pellet moistened with 15% ferric sulphate to pulp stumps for 15 seconds. This step can be repeated once if pulp is still bleeding.
5. Place thick mix of zinc–eugenol base in pulp chamber.
6. Restore with preformed metal crown.

Two-stage desensitizing pulpotomy

If a pulp does not stop bleeding following amputation of the pulp. Where inadequate local anaesthesia prevents a pulpotomy or when a tooth is exposed without local anaesthesia this technique can be used. Historically, devitalizing paste containing paraformaldehyde was used. The modern alternative is a steroidal antibiotic (e.g. Ledermix™), which can be placed over the exposure site and temporized. A ferric sulphate pulpotomy can then be completed at a second visit as previously described.

Pulpectomy

Non-vital pulps and pulps that do not stop bleeding following amputation of coronal pulp may be suitable for pulpectomy. In this technique, an attempt is made to remove radicular pulp tissue using both instruments and copious irrigation with sodium hypochlorite or chlorhexidine, following which pure zinc oxide paste is placed in the root canals. Whilst pulpectomy and root canal filling is the obvious choice for treating pulp pathology in mature permanent teeth (p. 287), the technique in the primary dentition is complicated by: • the long thin irregular root canals in primary molars • multiple 'blind channels' in molar pulps making complete pulp removal impossible • physiological resorption • exfoliation • difficulty in gaining adequate access to posterior teeth in young children • risk of damage to crown of developing successor.

In some cases tooth extraction may be preferred.

Review and follow-up

All teeth that have undergone pulp therapy should be reviewed at regular intervals, both clinically and radiographically.

PULP THERAPY IN IMMATURE PERMANENT TEETH

Pulp therapy may be required as a result of carious exposure or trauma. Carious exposure within a few years of eruption indicates high caries risk and careful consideration should be given to the overall treatment plan for the patient. In anterior teeth the exposure is usually due to trauma. In first permanent molars, pulp exposure is most likely due to caries. If the dentition is crowded, extraction may be the preferred option – an orthodontic opinion should be sought. Alternatively, it may be desirable to maintain temporarily whilst other teeth develop and erupt.

The pulp therapy technique to be employed in immature permanent teeth is dependent on two factors: • the degree of pulp pathology • stage of root formation.

Indirect pulp cap The aim is to remove bulk of carious dentine without pulp exposure and induce formation of secondary dentine. Works best in deep asymptomatic lesions. The technique is described on page 251.

Direct pulp cap Used in small exposures, iatrogenic, carious or following dental trauma. Contraindicated when evidence of irreversible pulpitis, e.g.: • spontaneous pain • tenderness on percussion • swelling • sinus • periapical or inter-radicular radiolucency • grossly carious or large exposure. Also contraindicated in immature incisors where pulp death cannot be treated by conventional root treatment.

Pulpectomy Where marked pulpitis is present or a tooth is non-vital and it has been decided to maintain a young permanent tooth, pulpectomy and conventional root canal therapy is the treatment of choice (p. 288). This option is not available if root formation is incomplete. Roots are usually complete about 3 years posteruption. Where root formation is incomplete, treatment options depend on tooth vitality (Figure 9.1).

Vital permanent teeth with open apices

A pulpotomy (removal of contaminated coronal pulp) is carried out and calcium hydroxide placed over the remaining healthy radicular pulp stumps. Aim to induce a calcific bridge but maintain a vital radicular pulp and induce completion of root formation (Figure 9.1a).

Non-vital permanent teeth with open apices

Most commonly arises following trauma to incisors at age 8–9 years with subsequent pulp necrosis. Root canal is wider at apex than at the coronal access area – conventional root canal therapy is not possible (Figure 9.1b). Barrier formation can be induced using non-setting calcium hydroxide.

Technique

1. Under rubber dam, gain access to root canal.
2. Local anaesthetic may be necessary as vital granulation tissue often present at apex.
3. Place file in canal and radiograph to determine working length (remember root formation incomplete – therefore correspondingly shorter).
4. Remove debris from canal, file wall with Hedström files and irrigate copiously with sterile saline.
5. When clean, fill canal with calcium hydroxide paste.
6. Review at 3–4 monthly intervals and change calcium hydroxide paste.

7. Aim is to induce formation of apical barrier (*apexification*). Degree of calcification can be determined either by tactile sensation or radiographically. Can take 6–18 months.
8. When complete, fill canal with gutta-percha using lateral condensation technique (p. 293).

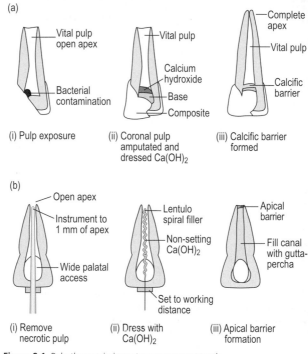

(a)

Vital pulp open apex

Bacterial contamination

(i) Pulp exposure

Vital pulp

Calcium hydroxide

Base

Composite

(ii) Coronal pulp amputated and dressed Ca(OH)₂

Complete apex

Vital pulp

Calcific barrier

(iii) Calcific barrier formed

(b)

Open apex

Instrument to 1 mm of apex

Wide palatal access

(i) Remove necrotic pulp

Lentulo spiral filler

Non-setting Ca(OH)₂

Set to working distance

(ii) Dress with Ca(OH)₂

Apical barrier

Fill canal with gutta-percha

(iii) Apical barrier formation

Figure 9.1 Pulp therapy in immature permanent teeth.

Mineral trioxide aggregate (MTA) A compound mixture of tricalcium silicate, tricalcium oxide and tricalcium aluminate (Portland cement) has been used to treat a number of endodontic problems including non-vital immature incisors. It is placed in the form of 'rods' using a long plugger into the apical area without the need to form a barrier and the tooth can be restored 4 hours later. Early results are promising but limited to case reports.

TRAUMATIC INJURIES

Trauma to children's teeth is a common occurrence, and one of the true emergencies likely to present in dental practice. In these circumstances, the child and parents/carers are likely to be anxious or distressed. Prompt and appropriate action by the dentist not only provides reassurance but can also influence markedly the results obtained.

Prevalence

The UK 2003 Child Dental Health Survey reported the incidence of trauma in central incisors as 4.1 per 1000 8 year olds, rising to 10 per 1000 at age 12 years.

Aetiology

Related to age and gender. Common causes include: • toddlers – trips and falls • older children – bicycle accidents • teenagers – contact sports, fights, alcohol.

Remember the possibility of non-accidental injury.

Predisposing factors

Increased overjet, incompetent lips.

Classification of trauma

Several classifications have been described, but generally more useful to describe damage in words. Presents as fractures, displacement, or fractures and displacement.

Fractures May involve: • enamel only • enamel and dentine without pulp exposure • enamel, dentine and pulp • root fracture.
Concussion Tooth traumatized but not loosened.
Subluxation Tooth is loosened in the socket but not displaced.
Extrusion Tooth displaced in occlusal direction.
Intrusion Tooth displaced apically into socket.
Lateral displacement: Tooth pushed laterally, buccally or palatally.
Avulsion Tooth totally displaced from socket.

In any patient presenting with dental trauma, the possibility of more serious underlying injury (e.g. concussion) should be considered (p. 423).

HISTORY

The basic principles of taking a history and conducting an examination outlined in Chapter 2 apply.

Specifically, establish: • when the injury occurred – time since injury influences the prognosis • where the injury occurred • how the injury occurred • whether loss of consciousness or not • any dizziness, amnesia • anti-tetanus vaccination status.

EXAMINATION
Extraoral
Note and diagrammatically draw swelling, bruising, laceration, limitation of movement. Examine the bony skeleton as described on page 424.

Intraoral
- Carefully remove adherent blood clot and debris.
- Count the teeth and account for any missing teeth or fragments of teeth. If soft tissue wounds are present, the possibility of fragments embedded within the tissues must be excluded (by radiograph).
- If tooth fracture is present, determine if pulp involved.
- Check occlusion. Disruption may indicate alveolar fracture.
- Palpate gently to determine tooth mobility – may be due to either displacement or fracture.
- Gently press the teeth using finger pressure before percussing the teeth if required – reaction to pressure is indicative of damage to the periodontal ligament. Where there is a history of indirect trauma (e.g. a blow to the chin) check the posterior teeth for fractures.

Special tests
Sensitivity (vitality) testing Of limited value in the immediate post-trauma period, but important in long-term follow-up. The vitality of any tooth that has been subject to trauma should be reviewed at 1 month post-trauma and then at 3–6-monthly intervals for at least 2 years.

Radiographs Radiographs are most important to establish:
- *Teeth* Root fractures or displacement. May require two radiographs at divergent angles to permit visualization. Periapical views are preferred. All injured teeth should be radiographed. Film holders should be used.
- *Lips* If fragments are suspected of being embedded in the lip, place film between lips and teeth, reduce exposure. Alternatively may use extraoral film held at right angles.
- *Bony fractures* If bony fractures are suspected, extraoral films are required (p. 55).

TREATMENT

Treatment is obviously dependent on the complexity of the injury and can be described as immediate, intermediate and long-term or permanent.

Objectives of treatment

Immediate • reassurance of patient and parent/carer • relief of pain • protection of pulp • suture of soft tissue lacerations • stabilization of fractured or mobile teeth.

Intermediate • pulp therapy • semipermanent restoration.

Long-term • crown • replacement of lost teeth • orthodontic therapy to close space • removable/fixed prosthodontics.

TREATMENT IN THE PRIMARY DENTITION

A major concern with injuries to primary anterior teeth is damage to the developing permanent successors which lie palatal to, and in close proximity with, the apex of the primary teeth. Most common injuries are loosening of teeth, intrusion or avulsion. Fractures are less common. Injuries occur most frequently in toddlers; treatment options are either extraction or observation without active treatment. Extraction is indicated where radiographs show follicular involvement or if apical pathology, occlusal interference is present. If it is decided to retain the tooth, regular review is required to ensure that the tooth remains vital, is shed normally and that the permanent tooth erupts. Damage to permanent teeth is most likely with avulsions and intrusions, particularly in children under 3 years.

TREATMENT IN THE PERMANENT DENTITION
Treatment of fractures

Enamel only Use a bur to smooth sharp edges. Review pulp vitality.

Enamel and dentine fracture Can be difficult to ensure that microexposure of pulp has not occurred. Even in absence of frank haemorrhage, assume microexposure if pulp can be visualized. In definite absence of exposure, cover dentine with hard-setting $Ca(OH)_2$ and restore using acid-etch composite technique. Composite placement is dependent on sufficient enamel remaining for retention. Preformed acetate crowns can be used as matrix, or can be built up freehand. Review pulp vitality. In the longer term, a post and core retained crown may be required. This should be delayed until late teens. Pulp necrosis is uncommon but is increased by: • failure to cover exposed dentine • concomitant displacement injury.

Fractures involving enamel, dentine and pulp Exposure of the pulp results in microbial contamination, and pulp therapy is required. The technique to be employed depends mainly on the degree of root formation.

Root formation complete

Pulp cap Where only a microexposure is suspected, pulp capping can be attempted, particularly if patient presents within a short time since injury. If unsuccessful, this can be followed up by conventional root canal therapy (p. 287).

Pulpotomy (p. 183) Also an option.

Pulpectomy Complete removal of coronal and radicular pulp, followed by conventional root canal therapy, may be indicated.

Root formation incomplete It is important to maintain a vital radicular pulp to encourage completion of root formation.

Pulpotomy Involves removal of the coronal pulp to eradicate infected pulp tissue but retain the radicular pulp, and is the treatment of choice (p. 183).

Root fractures

Prognosis is greatly influenced by the position of the fracture.

Fracture involving the gingival crevice Where a root fracture communicates with the gingival crevice, prognosis is poor. It may be possible to extract the coronal portion and root treat apical portion, extrude it and provide a post-crown.

Fracture not involving the gingival crevice If coronal portion is displaced, reposition and splint with functional splint for 3 weeks in the first instance. Regular review is required.

Longitudinal fractures Hopeless prognosis. Extract tooth and provide prosthetic replacement/close space orthodontically.

Treatment of displacement injuries

Pulp necrosis and root resorption are common following displacement injuries; degree of displacement and complete apices increase the risk.

Subluxation Advise soft diet and review.

Lateral displacement Reposition using local anaesthetic, grasping tooth between forefinger and thumb. Splint for 3–4 weeks. Review 1 year.

Extrusion Administer local anaesthetic and reposition in socket. Splint for 2–3 weeks. Review 1 year.

Intrusion
Incomplete root Leave to re-erupt for 1 month. If tooth fails to re-erupt, orthodontic extrusion.

Complete root Immediate orthodontic extrusion and simultaneous root canal treatment. Review 1 year.

Avulsion It is possible to successfully reimplant teeth which have been totally displaced from their sockets. Success is heavily dependent on: • the time the tooth has been out of its socket • how it has been stored • how the tooth (particularly root) has been handled.

Prognosis is best when the tooth is replaced within 30 minutes. After 2 hours, long-term retention is unlikely. Teeth stored dry; ankylose if reimplanted.

Reimplantation
Immediate treatment Examine tooth, rinse gently in sterile saline, avoid touching the tooth root, anaesthetize the socket, hold tooth between forefinger and thumb and reimplant. Splint for 1 week only. Prescribe antibiotics.

After 1 week Any requirement to remove the pulp is dependent on degree of root formation and time out of socket.

Complete root Extirpate the pulp before splint removal and dress with $Ca(OH)_2$, then root fill with gutta-percha.

Incomplete root If ideally stored (i.e. in milk or saliva) and reimplanted within 30 minutes the pulp may be left and reviewed weekly for the first month. If root resorption or apical rarefaction is seen $Ca(OH)_2$ therapy is required.

Tooth replanted after 30 minutes; the pulp should be removed before splint removal and root canal dressed with $Ca(OH)_2$. Replace every 3 months and root fill with gutta-percha after barrier formation (p. 183).

Most likely complication is root resorption. However, may act as suitable space maintainer until late teens when prosthetic replacement will be easier.

Splinting
Function of splint
• Immobilize loosened tooth. • Hold repositioned tooth in alignment. • Protect damaged structures when teeth in occlusion.

Types of splint
Can be fabricated *directly* (constructed in the mouth) or *indirectly* (made in laboratory).

Direct splints
Foil splint Constructed from foil moulded over teeth and cemented using zinc oxide–eugenol cement. Very useful in emergency.

Acid-etch splint Constructed from acrylic, epimine resin or composite. Easy to construct. Composite splints are strongest but liable to fracture. Wire inserts can be used where diastema is present, as can orthodontic brackets and wire.

Indirect splints
Removable acrylic splint Acrylic baseplate with Adams clasps on molars. Can incorporate posterior occlusal cover to relieve occlusion anteriorly and protect damaged structures.

Removable thermoplastic splint Vacuum-formed splint. Useful in overcoming retention problems in younger children where only central incisors have erupted.

Review
Pathology resulting from trauma to teeth is not always evident at initial presentation and may develop weeks, months or years later. Potential sequelae include: • pulp death • resorption, either internal or external • calcification and obliteration of root canal.

All teeth that have been subjected to trauma should be reviewed regularly both clinically and radiographically.

ORAL PATHOLOGY IN CHILDREN

HARD TISSUE PATHOLOGY

The most common disease to affect dental hard tissues is, of course, dental caries. Other pathology may result in abnormalities of eruption, tooth number, form, position or structure.

Abnormalities of tooth number
Supplemental teeth Duplication of teeth. Permanent upper lateral incisor is the most commonly involved. Usually extract one.

Supernumerary teeth Primary teeth 0.2–0.8%, permanent teeth 1–3%, more common in males and the maxilla. Most common in upper incisor region. May be:

Conical Usually in midline; either displaces the central incisor or prevents eruption. Also found high and inverted in the palate.
Tuberculate Often paired; most commonly on the palatal side of central incisors and prevent eruption.

Orthodontic assessment is recommended. Must establish position with appropriate radiographic technique. Can leave if not causing any problems. Do not remove before age 6 years. If intervention is essential, space requirements must be considered – often need to extract the primary canines. Delayed incisors may take some time to erupt and may require surgical exposure.

Hypodontia Fewer teeth than normal. Primary teeth <1%, permanent teeth 6%. Where the primary teeth are affected, one-third to one-half of permanent teeth are affected. In addition, teeth present may be smaller than average. Orthodontic assessment is recommended when planning restorative care.

Missing upper lateral incisors Can be unilateral or bilateral. If one side missing, the other side is often small and conical. Has an effect on the eruption of the permanent canine – greater chance of it being displaced palatally. Treatment options: • accept • restorative alone • space closure • space localize and restorative treatment.
Missing premolars Most commonly second premolar. Must decide on retention/extraction of the second primary molar – influenced by arch crowding and tooth condition. Remember, a retained primary molar may *infra-occlude*.
Missing lower central incisor If crowded, reasonable space closure may result following extraction of the primary tooth. If uncrowded, may wish to retain the primary tooth as an interim measure and then, when lost, consider adhesive bridgework. May require orthodontic alignment prior to this.

Abnormalities of tooth form
Dens-in-dente Must check for this (radiographically) if the lateral incisors are small and conical. Often requires extraction.

Dilaceration Abnormal angulation between the crown and root or within the root. May be related to intrusive trauma to primary dentition. May fail to erupt.

Abnormalities of tooth position

Impacted first molars　Impact behind second primary molar due to crowding or abnormality in tooth eruption such as orientation of the crypt. Treatment possibilities include keeping under observation but must maintain good oral hygiene. May self-correct if mild. Alternatively, attempt disimpaction using a separator or extract the second primary molar; this will, however, result in space loss.

Abnormal position of crypts　The crypt of any tooth can be displaced or rotated. Lower second premolar is most commonly affected. Little can be done at an early age.

Ectopic upper canines　Incidence 1–2%; 90% lie palatally or in line of arch. Early recognition is very important. By age 9 years should be palpable as a bulge high in the buccal sulcus. If not apparent by age 10 then carry out a clinical examination and appropriate radiographs. The prognosis is markedly improved if detected early. Extraction of the primary canine may help to encourage eruption in the correct position. Other options: • accept and review • extract • surgically expose and align orthodontically • transplant.

Transposition　In the upper arch this usually involves canine and first premolar. In the lower arch it is usually the canine and lateral incisor. Difficult to correct once established. If detected early in the lower arch attempts to align the lateral to the central incisor can be instituted before the canine erupts.

Abnormalities of tooth structure

Result from disturbances during the period of tooth formation.

Abnormal enamel

Enamel hypoplasia　Enamel is reduced in thickness or of deficient structure. Presentation ranges from pits and grooves to gross abnormalities.

Enamel hypomineralization　Enamel is of normal structure but not fully mineralized. Presents as changes in colour and translucency.

Local aetiology　Infection, trauma, irradiation, idiopathic. Usually affects only one or two teeth.

General aetiology　Environmental results from systemic disturbance during period of tooth formation. May occur pre-, peri-, or postnatally, e.g. rubella, syphilis, childhood infections, excess exposure to fluoride. The term molar–incisor hypoplasia has been used for defects of first permanent molars and incisors.

Hereditary　e.g. amelogenesis imperfecta or ectodermal dysplasia. Affects several or all teeth.

Amelogenesis imperfecta There are two common variants:
• *Hypomineralized type* Matrix formation normal, calcification is abnormal. Mainly autosomal dominant. • *Hypoplastic type* Matrix formation abnormal, but any matrix formed is normally calcified. Mainly X-linked.

Abnormal dentine

Dentinogenesis imperfecta Dentine consists of a reduced number of wide irregular tubules, with areas of atubular dentine. Loss of scalloping at ADJ. Teeth have opalescent bluish appearance. Teeth wear rapidly as enamel is lost.

Abnormal cementum

Hypercementosis May be associated with inflammation, over/underloading, Paget's disease.

Hypocementosis Associated with hypophosphatasia.

Bone pathology

Pathological conditions affecting bone are discussed on page 407.

SOFT TISSUE PATHOLOGY

Gingivitis is the most common disease to affect non-mineralized tissues in children. Other common conditions affecting soft tissue include aphthous ulcers, mucoceles, eruption cysts, papillomas and infections. These are discussed in Chapter 15.

The maxim that an abnormal lesion or suspicious area affecting the oral mucosa should be further investigated holds equally true for children.

CHILDREN WITH SPECIAL NEEDS

Special needs describes a wide range of conditions which result in patients requiring extra attention or special facilities in order to attain and maintain oral health.

Changes in the arrangements for the care of special-needs patients mean that those who may previously have resided in special centres or institutions are more likely to be accommodated in the community (*normalization*). It is important that these individuals continue to receive dental care. Special-needs patients are increasingly likely to seek care from general dental practitioners.

Various definitions of handicap and disability have been described. Can be usefully classified as:

Learning disability Varies in severity. Can be congenital (e.g. Down syndrome) or acquired (e.g. as a result of brain damage pre-, peri- or postnatally).

Physical disability Includes cerebral palsy, spina bifida, muscular dystrophy.

Sensory disability Blindness, deafness.

Medically compromised Describes patients who have an underlying medical condition which may either predispose to increased dental disease or which requires special precautions when carrying out dental treatment, e.g. cardiac disorders, haemophilia, transplants.

An individual patient may suffer a combination of these disabilities. Usually the complexity of providing dental treatment increases with the degree of disability.

Prevalence of disease
While the prevalence of dental caries in disabled children is similar to non-disabled children, levels of untreated disease (decayed component of dmf/DMF) are higher.

Risk factors
Special-needs children possess certain factors which increase the risk of dental disease.

Oral hygiene Significantly poorer in many special-needs groups, especially those with learning disabilities. Down syndrome patients are predisposed to periodontal disease.

Diet Difficulty in mastication may result in soft cariogenic foods being used. Feeding time may be prolonged, increasing exposure to sugar. Confectionery may be used as reward/pacifier by parents and carers.

Medication Long-term use of sweetened medicine. Drugs may predispose to xerostomia, increasing caries risk. Anti-epileptic drugs may lead to gingival hyperplasia.

Muscular function Decreased muscle tone may lead to drooling of saliva, chewing problems, retention of food, reduced self-cleansing. Increased muscle tone may lead to bruxism and toothwear.

Management of children with special needs
History The need for an adequate history, as in treating any patient, is obvious. Complicated by the need for more time and patience to obtain history. Need to involve parents, carers and

other health professionals concerned with care of the patient.
Liaison with the patient's physician is important.

Examination and treatment Technical aspects of patient care do
not differ greatly from non-special-needs patients. Most merely
require time and patience. However, given the many other problems
facing special-needs patients, dentistry is frequently given a low
priority.

Restorative care Essentially the same as for all patients. In more
severely disabled patients, sedation or general anaesthesia may be
required, particularly in cases of dental neglect requiring extensive
care (p. 107). The usual sequence of treatment under GA is:
• removal of plaque and calculus • restorative procedures
• extraction of teeth/surgery.

When operating under GA: • avoid treatment that cannot be
completed in one visit • use resorbable sutures • in cases of carious
exposure where there is any doubt as to prognosis, extraction is the
best option.

When the patient is rendered dentally fit, every effort should be
made to institute preventive care and minimize the need for future
general anaesthetics.

Factors hindering treatment

Availability of treatment Patient may have to travel long distances
and attend multiple clinics. May have to rely on ambulance
transport.
Access to dental premises Consider stairs, surgery design, facilities.
Attitude of parents/carers Parental anxiety may hinder treatment.
Parents may be extremely demanding.

Dental care should be incorporated into the patient's overall
care plan.

Prevention

Prevention of dental disease is paramount and should include:
• dietary advice to parents/carers • fluoride supplements
• appropriate arrangements for oral hygiene.

Toothbrushes can be modified to permit easier use in patients
with limited dexterity. Regular appointments with hygienists for
scaling may be useful.

Children with severe disability will require treatment by dentists
experienced in treating patients with special needs. However, whilst
challenging, the treatment of children with special needs should be
within the capability of most dental practitioners and provide a
rewarding experience.

CHAPTER 10

PERIODONTOLOGY

Structure of the periodontal
tissues   198

Aetiology and pathogenesis
of periodontal
diseases   199

Classification of periodontal
diseases   203

Examination and
diagnosis   204

Periodontal indices   208

Stages in periodontal
therapy   211

Hygiene phase
therapy   212

Periodontal surgery   220

Recall maintenance   224

Acute periodontal
conditions   224

Antibiotics in the
management of periodontal
diseases   227

Occlusion and periodontal
diseases   228

Furcation lesions   229

References   230

STRUCTURE OF THE PERIODONTAL TISSUES

The *periodontium* (*perio* = around, *odontos* = tooth) consist of the tissues which surround and support the teeth. Their function is to attach the tooth to the surrounding alveolar bone and to support the tooth during function. For descriptive purposes the periodontium can be divided into the *gingivae* and *periodontal ligament* (Figure 10.1).

GINGIVAE

Gingivae (singular = gingiva) are those parts of the masticatory mucosa that cover the alveolar process and surround the cervical portion of the teeth.

The gingivae are composed of connective tissue and epithelium, which can be divided into three histologically distinct areas:

Oral epithelium Continuous with epithelial lining of the attached gingivae. Composed of keratinized stratified squamous epithelium.
Sulcular epithelium Non-keratinized.

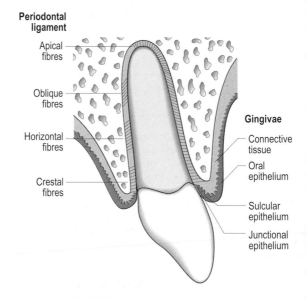

Figure 10.1 Structure of the periodontium.

Junctional epithelium Attached to the tooth by hemidesmosomes. Non-keratinized. Has larger cells with increased intercellular spaces.

Healthy gingivae have the following clinical features: • pale pink in colour • a stippled appearance • a well-defined 'knife edge' margin • scalloped outline • do not bleed on gentle probing with a periodontal probe.

PERIODONTAL LIGAMENT

Periodontal ligament is composed of collagen fibres, which form a branching plexus and are inserted into the cementum of the tooth root at one end and the alveolar bone at the other in the form of Sharpey's fibres. They are named according to the orientation of the fibre.

AETIOLOGY AND PATHOGENESIS OF PERIODONTAL DISEASES

In its widest sense, periodontal disease includes all pathological conditions of the periodontium but commonly refers to inflammatory diseases that are plaque-induced, i.e. *gingivitis* and *periodontitis*.

GINGIVITIS

> Gingivitis is an inflammatory response of the gingivae without destruction of the supporting tissues.

In the absence of adequate oral hygiene, dental plaque accumulates and the gingival tissue will progress from health to an established or chronic gingivitis over a 3-week period. The development of gingivitis is encouraged by both local and systemic factors. *Local factors* contributing to the development of gingivitis are those which encourage the accumulation of dental plaque or inhibit effective plaque removal and include calculus, crowded dentition, soft tissue factors, e.g. high fraenal attachment, restorations and prostheses. Systemic factors that influence the host response to plaque accumulation include pregnancy, puberty, diabetes mellitus and blood dyscrasias.

Inflamed gingivae have the following clinical features: • red in colour • swollen appearance • stippling is lost • increased flow of gingival crevicular fluid (GCF) • bleed readily on probing.

Gingivitis can have three possible outcomes, as described in Table 10.1.

PERIODONTITIS

> Periodontitis describes a group of inflammatory diseases that affect all the periodontal structures. It results in destruction of the attachment apparatus and development of a periodontal pocket.

The relationship between gingivitis and periodontitis is complex. Whilst plaque accumulation almost always leads to gingivitis, it does not invariably lead to periodontitis. Why only a proportion of sites with gingivitis progress to periodontitis and why this is more likely in some individuals than in others has been the subject of much research.

Breakdown of the periodontal ligament and the development of a periodontal pocket is an unpredictable event. When it occurs, the rapidity with which connective tissue attachment is destroyed varies both between individuals and at individual tooth sites within the same mouth.

FACTORS PREDISPOSING TO PERIODONTITIS
Microbiological factors
The precise manner by which plaque organisms induce breakdown of the periodontal tissues is not known. The 'non-specific plaque

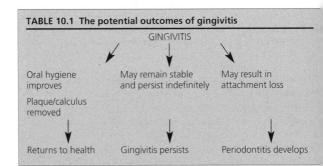

TABLE 10.1 The potential outcomes of gingivitis

GINGIVITIS

Oral hygiene improves	May remain stable and persist indefinitely	May result in attachment loss
Plaque/calculus removed		
Returns to health	Gingivitis persists	Periodontitis develops

hypothesis' postulates that periodontal disease is the result of toxin production by a range of bacterial species and more than 300 species of micro-organisms have been isolated from periodontal pockets. There is evidence, however, that certain Gram-negative anaerobic bacteria are isolated more commonly at sites of active periodontal destruction (Table 10.2). These organisms accumulate as a biofilm and interaction and synergism between organisms is important in the pathogenesis of disease. Virulent micro-organisms capable of initiating or propagating attachment loss, if present at a critical minimal infective dose, in susceptible individuals, or at susceptible periodontal sites in susceptible individuals, have the ability to breach the host defence mechanism, exposing the host tissues to toxic bacterial components. As a result host cells (e.g. monocytes and fibroblasts) are stimulated by bacterial components such as *lipopolysaccharides* (LPS) to produce cytokines. These are powerful chemical messengers which stimulate inflammatory responses and catabolic processes such as bone resorption and collagen destruction via enzymes know as matrix metalloproteinases (MMPs).

Host factors

Bacterial plaque produces many substances which can cause damage to the periodontium. The tissues rely on several host defence mechanisms to protect against plaque irritants. These include: • polymorphonuclear neutrophils (PMNs) • the complement system • the cellular and humoral immune responses • various chemical mediators of inflammation.

In response to plaque accumulation, gingival crevicular fluid (GCF) permeates through the junctional epithelium. This transudate is rich in neutrophils that can neutralize potential pathogenic agents by phagocytosis. It has been suggested that defects in neutrophil function may account for certain forms of periodontal disease. Within the neutrophils, lysosomes (cytoplasmic organelles) contain powerful enzymes such as elastase and collagenase, which can digest bacterial products. However,

---

TABLE 10.2 Bacteria most commonly associated with periodontal disease

Porphyromonas gingivalis
Prevotella intermedia
Actinobacillus actinomycetemcomitans
Fusobacteria
Treponema spp.

these substances may also be released into the gingival tissues, causing localized tissue damage.

Much interest has focused on the chemical mediators of inflammation and on both bacterial and host-derived enzymes as potential markers of active periodontal destruction.

Genetic factors and periodontitis

There is currently interest in the contribution of host genetics to the development of periodontitis. Studies suggest that there is a host genetic component of susceptibility for several rare forms of syndromic periodontitis associated with conditions such as Papillon–Lefèvre, Ehlers–Danlos or Chédiak–Higashi syndromes. With the exception of these syndromic forms of periodontitis, specific genes have either not yet been identified or rigorously demonstrated to have a causal relationship with commonly occurring forms of periodontitis. There is no evidence of any simple pattern of genetic transmission that would support an aetiological role for a single gene mutation in chronic periodontitis.

Smoking

Cigarette smoking is a significant risk factor for both periodontitis and acute necrotizing ulcerative gingivitis (ANUG). Several mechanisms have been suggested as an explanation of how smoking predisposes to periodontal disease. The vasoconstrictive effects of nicotine may interfere with host response mechanisms and with both neutrophil and fibroblast function. Smoking may also influence the microbial composition of dental plaque. Those who smoke are 2.5–4 times more likely to develop periodontitis. Smokers also respond less well to periodontal therapy. There is good evidence that smokers experience significantly less reduction in pocket depths following periodontal therapy than non-smokers. Studies show that probing depth reduction and clinical attachment level improvements in smokers are 50% to 75% those of non-smokers following non-surgical and surgical periodontal therapy.

Stopping smoking benefits periodontal health and improves the outcome of treatment. Members of the dental team have a key role to play in educating patients on the effects of smoking on oral health and on the benefits of smoking cessation (p. 163).

Systemic disease and periodontitis

Systemic disease and periodontitis may interact in two ways. Systemic disease may predispose to periodontitis. This is an important and established factor in the aetiology of periodontitis. Systemic diseases that impair the host defence mechanism may increase the risk of periodontitis. Many systemic conditions associated with or predisposing to periodontal attachment loss have, as a common attribute, defective neutrophil function, e.g. agranulocytosis, cyclic neutropenia. Patients with uncontrolled diabetes, Down syndrome and human immunodeficiency virus (HIV) are all at increased risk of periodontitis.

The second aspect of the relationship between periodontitis and systemic disease focuses on periodontitis as a predisposing factor for systemic disorders. Research has suggested that periodontitis may predispose to cardiac disease and preterm low birth weight babies, though studies on these topics have given conflicting results and the significance of these relationships awaits determination.

CLASSIFICATION OF PERIODONTAL DISEASES

Numerous classifications of periodontal diseases have been suggested. That in most common usage is described in Table 10.3.[1]

Gingival diseases

These are divided into those conditions which are either dental plaque induced or not primarily associated with dental plaque.

Examples of plaque-induced gingivitis include gingivitis with or without local contributing factors such as tooth anatomical factors, dental restorations and appliances. General factors contributing to gingivitis include hormonal changes in puberty and pregnancy.

TABLE 10.3 Classification of diseases that may affect the periodontium

I Gingival diseases
  A Dental plaque-induced gingival diseases
  B Non-plaque-induced gingival diseases
II Chronic periodontitis
  A Localized
  B Generalized
III Aggressive periodontitis
  A. Localized
  B Generalized
IV Periodontitis as a manifestation of systemic disease
V Necrotizing periodontal diseases
VI Abscesses of the periodontium
VII Periodontitis associated with endodontic lesions
VIII Developmental or acquired deformities and conditions

Conditions not primarily associated with dental plaque include bacterial and viral infections directly affecting the gingival tissues, e.g. primary herpetic gingivostomatitis.

Chronic periodontitis

Replacing the term 'adult periodontitis', this term describes the most commonly presenting form of periodontitis. It may be localized affecting just some teeth or tooth sites, or more generalized. The term chronic periodontitis does not imply that the condition is resistant to treatment.

Aggressive periodontitis

These forms of periodontitis represent highly aggressive forms of the disease with extensive destruction of the tooth-supporting apparatus. These forms of disease were previously known as 'early-onset' periodontitis, and encompass conditions formerly known as localized juvenile periodontitis and rapidly progressive periodontitis. Two forms of aggressive periodontitis are described – localized and generalized.

Periodontitis as a manifestation of systemic diseases

This term describes periodontitis associated with underlying conditions such as blood disorders affecting the periodontal tissues or associated genetic disorders, e.g. Down syndrome, Ehlers–Danlos syndrome and Chédiak–Higashi syndrome.

However, neither diabetes nor smoking is included in this section of the classification system as they are considered to act as modifiers of all forms of periodontal disease.

Necroting periodontal diseases

These include necrotizing ulcerative gingivitis (p. 224) and necrotizing ulcerative periodontitis.

EXAMINATION AND DIAGNOSIS

The features of taking a history and examination described in Chapter 2 are relevant. However, the specific features relating to the diagnosis of periodontal disease should be noted and recorded (Table 10.4).

TABLE 10.4 Features to be noted during a periodontal examination

Visual	Deposits – supragingival plaque, calculus
	Gingivae – erythema, hyperplasia, recession
	Occlusal abnormalities
Probing	Pocket depths
	Bleeding on probing
	Subgingival calculus
	Furcation defects
Palpation	Mobility

EXAMINATION
Oral hygiene

Determination of the patient's oral hygiene status is crucial. The presence of supragingival plaque and calculus deposits should be noted in terms of distribution within the mouth and the quantity present. However, whilst plaque and calculus deposits give some indication of the patient's level of oral hygiene, the presence of gingival inflammation (gingivitis) provides a better indication of the patient's long-term plaque control.

Plaque When present in small amounts, plaque is not always apparent solely by visual examination, and it is necessary to run a probe around the gingival margin to enable trace amounts to be visualized. Use of a probe is also required to detect plaque in interproximal spaces.

Calculus Formed by mineralization of plaque, this is described according to its relation to the gingival margin.

Supragingival calculus Formed above the gingival margin, it accumulates most readily adjacent to the orifices of the major salivary glands: on the lingual aspects of the lower incisor teeth, and the buccal aspect of maxillary molars. It is light yellow in colour and is best visualized by drying the teeth. It is composed of calcium phosphate crystals – brushite, whitlockite, octacalcium phosphate and hydroxyapatite. It is relatively easily removed by scaling.

Subgingival calculus Dark brown or green in colour, subgingival calculus is located beneath the gingival margin. Present either in sheets covering the entire root surface or in discrete clumps, it is detectable only by tactile means or by using an air syringe to deflect the gingivae. The ball end of the CPITN probe (p. 209), used with light touch, is the most effective means of determining the location of subgingival calculus, which appears as a rough area or catch on the root surface. A sound knowledge of root surface anatomy is required to enable accurate probing. Subgingival calculus may come to lie supragingivally following gingival recession. It is firmly adherent to the root surface and its removal requires careful scaling technique.

Gingival health The condition of the gingivae should be recorded. This should take account of the distribution and severity of:

Erythema The degree of redness, an indication of gingivitis. Note areas of haemorrhage.
Hyperplasia Any gingival swellings, or areas of overgrowth.
Recession Measured as the position in millimetres of the gingival margin below the amelocemental junction.

Pocket depths A periodontal probe should be used to determine pocket depths. A note should be made of the teeth and surfaces affected and can be recorded as the average and worst depths. The patient's periodontal status can be summarized using the Basic Periodontal Examination (BPE), page 208.

Bleeding on probing The presence of bleeding on probing is a crucial indicator in periodontal examination and diagnosis, as it is the most reliable indicator of disease activity. Careful note should be made of the pockets that bleed on probing and the severity of the haemorrhage.

Furcation lesions Probing also enables furcation lesions to be detected. A furcation lesion occurs in multirooted teeth when the loss of periodontal attachment has reached the area where the roots diverge. When this occurs, it becomes increasingly difficult to ensure that all subgingival deposits are removed from the furcation and for the patient to keep this area clean.
    Furcation lesions can be graded as:

Grade 1 Bone loss up to one-third of the tooth width, i.e. about 3 mm of horizontal attachment loss.
Grade 2 Bone loss between one-third and two-thirds of the tooth width.
Grade 3 A 'through and through' lesion.

Tooth mobility All teeth should be carefully palpated to determine mobility. Move the tooth between an instrument handle and an index finger in a buccolingual direction (and mesiodistal direction when no adjacent tooth is present). The amplitude of movement of the crown tip from its most extreme lingual (or distal) position should be observed.

Visible mobility should be scored as follows (Miller's Index):

Score 1 Mobility up to 1 mm.
Score 2 Mobility of 1–2 mm.
Score 3 Mobility over 2 mm and/or rotation or depression.

Occlusion Any abnormalities of occlusion should be noted. Features to be observed include: • premature contacts • overerupted teeth • deep traumatic overbites.

DIAGNOSIS

Having recorded these factors, together with information on the patient's presenting complaints, age, medical and social history, a provisional diagnosis can be made.

Additional information may be obtained from: • radiographic examination • pulp vitality tests • study models • biopsy • microbiological and haematological investigations.

Radiographs in the diagnosis of periodontal disease

Radiographs are essential in the diagnosis and management of periodontal disease, but, as with all radiographs, should be used only to supplement clinical examination (Chapter 4).

The following information should be noted:

Bone levels • degree of bone loss – mild, moderate or severe • distribution of bone loss – localized or generalized • pattern of bone loss – vertical, horizontal or both.

Furcation defects • teeth affected.

Crown : root ratio • relative length of the root to the crown – particularly relevant in incisors.

Root morphology

Restorations • overhanging margins • deficient margins • recurrent caries.

Periapical pathology – perio-endo lesions.

A definitive diagnosis should be made before formulating a treatment plan.

PERIODONTAL INDICES

Traditionally, oral hygiene was recorded as good, satisfactory, or poor. Currently, numerous indices are available. Many were developed for use in clinical trials and are of limited use in individual clinical treatment. The most commonly used are:

Debris index (Green & Vermillion 1964[2])

0 = No plaque
1 = Plaque covering 1/3 tooth
2 = Plaque covering 2/3 tooth
3 = Plaque totally covering tooth

Plaque index (Silness & Loe 1964[3])

0 = No plaque detected
1 = Looks clean but material can be removed from gingival 1/3 with probe
2 = Visible plaque
3 = Tooth covered with abundant plaque

Modified gingival index (Loe 1967[4])

0 = Healthy gingivae
1 = Gingivae look inflamed, but don't bleed when probed
2 = Gingivae look inflamed and bleed when probed
3 = Ulceration and spontaneous bleeding

THE BASIC PERIODONTAL EXAMINATION (BPE)

The Basic Periodontal Examination (BPE) is derived from the Community Periodontal Index of Treatment Needs (CPITN), which was developed as a screening tool to enable the prevalence of periodontal disease in a community to be summarized.

The index comprises six codes (0–4 and *). An individual patient's periodontal status can be summarized by six numbers. For examination purposes the dentition is divided into sextants as shown below:

17–14	13–23	24–27
47–44	43–33	34–37

The use of a CPITN probe (Figure 10.2) is mandatory. This has a ball end 0.5 mm in diameter. A colour-coded area extends from 3.5–5.5 mm. A probing force in the order of 20–25 g is recommended. This corresponds to gentle pressure; pain during probing indicates that too much force is being applied.

The CPITN probe is gently inserted into the gingival pocket and the depth of penetration read against the colour-coded band. At least six points on each tooth should be examined by gently 'walking the probe' around the tooth.

For each sextant only the highest score is recorded. Any sextant containing only one tooth is recorded as missing and the score for that tooth included in the adjacent sextant.

A simple box chart is used to record the score for each sextant.

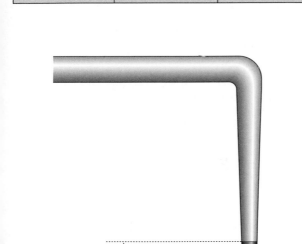

5.5 mm

3.5 mm

0.5 mm

Figure 10.2 Community Periodontal Index of Treatment Needs (CPITN) probe.

BPE codes

Code 0   Healthy gingival tissues with no bleeding after probing.

Code 1   Bleeding on probing, plaque present, but no calculus or defective restoration margins, pockets <3.5 mm.

Code 2   Bleeding on probing, calculus detected or defective restoration margins but pockets <3.5 mm.

Code 3   Pocket within the colour-coded area, i.e. pocket >3.5 mm–<5.5 mm.

Code 4   Colour-coded area disappears, indicating pocket >5.5 mm.

Code *   Denotes the presence of furcation involvement or attachment loss >7 mm.

The BPE, whilst useful as a guide to a patient's overall periodontal status, is insufficiently sensitive for monitoring individual patient treatment over a period of time because only the worst score is recorded in each sextant. Codes for Periodontal Treatment Assessment have been proposed. These categorize a patient's periodontal treatment needs into three levels of complexity and are designed as a guide to the need for specialist periodontal care. In summary BPE codes 1–3 are deemed suitable for non-specialist periodontal care. Code 4 and * frequently suggest that the complexity is such that the patient may need referral for specialist periodontal care. This is particularly so if the patient is young and suffering from aggressive forms of periodontitis, or has a complicating medical history, e.g. uncontrolled diabetes.

POCKET CHARTS

The data resulting from a comprehensive periodontal examination can be recorded on a pocket chart. This usually includes the following details: • missing teeth • position of the gingival margin • pocket depth • loss of attachment • bleeding on probing • furcation lesions • mobile teeth.

The information recorded at the initial visit is important in diagnosis, treatment planning and determining prognosis. The chartings recorded during and after hygiene phase therapy indicate treatment success and highlight specific problems or areas requiring further therapy.

Other periodontal terms

False pocket Where increased probing depth is due to gingival enlargement without loss of attachment of the periodontal ligament.

True pocket Where increased probing depth results from destruction of the periodontal ligament.

Recession Where the gingival margin lies apical to the amelocemental junction.

CAUSES OF GINGIVAL RECESSION

- As a natural consequence of ageing.
- Due to plaque-induced gingival inflammation.
- Prominent position of tooth in the dental arch, e.g. buccal aspect of upper canine.
- Underlying bony dehiscence.
- Trauma:
  - toothbrushing
  - deep overbite
  - denture-induced trauma
  - other habit.
- High fraenal attachment.
- Following periodontal treatment.

STAGES IN PERIODONTAL THERAPY

Following examination and diagnosis, periodontal therapy is usually carried out in the following stages.

1. **Hygiene phase**
   This stage of therapy comprises:
   - dental health education and instruction in plaque control
   - elimination of obstacles to effective oral hygiene, including defective restoration margins, grossly malpositioned teeth and teeth of hopeless prognosis
   - non-surgical subgingival scaling and root planing.
2. **Reassessment**
   Conducted 4–6 weeks after the completion of hygiene phase. A further full periodontal assessment is carried out including plaque, gingivitis and pocket charts. This indicates the success of therapy and highlights specific problems or areas requiring further therapy.

3. **Corrective phase**
   Disease that persists following the hygiene phase is treated by further root planing or surgery.
4. **Supportive periodontal care/maintenance phase**
   Long-term follow-up is required to monitor the success of therapy. Patients should be reviewed at regular intervals to monitor oral hygiene and permit early detection of recurrent disease. Careful probing of all tooth surfaces is required to detect bleeding pockets, the only currently reliable indicator of active periodontitis.

HYGIENE PHASE THERAPY

ORAL HYGIENE INSTRUCTION

Successful prevention and treatment of periodontal disease is heavily dependent on the ability of the patient to maintain an adequate standard of plaque control. Thus the ability to motivate the patient to improve oral hygiene is of paramount importance.

Oral hygiene instruction should be tailored to the circumstances and needs of the individual patient.

Begin by explaining the nature of periodontal disease, the role of dental plaque and the need to improve cleaning in areas particularly difficult to reach, e.g. lingual aspect of lower molars.

- Models and information leaflets may be of value in aiding patient understanding.
- Visualization of plaque can be enhanced by the use of disclosing agents and a hand-held mirror.
- Rather than recommend a standardized toothbrushing regimen, it is more important to establish deficiencies in current practice and offer advice tailored to the needs of the individual patient.

Disclosing agents

Tablet For patient home use.

Solution Better for use in the surgery as solution can be used to disclose specific areas.

Toothbrushing technique

Numerous toothbrushing techniques have been described, of which the modified Bass technique is probably the simplest and most effective. The head of the toothbrush should be angled so that the filaments are at 45° to the long axis of the tooth and should be placed at the gingival margin to allow the tips of the filaments just to enter the gingival crevice. A back-and-forth movement should be used to facilitate plaque removal (Figure 10.3). It should be stressed that accessing the 'awkward' areas is more important than continually cleaning the more easily accessible surfaces. Scrub techniques and toothbrushes with hard filaments should be avoided as these can cause gingival recession.

The decreasing cost of electric toothbrushes has increased their popularity. While previously their use was recommended mainly for special-needs patients or those with particular dexterity problems, their use can now be more widely recommended. Powered toothbrushes have the advantage of a smaller head than conventional brushes. However, irrespective of whether patients choose to use either a manual or a powered brush, spending

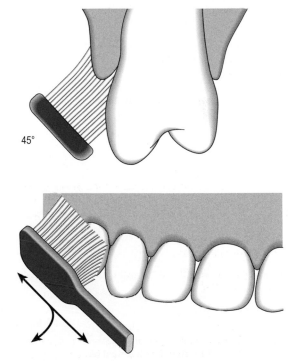

Figure 10.3 Modified Bass toothbrushing technique.

sufficient time brushing, and ensuring that the difficult-to-reach areas are clean, is the key to prevention of periodontal problems.

Interproximal plaque control Whilst plaque most readily accumulates in the interproximal region immediately beneath the contact area, this is the region least likely to be reached by toothbrush filaments. For this reason patients must also be instructed in interproximal plaque control techniques. A variety of aids for between-tooth cleaning are available (Table 10.5). Patients require individual tuition in the use of interproximal aids if they are to use them effectively.

It is however, very important not to 'overload' the patient with a vast armamentarium of tooth-cleaning devices. Only when the patient achieves a satisfactory level of toothbrushing should interproximal aids be introduced. When promoting improved plaque control, it is important to warn patients that, initially, bleeding on cleaning will be apparent due to existing gingivitis, but that this will decrease rapidly as plaque control improves. This is important as, without this advice, the treatment may appear only to worsen the presenting complaint!

TABLE 10.5 Oral hygiene aids	
Toothbrushes	The most important features are the size of the head, medium texture filaments and rounded ends to the bristles
Electric toothbrushes	May be of particular benefit in patients with reduced manual dexterity
Single tufted brushes	Cleaning around lone-standing teeth, partially erupted third molars, proximal spaces adjacent to saddle areas in partially dentate patients. Also useful in localized areas of recession and exposed portions of dental implants
Floss	Waxed or unwaxed. Waxed may be easier for first-time users
Tape	Broader than floss, it passes between teeth more easily. May be beneficial where interproximal restorations are present
Superfloss	Used for cleaning under bridge pontics
Floss threader	Used to pass floss beneath pontics, cheaper than using Superfloss
Interproximal (bottle) brushes	The method of choice for interdental cleaning when space permits. Available in a range of sizes; choose the largest size which passes between the teeth without causing discomfort
Wooden sticks	Not as effective as interproximal brushes

CHEMICAL PLAQUE CONTROL

Whilst periodontal disease is bacterial in origin, the use of chemicals and drugs in the prevention of plaque accumulation is of limited use in the long-term inhibition of periodontal disease.

Reasons for chemicals being of limited use include:

- non-specific plaque hypothesis – unlike other diseases of bacterial origin, periodontal disease is caused by a range of bacterial species
- the organisms involved are commensal in origin and thus there is no logical end point to treatment
- the organisms are located subgingivally where mouthwashes do not penetrate
- many agents lack sufficient substantivity and do not remain active long enough to exert a pharmacological effect.

Other concerns relate to the indiscriminate use of antimicrobials and the contribution this may make to increasing microbial resistance to therapeutic agents.

 Long-term prevention of periodontal disease is dependent on adequate mechanical plaque control.

A range of mouthwashes are available for the chemical control of plaque. However, their use should be regarded as short term until the patient is able to reintroduce or master adequate mechanical plaque control. The most effective antiplaque agent is *chlorhexidine gluconate*.

Chlorhexidine gluconate
Indications for use

- After oral surgery to reduce postoperative infection, pain and inflammation.
- In the management of periodontal problems as part of a palliative care programme.
- To help prevent drug-induced gingival overgrowth.
- For patients with fixed intraoral appliances, e.g. intermaxillary fixation devices.
- To prevent secondary infection in ulcerative conditions, e.g. ANUG, viral infection.

Other chemicals commonly used as antiplaque agents include quaternary ammonium compounds, e.g. cetylpyridinium chloride

(CPC) • phenols • triclosan – a *bis*-phenol, non-ionic germicide. Used in both mouthwashes and toothpastes, its activity can be enhanced by combination with zinc citrate or incorporation of copolymers.

SCALING AND ROOT PLANING

Root planing involves removal of subgingival plaque, calculus and infected cementum.

Removal of both sub- and supragingival deposits are essential elements of hygiene phase therapy, a process known as scaling and root planing. This can be achieved using either hand instruments or ultrasonic scalers. It is important that instruments are used correctly to ensure a smooth root surface.

Hand instruments

Scaling instruments can be classified as chisels, sickles, hoes, curettes and files (Figure 10.4). However, within these fundamental groups a wide variety of instruments are available. Scalers are usually paired, whereby one instrument is the mirror image of its partner, to ensure that the cutting edge of the scaler conforms to the tooth curvature at all times (Table 10.6).

The blade of the scaler is made of either stainless steel or tungsten carbide. To be effective, instruments should be sharpened regularly. Stainless steel instruments are sharpened using an Arkansas stone; for tungsten carbide instruments a diamond file is used. Blunt scalers may fail to remove subgingival calculus and only burnish it smooth on the root surface, making subsequent detection and removal difficult.

A modified pen grasp should be used – the scaler is grasped between the thumb and forefinger and the shank of the instrument is rested against the middle finger, which acts as the finger rest and also as the fulcrum around which the force is applied. This should be placed on tooth or bone close to the point of application of the force.

When scaling: • great care must be taken not to lacerate the soft tissues • avoid gouging or creating grooves on the root surface, which allow proliferation of subgingival plaque and decrease the chances of healing • a systematic approach to scaling is required to ensure that all tooth surfaces are cleaned.

The recommended operator and patient positions when using hand instruments are described in Table 10.7.

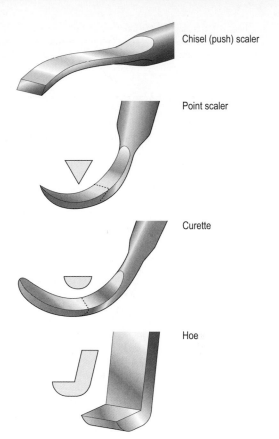

Chisel (push) scaler

Point scaler

Curette

Hoe

Figure 10.4 Scaling instruments.

Ultrasonic scalers

Ultrasonic scalers are composed of an electric power generator, a handpiece and an insert with a working tip. Electrical energy is converted to mechanical energy, causing the tip of the instrument to oscillate about 25 000 times per second through an amplitude of 0.006–0.1 mm. A fine water jet is directed onto the vibrating tip, not only acting as a coolant but also causing the formation and violent collapse of microscopic bubbles (the cavitation effect). The scaling action results from both the mechanical movement of the tip and the flushing and cavitation effect of the water spray.

TABLE 10.6 Scaling instruments

Instrument	Description	Area of application
Chisel (push) scaler	Chisel head, angled at 45°	Applied from labial aspect to remove gross supragingival deposits from approximal surfaces of mandibular anterior teeth
Point scaler (includes sickle scalers and jacquettes) (also known as trihedral scalers)	Triangular in cross-section and have two cutting edges which converge to a sharp point	All buccal and lingual embrasure areas, supragingival and 2–3 mm subgingival Manipulated with wrist movement so that the point always moves towards and into the embrasure
Hoes	Have a blade set at 100° angle to the shank and cutting edge is beveled at 45° A set of 4 is required to give access to all tooth surfaces	Allows access to deep pockets. Used in a series of short pull strokes to remove subgingival deposits
Curettes	Curved spoon-shaped blade with two cutting edges that meet to form a rounded toe	Supra- and, especially, subgingivally throughout the mouth. Used following hoes in root planing
Periodontal files (Hirschfeld files)	Has multiple straight cutting edges at the working end of the instrument	Used to roughen the surface of burnished calculus, or to 'crush' calculus to facilitate its removal with other instruments

A variety of working tips are available. Ultrasonic scalers are best used for removing gross supragingival deposits and heavy staining and can also be used subgingivally.

As much of the instrument tip as possible should be held in contact with the tooth (to avoid gouging), and should be kept in motion at all times with a light brushing stroke. The lowest possible power setting consistent with satisfactory resonance should be used. Efficient high-volume aspiration is essential when using an ultrasonic scaler to remove the water and reduce aerosol production.

TABLE 10.7 Scaling technique – operator and patient positions

Teeth	Operator position (12 o'clock = directly behind patient)	Patient position
	7 o'clock, facing patient	Semi-upright, patient's head between operator's shoulder and elbow
33–43 buccal	Direct vision	
33–43 lingual	Reflected vision	
	11 o'clock, behind patient	Patient supine
34–38 lingual	Direct vision	
44–48 buccal	Direct vision	
34–38 buccal	Direct vision	
44–48 lingual	Direct vision	
13–23 buccal	Direct vision	
13–23 palatal	Reflected vision	
14–18 buccal	Direct vision	
14–18 palatal	Reflected vision	
24–28 buccal	Direct vision	
24–28 palatal	Direct and reflected vision	

Avoid ultrasonic scalers in patients fitted with a cardiac pacemaker.

Healing following scaling and root planing

Reduction in pocket depth occurs by two principal mechanisms.
• Recession of the gingival margin due to resolution of inflammation and subsequent reduction in swelling and hyperplasia. • Reattachment to the root surface. This occurs primarily by the formation of a long junctional epithelial attachment. Epithelial cells grow from the gingival sulcus to repopulate the pocket lining and attach by hemidesmosomes to the root surface. This is most likely to occur in the absence of inflammation; hence the need for scrupulous plaque control and complete removal of deposits from the tooth root to leave a smooth, plaque- and calculus-free surface.

Whilst the periodontal ligament contains precursor cells that have the ability to form a connective tissue reattachment, the restitution of a true periodontal ligament following treatment occurs only in limited circumstances. This may be encouraged by the use of guided-tissue regenerative techniques (p. 230).

Polishing

Well-polished, smooth tooth surfaces retain plaque less well than rough surfaces and thus it is useful to polish teeth after removal of plaque and calculus. • Gross stains should be removed using hand or ultrasonic instrumentation. • A small webbed rubber cup held in a special contra-angled handpiece and run at slow speed should be used. • The polishing cup is placed above the gingival margin and smoothly pulled coronally. • Do not repeatedly polish the same tooth surface as it is important to avoid overheating. • Use a fluoride-containing paste.

An often overlooked benefit of polishing teeth is the sense of well-being it promotes in the patient, thereby providing a greater incentive to carry out home care procedures.

PERIODONTAL SURGERY

> Periodontal surgery can be defined as any procedure involving the periodontal tissues requiring the use of a scalpel.

A wide variety of surgical techniques and procedures have been described. Periodontal surgery aims to reduce pocket depth and/or restore gingival contour to a state that can be maintained free of inflammation by the patient.

When is periodontal surgery carried out? Periodontal surgery should ideally be performed only after hygiene phase therapy has been completed. There are several reasons for this. • When pockets are due mainly to gingival hyperplasia, improvement in oral hygiene may result in resolution of inflammation and reduction in swelling, so surgery is avoided. • Reduction in inflammation means that haemorrhage at operation is less of a problem. • Where pockets are shallow (<5 mm), resolution following scaling and root planing may obviate the need for surgery. • Flap surgery is contraindicated in patients who are unable to maintain adequate levels of plaque control or who continue to smoke tobacco.

Periodontal surgery can be classified as gingivectomy, flap procedures or mucogingival surgery.

GINGIVECTOMY

Gingivectomy involves the excision of excess gingival tissue.

Indications Gingival hyperplasia • epulides, pericoronal flap
• elimination of subgingival restoration margins • recontouring
following acute necrotizing ulcerative gingivitis.

Technique

- The depth and morphology of the pockets or tissues to be eliminated are established by probing and can be marked using pocket-marking tweezers.
- Excess tissue to be removed is excised in toto by an incision made at an angle of 45° to the long axis of the tooth, so that the blade impacts against the tooth slightly apical to the base of the pocket.
- Sterile swabs are used to control haemorrhage before a periodontal dressing (e.g. CoePack®) is placed to protect the wound area.

FLAP PROCEDURES

Involve the elevation of a flap to permit access to the root surface.

The basic principles of flap design must be followed: • must be sufficiently large to expose any underlying bone defects • base must be wide enough to maintain adequate blood supply • incisions must allow movement of the flap without tension • important vessels and nerves must be preserved.

There are two basic types: replaced flap and repositioned flap.

Replaced flap

Here the flap is sutured in or near its original position. Also known as open flap curettage or modified Widman flap.

Indications • Allow access to root and alveolar bone to enable removal of subgingival deposits and granulation tissue where pockets persist following hygiene phase therapy. • Reduce pockets by encouraging a new epithelial and/or connective tissue reattachment at a more coronal level. • Used in osseous regenerative procedures such as guided tissue regeneration.

Technique

- An intracrevicular incision is made around the necks of the teeth with the scalpel parallel to the long axis of the teeth. Care should be taken to preserve as much tissue as possible. (In the modified Widman flap, the pocket-lining epithelium is also excised via an inverse bevel incision.)
- Vertical relieving incisions are required buccally if pockets are deep. Flaps should be sufficiently extensive to expose the marginal bone.
- Subgingival calculus deposits and granulation tissue should be removed.
- The flaps are replaced with interrupted sutures, taking care to achieve approximation of wound edges interdentally where possible.

Repositioned flap

Here, the flap is repositioned apically, coronally or laterally following surgery. Apical repositioning is the most common.

Indications • Eliminate pockets by positioning the gingival tissue apically • Increase the zone of keratinized gingivae. • Expose additional root for restorative procedures, i.e. crown lengthening.

Technique

- Buccal and lingual/palatal flaps are raised using either intracrevicular or inverse bevel incisions.
- The flap is reflected and dissected from the alveolar process in order that it is sufficiently mobile to enable repositioning.
- Any adherent granulation tissue or subgingival calculus deposits are removed.
- The flap is sutured in the desired position and may be held in place by the placement of a periodontal pack.

MUCOGINGIVAL SURGERY

> Procedures that involve alteration of mucogingival relationships.

Are concerned with: • increasing the width of attached gingivae • eliminating pull on the free gingival margin by fraenulae or muscle pull • covering gingival clefts or recession.

Unlike the alveolar mucosa, the attached gingivae are covered by stratified squamous epithelium and thus are designed to withstand frictional forces encountered in eating, toothbrushing, etc. Whilst in the past it was thought that a minimal width of attached gingivae was necessary to prevent periodontal disease, it is now accepted that the presence of the attached gingivae is not crucial for the maintenance of gingival health, provided the patient can keep the area clean. Thus mucogingival procedures are carried out less frequently than in the past.

Techniques can be classified as:

Fraenectomy

Involves excision of the fraenum or high muscle attachments and is used: • to dissipate pull on the gingival tissues and prevent recession • to enable easier access for tooth cleaning • before orthodontic treatment to enable approximation of upper central incisors where an interdental fraenal attachment may prevent closure of a midline diastema.

Laterally repositioned flaps

Used to cover isolated areas of recession.

Free gingival grafts

Used to cover isolated areas of recession.

Care and instructions following periodontal surgery

> **Crucial to the success of all periodontal surgical procedures is the maintenance of a plaque-free environment during the healing process.**

In order that sutures or periodontal dressings are not disturbed in the immediate postoperative period, mechanical plaque control in the area of surgery should be suspended and replaced with the twice-daily use of 0.2% chlorhexidine gluconate mouthwash. Patients should be encouraged to rinse vigorously, ensuring the solution reaches the interdental areas. Patients should be advised to use appropriate analgesics (paracetamol or ibuprofen) to relieve postoperative discomfort. Alcohol, very hot drinks, or excessive exertion should be avoided in the 24 hours following surgery.

Sutures and any packs or dressings are normally removed 1 week postoperatively. The use of chlorhexidine should be encouraged for a further week to 10 days, before mechanical interproximal cleaning is reintroduced.

Patients should be reviewed at regular intervals to monitor healing and reinforce the need for scrupulous plaque control.

Complications of periodontal surgery

Periodontal surgery almost invariably results in a degree of gingival recession. This has a number of consequences: • the increased exposure of the root surface may lead to dentine hypersensitivity • the increased tooth length may have implications for aesthetics in anterior teeth • the exposed root surface is more vulnerable to root caries.

RECALL MAINTENANCE

When active periodontal therapy is complete, a recall and maintenance programme is required. This aims to monitor plaque control and check for recurrent periodontal disease, best indicated by bleeding on probing. In general, recall intervals should initially be short (6–8 weeks) and then gradually extended provided the periodontium remains stable. The precise recall interval should be tailored to the patient's individual circumstances.

ACUTE PERIODONTAL CONDITIONS

ACUTE NECROTIZING ULCERATIVE GINGIVITIS

An acute ulcerative condition affecting the marginal gingivae.

Is painful, of sudden onset and leads to loss of the interdental papillae.

Clinical features: • Interproximal necrosis – begins at tips of the papillae; may spread laterally to involve all of gingival margin

• ulceration – grey slough, easily removed to leave raw bleeding surface • pain • halitosis • metallic taste. If severe:
• lymphadenopathy • fever • malaise.

Site • Most commonly affected sites are incisor region and partially erupted third molars.

Occurrence: • Second and third decades (mostly 18–26 year olds) • males = females • more common in winter.

Predisposing factors: • Inadequate oral hygiene • smoking • stress • impaired host resistance.

Diagnosis Usually on clinical grounds but can be confirmed by a smear which shows • neutrophils • spirochaetes • fusiforms.

Treatment
Immediate
Local treatment • Mechanical debridement; ultrasonic scaler will remove debris and has the advantage of oxygenating area • oral hygiene instruction.

Systemic treatment • Metronidazole, especially if fever or pyrexia present; 200 mg three times daily for 3 days.

Follow-up treatment
Further investigations are indicated if ANUG fails to resolve or patient suffers recurrent bouts of ANUG. May indicate underlying immunosuppression (e.g. HIV). Occasionally gingival recontouring is required to correct gingival morphology and eliminate interdental craters.

PERIODONTAL ABSCESS

> An acute collection of pus within a gingival or periodontal pocket.

Predisposing factors The presence of subgingival plaque; also frequently associated with a deep periodontal pocket. Clinically requires differentiation from an abscess, which is pulpal in origin (a periapical abscess). Deduced from clinical features, radiographs and vitality tests (Table 10.8). Diagnosis is complicated by heavily restored or multirooted teeth.

Remember, can originate from both periapical and periodontal sources – a combined *perio-endo lesion*.

TABLE 10.8 The differentiation of abscesses that are periodontal and periapical in origin

	Periodontal abscess	Periapical (dental) abscess
Pain	Acute onset	History of toothache
Swelling	Usually localized, extraoral swelling unlikely	Over tooth apex, more likely to be extensive
Pocket	Always present; more likely in presence of periodontal disease	± pocket
Sinus	Frequently on attached gingivae	Tracks to apex
Percussion	TTP, worse laterally	TTP, especially in axial direction
Restoration status	More likely if tooth caries-free/unrestored	More likely in heavily restored tooth
Vitality	Tooth vital	Tooth non-vital
Radiographs	Little evidence in early stages; bone loss	Loss of lamina dura in periapical area (after 10 days or so)

TTP, tender to percussion.

Treatment of periodontal abscess

1. Establish drainage
   a. most frequently via gingival sulcus
   b. occasionally requires incision if fluctuant
2. Microbiological sample for culture and sensitivity
3. Subgingival scaling to remove
   a. foreign objects
   b. subgingival calculus (there is evidence that restricting scaling to the superficial aspects of the pocket results in better healing – periodontal ligament fibres are not destroyed)
4. Irrigate with sterile saline or chlorhexidine
5. If drainage can be achieved via the the periodontal pocket, the systemic antibiotics/antimicrobials are often unnecessary. However, if systemic involvement, e.g. cellulitis, pyrexia: amoxicillin 250 mg three times

daily for 7 days or metronidazole 200 mg three times daily for 5 days should be prescribed.
6. Review in 2–3 days
7. Treatment for underlying problem.

PERIO-ENDO LESION

Occurs when an infection involves both pulp and periodontal ligament space simultaneously.

May arise as a result of: • infection in a necrotic pulp draining via the periodontal ligament (usually in the presence of existing periodontal disease) • toxins from pulp reaching periodontal ligament via lateral or accessory canals, especially in the furcation region • the root having been perforated by a pin or post.

Treatment Endodontic treatment should be carried out *before* periodontal treatment, as resolution of the endodontic problem is a necessary prerequisite for periodontal healing.

ANTIBIOTICS IN THE MANAGEMENT OF PERIODONTAL DISEASE

Whilst antibiotics are beneficial in the management of acute periodontal infections, they have a limited role in the long-term treatment of periodontitis. The non-specific nature of the bacteria that cause chronic periodontitis, the rapid repopulation of periodontal pockets following therapy and the fact that most periodontopathogens can be found in healthy mouths mean that systemic antibiotics are not indicated in the routine management of chronic periodontitis.

When used, antibiotics can be given *systemically* or delivered *locally*.

Systemic antimicrobials Prescription of a tetracycline in cases of aggressive early-onset forms of periodontitis has been advocated. Some authorities have advocated a combined regimen of metronidazole and amoxicillin.

Locally delivered antimicrobials designed for direct insertion into the periodontal pocket are available. They consist of acrylic fibres or gel impregnated with either a tetracycline or metronidazole. A chlorhexidine-impregated chip (PerioChip®) is also available for local insertion in a periodontal pocket. These devices may be of some benefit in persistent, isolated pockets, in patients with good oral hygiene. They should be used in conjunction with root planing.

Concerns over increasing microbial resistance to antibiotics means very careful consideration should be given to the potential benefits in a given case before resorting to antimicrobial therapy.

Host modulatory therapy In addition to their bacteriostatic effects, tetracyclines are known to inhibit proteolytic enzymes such as collagenase. This has led to their use in subantimicrobial doses as an adjunct to scaling and root planing (Periostat®). The recommended dose of, e.g., doxycycline is 20 mg twice daily for 3 months up to a maximum of 9 months of continuous dosing. At this dose the doxycycline is said to limit the effects of collagenase in periodontal breakdown, but must be used in conjunction with scaling and root surface debridement of the highest standard.

OCCLUSION AND PERIODONTAL DISEASES

A primary function of the periodontal tissues is to support the tooth when a load is applied. If subjected to excessive force, resorption of the surrounding alveolar bone may ensue.

Contrary to previous suggestions, trauma from occlusion cannot *induce* periodontal tissue breakdown. However, in the presence of pre-existing periodontal disease, excessive occlusal loading may increase the rate of periodontal destruction.

Occlusal trauma is damage to the supporting tissues caused by excessive occlusal stresses. This can arise from a number of sources:

Habits Bruxism, tooth grinding, pencil/fingernail chewing.

Dental treatment Lack of posterior support due to loss of molar/premolar teeth, poorly designed dentures, poorly contoured restorations, orthodontic treatment.

Occlusal disharmony Due to tooth drifting, overeruption creating interferences and preventing smooth closure to intercuspal position.

Lack of periodontal support Due to periodontal disease.

Treatment of occlusal trauma Involves removal of the excess load and concurrent treatment of the coexisting periodontal disease. This may involve selective tooth grinding, provision of a biteguard, or splint.

SPLINTS

> Splint – a means of increasing tooth support by joining to an adjacent tooth or teeth.

Current indications are limited to: • tooth mobility interfering with mastication or causing patient discomfort • retaining teeth that have been realigned by orthodontic therapy.

Splints may be removable or fixed (Table 10.9).

FURCATION LESIONS

> A furcation lesion describes loss of periodontal attachment extending to the bi- or trifurcation of multi-rooted teeth.

When bone loss involves the inter-radicular area, removal of subgingival deposits and subsequent maintenance by the patient can be difficult.

In addition to scaling and root planing, the following procedures may be considered necessary depending on the severity of the furcation defect.

Furcation-plasty

A flap is raised and the tooth and/or bone is recontoured to facilitate self-cleansing. Use is restricted to buccal and lingual defects. Dentine hypersensitivity may be a problem.

TABLE 10.9 Classification of splints

Removable
Partial denture – connectors give additional support to mobile teeth
Acrylic occlusal splint (or biteguard) – worn at night only

Fixed
Multistrand wire splint – attached with unfilled composite resin, this is the splint of choice. Its use may not be possible where there is a deep overbite or diastemas between the teeth
Composite strands – attached with resin
Etch-retained metal splints – e.g. Rochette and Maryland splints. Prone to failure due to inflexible nature

Root resection

Involves sectioning of the tooth and removal of one or two roots. The root to be retained should be endodontically treated and then restored with a crown or as an abutment for a double crown.

Tunnel preparation

Used in lower molars. The interdental space is widened surgically so that, when healing is complete, an interproximal brush can be passed between the roots, underneath the crown. Where space is limited, complete separation of the roots (*hemisection*) followed by placement of a double crown (where the roots are crowned and joined by an occlusal pontic) may facilitate creation of sufficient space to accommodate an interproximal hygiene aid.

Guided-tissue regeneration

This surgical technique involves elevation of a mucoperiosteal flap and curettage of granulation tissue and subgingival deposits. A polytetrafluoroethylene (PTFE) membrane (e.g. Gore-tex®) is then sutured under the flap to cover the bony defect. The membrane acts as a barrier to prevent epithelial downgrowth and allows the formation of a connective tissue reattachment and encourages bony infill of the defect. The membrane is then surgically removed 6 weeks later. Resorbable membranes (collagen, polylactid) negate the need for a re-entry procedure.

It should be remembered that successful management of furcation defects is dependent on optimal home care, and the above procedures are time consuming and technically demanding. For this reason, cases should be selected with care. Where the tooth in question is non-essential, scaling and root planing as a palliative measure may be preferable to complex treatment options.

REFERENCES

1. Armitage GC 1999 Development of a classification system for periodontal diseases and conditions. Annals of Periodontology 4:1–6
2. Greene JC, Vermillion JR 1964 The simplified oral hygiene index. Journal of the American Dental Association 68:7–13
3. Silness J, Loe H 1964 Periodontal disease in pregnancy. II Correlation between oral hygiene and periodontal condition. Acta Odontologica Scandinavica 22:121–135
4. Loe H 1967 The Gingival Index, the Plaque Index, and Retention Index system. Journal of Periodontology 38:610–616

CHAPTER 11

OPERATIVE DENTISTRY

This chapter discusses
operative dentistry, fixed
prosthodontics and
endodontics

Diagnosis of pulpal
pain   232

Treatment planning   235

Occlusion   239

Principles of cavity
preparation   242

Management of the deep
carious lesion   251

Alternative cavity
preparation
techniques   253

Crowns   253

Veneers   263

Inlays and onlays   268

Fixed bridges   271

Fixed–movable
bridges   277

Adhesive bridges   278

Tooth wear   280

Bleaching   284

Microabrasion   288

Endodontics   288

Surgical endodontics   296

Relationships within
restorative dentistry   298

DIAGNOSIS OF PULPAL PAIN

TYPES AND FEATURES OF PULPAL AND RELATED PAIN

Reversible pulpitis Pain of short duration (seconds) on response to hot, cold or sweet things. Relieved by analgesics. Poor pain localization.

Irreversible pulpitis Pain of long duration (seconds–minutes), often worse with hot stimuli, may be throbbing and dull in nature, better pain localization than reversible pulpitis, not always relieved by analgesics.

Periapical periodontitis Dull, throbbing, often constant pain; frequently kept awake, patient can usually localize pain to a particular tooth, tender to chew on tooth, poor relief by analgesics.

HISTORY

Pain history is *essential* in the diagnosis of pulpal pain.
Important features are:

Pain quality
Sharpness Sharp pain can indicate, e.g. exposed dentinal tubules, fractured cusp.
Dullness May indicate pulpal hyperaemia.
Throbbing Throbbing pain, particularly if constant, may indicate an irreversible pulpitis.

Duration
Short (i.e. a few seconds) can indicate a reversible pulpitis but may indicate pain of non-dental origin, e.g. trigeminal neuralgia (p. 475).
Constant Often indicates irreversible pulpitis or one of its sequelae.

Stimuli
Reaction to heat Often irreversible pulpitis reacts to heat but not cold.
Reaction to cold Often reversible pulpitis, exposed dentine or cracked cusp. These conditions also often react to heat.
Reaction to pressure May indicate periapical or periodontal abscess. Reaction to *release* of pressure may indicate a cracked cusp.

Reaction to sweet stimuli Frequent occurrence in reversible pulpitis or with exposed dentine

Site and radiation

History should indicate the primary site of pain and where it radiates. Pain in teeth adjacent to the tooth the patient suspects as the cause of pain or opposing arch is common. Referred pain from non-dental causes (e.g. sinusitis) should be borne in mind.

Pain localization is particularly difficult in low-grade reversible pulpitis and in children.

Timing

Pain pattern day and night is important. Pulpal pain is often worse at night.

A pain history gives the dentist a guide as to the source of pulpal pain. It does not produce a diagnosis on its own.

CLINICAL EXAMINATION

In dealing with pulpal pain, the examination should be conducted as follows:

Visual

Look for: • obvious cavities • cracked cusps • fractured restorations • swelling • sinus tracts.

Probing

To aid visual examination.

Percussion

When coupled with pain history, tenderness on percussion is an important feature of irreversible pulpitis, periapical periodontitis and periapical abscess. Percussion should be in an apical and lateral direction and several 'control' teeth should be percussed to check responses.

SPECIAL TESTS

Special tests are extremely useful in confirming suspicions from a pain history and examination.

Vitality testing

Use heat, cold, electric stimuli. Important to use 'control' teeth. May indicate normal, exaggerated or no response to stimulus.

Laser Doppler

Measures pulpal blood flow and gives an indication of pulpal vitality, not routinely used.

Radiographs

Periapical radiographs Indicate bony change apically, although they also show proximity of restorations/caries to the pulp and may give an indication of previous indirect or direct pulp capping.

Bitewing radiographs Also indicate proximity of restorations/caries to the pulp.

Multi-rooted teeth may need two or more radiographs at different angles to show problems.

Transillumination

May indicate caries mesially or distally on anterior teeth.

Tooth 'slooth'

An aid to localizing cracked cusps.

PROBLEMS IN DIAGNOSING PULPAL PAIN

To the inexperienced dentist, pain history and examination may be extremely confusing and resultant diagnosis difficult. This is particularly true when:

The mouth is heavily restored Multiple crowns, endodontically treated teeth, etc., may 'hide' the diagnosis. Less radio-opaque restorative materials make radiographic diagnosis of caries difficult.

Multiple pathology In a neglected mouth multiple problems may be apparent, making it difficult to localize the source of an individual's pain at a particular time.

Non-organic pain Symptoms of atypical facial pain may be confused with pulpal pain.

Dual pathology Where symptoms are arising from more than one tooth simultaneously.

Anxious patient May be withdrawn. Can be difficult to obtain a satisfactory history. Additionally, there may be exaggerated responses to examination.

In the diagnosis of pulpal pain, intervene only on the evidence of more than one symptom or sign. If unsure of the diagnosis in a particular case, more evidence should be gathered by further special tests or repeating history or examination. *Irreversible* dental treatment should *not* be embarked upon until the diagnosis is established.

TREATMENT PLANNING

HISTORY TAKING

The general features of history taking and treatment planning are discussed in Chapter 2. This section discusses features specific to treatment planning in fixed prosthodontics and endodontics.

Factors required in history

Patient complaints • Pain history of critical importance (p. 232) • swelling • failed or fractured restorations • aesthetic or speech problems • tooth wear.

History of treatment to teeth • When were restorations placed? • How many times have they failed? • Has tooth caused symptoms before? • How long has tooth been wearing away?

General dental history • How heavily restored is the dentition? • Have dentures been worn? • Has there been orthodontic therapy? • What treatments have been tried for present complaint? • Is the patient dentally motivated? Oral hygiene habits?

Medical history In fixed prosthodontics and endodontics, relevant medical problems may alter proposed treatment (p. 13).

Social history When contemplating prolonged or complex treatment, the patient's ability to attend and withstand long appointments is important, as is mobility. Financial considerations may also impact on treatment options. Sometimes specific family history of dental disease is important, e.g. aggressive periodontitis.

EXAMINATION

Extraoral examination

In fixed prosthodontics and endodontics, extraoral examination may reveal important points: • presence of swelling • signs of craniomandibular disorders, e.g. joint clicking, masseteric hypertrophy, tenderness in joints or muscles of mastication • smile lines, general aesthetics of current teeth and anterior restorations • trismus. In severe trismus, access to undertake restorative procedures may be impossible.

Intraoral examination

Mucosa Mucosal health is important. Features of particular relevance in fixed prosthodontics include lichenoid eruptions adjacent to restorations and desquamative gingivitis.

Periodontal health Oral hygiene, gingival condition, periodontal status, mobility and drifting of teeth, furcation involvement, recession and sensitivity should be assessed and charted (p. 204).

Caries Caries should be carefully charted. Note tooth surface affected. Differentiation should be made between active, recurrent, root surface and arrested caries. Individuals with rampant uncontrolled caries should be identified.

Restorations Existing restorations should be carefully probed and charted to determine marginal leakage, recurrent caries, contour, occlusal relationship with other teeth, fracture, debonding and cleansability.

Tooth wear Both physiological and pathological tooth wear should be noted.

Occlusion Particular attention should be paid to the functional occlusion, tilted and overerupted teeth.

Symptomatic teeth Examination and diagnosis of pulpal pain has been discussed previously (p. 232).

Endodontic status Suspicious or key teeth should be confirmed as apically healthy or unhealthy, vital or non-vital. Evidence of previous root canal treatment and its quality should be noted.

Saddles Edentulous saddles should be noted and particular interest paid to abutment teeth.

Removable prostheses If present, these should be examined in detail both in and out of the mouth (p. 301).

It is extremely important to chart restorations and essential treatment needed in the patient's case record in order that a treatment plan can be formulated.

Radiographic examination

Comprehensive radiographic examination is an essential feature in fixed prosthodontics and endodontics to determine: • caries • apical pathology • endodontic success or failure • problems with posts, e.g. perforation, short post • overhanging restoration margins • failing restorations • periodontal bone support • root fractures.

Radiographs should be taken using doses of radiation according to the 'as low as reasonably practicable' (ALARP) principle (see Chapter 4).

Useful radiographs in fixed prosthodontics: • periapicals • bitewings • occlusals.

Useful radiographs in endodontics: periapicals.

Additional in the dentate patient

Special tests are frequently required: • percussion testing of teeth
• vitality testing • radiographs • study casts • full occlusal analysis
• diagnostic wax-up of potential prostheses or rehabilitation.

DIAGNOSIS IN THE DENTATE PATIENT

Good history taking and sound clinical examination techniques
ease diagnosis and allow for appropriate patient management. The
possible diagnoses in dentate patients are numerous. Most patients
will fall into one or more of the categories listed in Table 11.1.

Great care should be taken in 'categorizing' patients since an
individual's dental needs may vary throughout life.

MANAGEMENT

Prioritization of treatment is the key to effective treatment
planning in fixed prosthodontics and endodontics. *Control of pain
is the first priority.*

Thereafter, a suggested sequence of treatment is:

Initial treatment

Control aetiology of problem e.g. for caries give advice on diet, oral
hygiene, use of topical fluoride.

Stabilization phase • Extract unrestorable teeth • restore by simple
means (usually intracoronal restorations) all restorable teeth
• simple endodontic treatment to key teeth.

TABLE 11.1 Potential categories of dentate patient

- Dental pain
- Non-dental pain
- Caries
- Tooth wear
- Periodontal diseases
- Previous misdiagnosis, e.g. treated for periodontal problem when problem may be endodontic
- Iatrogenic problems, e.g. previous failed crowns or endodontics
- Routine, e.g. symptom-free patient attending for check-up
- Aesthetic problem, e.g. tooth discoloration
- Occlusal problem
- Functional problem, e.g. insufficient teeth to chew adequately
- Traumatic problem, e.g. broken teeth following acute trauma
- Management problem, e.g. dental phobic

Reassess response to treatment • Assess patient's motivation, oral
hygiene, diet • reassess problem teeth • reassess treatment plan –
in some poorly motivated patients, complex treatment will
inevitably fail due to poor oral hygiene • in some patients no
further treatment is required.

Definitive treatment

This includes: • premolar and molar endodontics • endodontic
retreatment • provision of post cores • crown and bridgework
• removable prosthesis construction • implants.

In the formulation and carrying out of treatment attempt to:
• keep treatment as simple as possible • construct treatment plans
where there is scope to reassess and change plan • know your own
professional limitations • know your patient's limitations.

Management options in operative dentistry

Who? The dentist must decide who is the most appropriate
person to devise and carry out treatment on the dentate
patient. A hygienist or therapist is invaluable for delivering
some aspects of care and specialist help should be sought for
difficult cases.

What? Taking history, examination and diagnosis into account,
decide what to do given varying possible treatment options, e.g.
consider bleaching/veneer/crown/do nothing for a discoloured
tooth.

When? Timing of treatment is important. Clearly, pain
management is carried out as soon as possible. On the other
hand, complex crown and bridgework often has time and
financial implications for the patient and may have to be
delayed.

Where? Patients with medical problems may require treatment in a
hospital setting. In elderly patients mobility can be a problem.

How? Complex crown and bridgework, molar endodontics,
retreatment endodontics, etc., are difficult and demanding for
both dentist *and* patient. The dentist should be capable of
carrying out these procedures if attempting a treatment plan
involving them. Referral to specialists should be sought if
treatment is beyond an individual's limitations.

When planning treatment in operative dentistry the dentist
should take into account not just the teeth but the individual
patient's total oral health and general health needs.

OCCLUSION

Occlusion is the relationship of cusps or masticating surfaces of maxillary and mandibular teeth.

Retruded contact position Position of the mandible when the condyles are in their most retruded position in the glenoid fossa and there is occlusal contact of the teeth.
Intercuspal position The position of maximum intercuspation of the teeth.
Stable occlusion An occlusion in which overeruption, tilting and drifting of teeth cannot cause new occlusal interferences. (Sometimes a degree of occlusal instability is acceptable.)
Occlusal harmony The absence of occlusal interferences, which allows mandibular movement in all excursions (with the teeth together), and does not result in discomfort, strain or harm to the teeth or masticatory apparatus.

How key teeth move across each other is important. In fixed prosthodontics, a *functional* rather than a *morphological* (Angles class) approach to occlusion is required.

Border movement of the mandible

Bennett movement Condyle on working side moves laterally.
Bennett shift Condyle on non-working side moves forwards and mesially.
Working side describes the side *towards* which the mandible deviates in lateral excursive movements.
Non-working side describes the side *away from* which the mandible deviates in lateral excursive movements.
Occlusal interferences may encroach on or expand border movements. Can occur, e.g. by tooth extraction or overcontouring of a restoration.

Mandibular border movements are shown in Figures 11.1 (lateral view) and 11.2 (view from above):

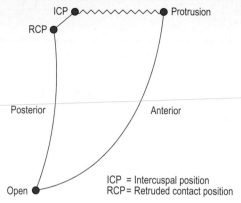

Figure 11.1 Mandibular border movements (lateral view).

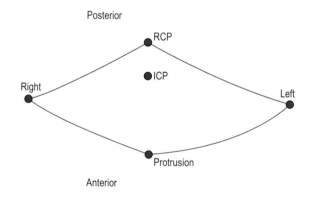

Figure 11.2 Mandibular border movements (view from above).

Retruded contract position (RCP)
- In 10–20% of population RCP = intercuspal position (ICP).
- In 80–90% of population RCP ≤2 mm posterior to ICP.

MANDIBULAR MOVEMENTS

Mandibular movements are defined as protrusive, retrusive and lateral (left and right).

Protrusive movement

Usually incisor teeth guide protrusion except in anterior open bite or Class III incisor relationships. Incisor relationship determines length and angle of protrusion, e.g. Class II division 2 occlusion with deep overbite results in nearly vertical protrusion. When building restorations, usually want to reproduce incisor relationship. In other circumstances, e.g. very worn teeth, restorations change incisor relationship and therefore protrusion.

Retrusive movement

Retrusion is the slide from ICP to RCP. Any disturbances of an even slide may require adjustment.

Lateral movement

Ideally *canine guided* occlusion with no contact on non-working side. In some cases '*group function*' (pairs of bicuspid teeth) may guide the working side.

OCCLUSAL INTERFERENCES

An occlusal interference results from contact between teeth in one of the excursions so that the smooth movement of the mandible is interrupted or unfavourable guidance (e.g. non-working contact) occurs.

   Interferences are difficult to detect as periodontal proprioceptors condition the mandible to move so that interference is avoided.

EXAMINATION OF THE OCCLUSION

Examination of the occlusion should be a routine procedure in fixed prosthodontics. However, certain aids help in full occlusal assessment (which is often reserved for complex occlusions, tooth wear cases or when contemplating occlusal rehabilitation).

Aids to occlusal examination • Articulating paper • occlusal indicator wax (0.5 mm thick) • plastic strips (Mylar 40 µm thick; Shimstock 8 µm thick) • study casts • diagnostic wax-up • facebow mounting.

Features to be noted in occlusal examination • Degree of occlusal stability • type of lateral guidance • patient complaints (especially myofascial pain dysfunction syndrome [MPDS], chronic dental pain, mobile teeth) • degree of difficulty in making mandibular movements • presence of occlusal interferences • overerupted and tilted teeth • does RCP = ICP? • smoothness and slide from RCP to ICP • presence of non-working contacts • tooth wear/faceting • tooth mobility in excursive movements.

OCCLUSAL AIMS IN FIXED PROSTHODONTICS

To leave a stable occlusion with no additional occlusal interferences.

Use of an articulator that is *semiadjustable* and allows the maxillary cast to be related to an approximation of the *terminal hinge axis* is essential in advanced crown and bridgework. This type of articulator has variable condylar guidance in at least a straight line and permits adjustment to incisal guidance.

Terminal hinge axis describes an axis passing through the lower part of the condyles, about which the condyles rotate when they are in their uppermost, centred position in the glenoid fossae.

PRINCIPLES OF CAVITY PREPARATION

OBJECTIVE OF CAVITY PREPARATION

• Removal of carious tissue. • Minimize pulpal and/or periodontal damage. • Cavity should be prepared such that restorative material to be used can restore function and appearance of the tooth and is retained in the tooth.

Basic principles of cavity preparation

Caries is a dynamic disease process involving the gain/loss of mineral from the tooth (p. 152). The first stage of management is always a preventive approach that focuses on the use of dietary advice and topical fluoride. However, once the carious process involves dentine most clinicians consider using an interventive approach to remove the carious tissue.

> ⚠ The fundamental guiding principle of cavity preparation is that the preparation should only be as large as the carious lesion. Radiographs should be examined carefully using good illumination and ideally magnification to assess the extent and depth of the lesion.

Although cavities vary widely, the following basic steps are common to the preparation of most cavities:

1. Outline form
Outline form encompasses the carious lesion, grossly unsupported enamel, and is made up of smooth angles rather than sharp edges.

2 & 3 Resistance and retention forms
These are considered together as they are achieved simultaneously.

Resistance form refers to the features of the cavity design that resist occlusal forces.
Retention form refers to the features of the cavity design that resist displacement of the final restoration.

Retention form may vary depending on the material that will fill the cavity, e.g. a cavity to be filled by resin composite gains additional retention via micromechanical retention from acid etching of enamel. Therefore such a cavity requires less retention than a cavity that will be restored by a material such as amalgam.

4. Management of remaining caries
Removal of existing caries should be undertaken with the following principles in mind: • The cavity margin must be caries free. • Great care should be taken to remove all caries and stained dentine from the amelodentinal junction to prevent lateral spread • Stained but hard dentine may be left in the deepest parts of the cavity. • Soft dentine should be removed.

5. Enamel margin finishing
In most cavities the cavosurface angle (CSA, solid-line angle between cavity wall and tooth surface) should be around 90°. Cavity margins should be closely inspected and grossly unsupported enamel removed. However, the marginal strength of the restorative material for a particular cavity is a major factor in determining the best CSA and the amount of unsupported enamel to be removed.

6. Cavity toilet
After mechanical cavity preparation is complete, residual debris should be dislodged with a hand instrument, the cavity cleaned with water, isolated and dried.

CLASSIFICATION OF CAVITIES

Black's classification is a simple and convenient way of classifying cavities based on the tooth surfaces affected. However, it must always be remembered that the shape of any cavity is primarily dictated by the extent and spread of the carious process. Recently, it has been suggested that a Class VI cavity be added to this classification. This lesion involves wear of the incisal tips of anterior teeth (Table 11.2).

Class I cavity

Primary occlusal caries is usually operatively managed using a preventive resin or enamel biopsy approach which is then restored with composite resin and the surrounding fissures sealed. More extensive cavities and replacement restorations are often managed with a more traditional occlusal amalgam restoration due to concerns over the longevity and wear resistance of composite.

Preventive resin preparation/enamel biopsy

- Initial preparation made with small pear-shaped bur
- Only access areas of fissure system that appear carious
- If no caries found, cavity can be 'aborted' and sealed
- Remove any carious dentine using small rosehead burs
- Remove only friable enamel margins – firm enamel will be supported with composite
- Do not bevel occlusal cavity margins – this will result in thin layer of composite which will fracture, stain and wear
- Etch cavity margins, wash and dry

TABLE 11.2 Black's classification of cavities

I	Cavity originating in anatomical pit or fissure
II	Cavity originating on mesial or distal aspect of molar/premolar teeth
III	Cavity originating on mesial or distal aspect of incisors/canines not involving incisal edge
IV	Cavity originating on mesial or distal aspect of incisors/canines involving incisal edge
V	Cavity originating in cervical third of buccal/lingual/palatal aspects of teeth (excluding anatomical pits)
VI	Cavities involving wear of incisal edges of upper and lower anterior teeth

- Apply dentine bonding agent if dentine exposed
- Restore cavity with composite (flowable composite may help; apply composite incrementally if cavity large)
- Seal remaining fissure system

Class I cavity – amalgam

- Often begins as enamel biopsy until 'occult' caries found at ADJ
- Initial preparation made with small pear-shaped bur
- CSA 90–110°
- Remove all undermined enamel – will not be supported
- Use lining that will seal underlying dentine such as GIC – alternatively, seal cut dentine with a dentine bonding agent
- Restore with amalgam and carve

Class II cavity

There are a number of different ways to approach an approximal carious lesion. These include:

- Occlusal via marginal ridge – most commonly
- Bucally/lingually – when teeth are tilted
- Directly – when adjacent tooth missing
- Occlusally leaving marginal ridge intact – tunnel preparation.

Occlusal approach – composite

Most commonly used – aim to produce scoop form to cavity using pear-shaped bur.

- Remove any remaining carious dentine using small rosehead burs
- Remove all friable enamel – may leave unsupported enamel
- Bevel approximal enamel surface
- Line or seal exposed dentine with dentine bonding agent
- Apply matrix band and wedge
- Restore with composite in triangular-shaped increments, taking care not to join buccal and lingual cusps

Occlusal approach – amalgam

- Form of cavity is a scoop-box – slightly narrower occlusally than gingivally
- CSA 90–110°
- Remove all undermined enamel – will not be supported
- Place small vertical retention grooves using small rosehead bur in buccal and lingual walls of approximal box just inside ADJ
- Use lining that will seal underlying dentine, but avoid blocking out retention grooves
- Alternatively, seal cut dentine with a dentine bonding agent
- Apply metal matrix band and wedge
- Restore with amalgam and carve

Alternatives

Traditional MO/DO amalgam

Much operative dentistry involves the replacement of previous restorations

If preparation involves an occlusal lesion giving MO/DO cavity then additional approximal retention grooves are unlikely to be needed

Tunnel preparation

- Aims to preserve marginal ridge by approaching approximal caries more obliquely
- Main advantage is that overall strength of tooth is preserved
- Cavity usually restored with a glass ionomer/cermet base and 'occlusal' composite
- Technically difficult and needs magnifying loupes to prepare
- Concerns over ability to clear ADJ of caries coronally
- Fracture of marginal ridge long term, particularly in premolars.

Direct access

- Only restore when preventive approaches fail to arrest caries
- Treat as for smooth surface caries (Class V).

Class III cavity

- Cavity preparation
- Preferably use palatal/lingual approach as buccal enamel left intact

- Use labial approach only when direct access is possible (due to anterior tooth crowding)
- Remove friable enamel, but leave unsupported enamel as this will be supported by composite
- Restoration placement
- Pretreat cavity surface with acid etching of enamel/dentine bonding/application of unfilled resin
- Place matrix strip so that it extends below contact area
- Adapt matrix to cervical margin as this is area where excess composite is difficult to remove
- Matrix supported palatally/lingually by finger and material placed/injected into cavity
- Once restoration placement complete, strip is moved over labial surface and material cured
- May need to use wedge for closer cervical adaptation
- Finishing and polishing
- Excess can be removed by hand instruments/composite finishing burs
- Series of polishing discs are useful in gaining aesthetic polish
- Contact areas may be finished using interproximal finishing strips
- Final gloss can be added with polishing cream (e.g. Enhance)

Alternative

Large or aesthetically critical cavities can be restored using a 'composite layering' technique. Many manufacturers produce composites with a large range of dentine and enamel shades. Restore the bulk of the missing dentine with a dentine shade composite or alternatively use GIC. Restore the remainder of the cavity using an enamel shade with a matrix strip.

Class IV cavity

Class IV cavities are usually caused either by trauma or the collapse of a large interproximal lesion affecting an anterior tooth. Tooth wear can also produce 'Class VI' lesions affecting the entire incisal edge.

- Cavity preparation
- May need little or no preparation
- A long labial bevel may help with retention and allow the composite and tooth to blend together naturally

- Restoration placement
- Pretreat cavity surface with acid etching of enamel/dentine bonding/application of unfilled resin
- Place matrix strip so that it extends below contact area
- Alternatively, use a pre-formed transparent matrix, such as an Odus Pella crown form
- Adapt matrix to cervical margin carefully as this is area where excess composite is difficult to remove
- Apply composite in 1–2 mm thick increments and cure from both labial and palatal aspects
- Use matrix to apply final increment
- Finishing and polishing
- As for Class III (p. 247)

Alternative technique

Where there is extensive loss of tooth tissue an alternative approach is to carry out a diagnostic wax-up on a plaster model. A silicone putty matrix is made using a small sausage of impression putty, adapted to the palatal surface of the wax-up. This matrix is then used to provide support while the palatal surface of the composite restoration is developed. Once this has been completed, the remainder of the restoration can be 'filled in' by hand, using clear interproximal strips.

Class V cavity (cervical caries)

- Only restore when preventive approaches fail to arrest caries
- Access lesion; extend until the ADJ is caries free
- Gingival margin outline often subgingival
- May need retraction cord/electrosurgery to control haemorrhage or gain adequate subgingival access
- Many alternative restorative materials including amalgam, composite, GIC, cermet, resin-modified GIC and compomer
- Clinical trials suggest that GIC has greatest longevity
- If amalgam used may need undercuts occlusally and gingivally (use small rosehead burs)

CORE RESTORATIONS

Badly broken down teeth may require an extensive multisurface restoration known as a core. These often provide the foundation for a crown, as the remaining natural tooth substance is severely compromised and requires protection against occlusal loads and potential fracture.

Various types of cores can be used depending on whether the tooth is vital or is root filled:

Vital teeth

Slots and grooves

Slots and grooves approximately 1–2 mm deep can be placed in sound, caries-free dentine. Restorative materials can lock into these to provide additional retention.

Adhesive approach

Dentine adhesives can be used to provide additional retention for composite restorations and similar adhesives are available for amalgam (e.g. amalgambond). An alternative approach is to use Panavia as a lining material; this will bond to enamel and dentine and the technique involves packing amalgam directly onto wet Panavia. As the amalgam is placed it will exclude oxygen and the Panavia will set. If this approach is used remember to place a thin smear of petroleum jelly on the inside of any metal matrix band as the Panavia will also bond to this.

Dentine pins

Either stainless steel, titanium or gold plated. Pins are threaded and pin hole is slightly smaller than diameter of pin so that elasticity of dentine 'grips' pins. Many clinicians now tend to avoid dentine pins wherever possible, as pulpal exposure or perforation into the periodontal ligament is an ever present threat.

Technique

- Pin should be placed in largest bulk of sound dentine available, not at ADJ (enamel will craze and chip); usually place 1 mm inward from ADJ
- Use low revs and water coolant during pin hole preparation
- Pin must not be placed in pulp or PDL (knowledge of dental anatomy essential)
- If using more than one pin they should be as far apart as possible
- Pins may be bent towards centre of restoration, after placement
- Correct packing of restorative material around pins is essential to develop retention.

Non-vital – root-filled teeth

Nayaar core/Coronal-radicular amalgam core/Amalcore (terms used interchangeably).

Used for core placement in root-filled premolar and molars.

Technique remove coronal gutta-percha to a depth of 3–4 mm and place restorative material into coronal pulp chamber before building up rest of core.

Post crowns – see page 258.

CHOICE OF RESTORATIVE MATERIAL

The following is offered as a guide:

Amalgam
Large/multisurface restorations in molars (high occlusal loads)
Repair of existing amalgam restorations

Composite
Fissure sealants
Class I and II restorations in posterior teeth
Class III restorations
Class V restorations in aesthetically critical areas
Class IV restorations (consider layering techniques)

Glass ionomer cement
Root caries
Class III restorations in high caries risk patients (e.g. xerostomia)

Compomers
Non-carious cervical lesions

Resin modified glass ionomer cement
Liners and bases
Luting cements.

MANAGEMENT OF THE DEEP CARIOUS LESION

A deep carious lesion occurs when caries lies in close proximity to the dental pulp.

When a cavity is considered deep but the pulp is not exposed, hard stained dentine may be left over the pulpal area. Removal of this frequently results in pulpal exposure.

TECHNIQUES FOR MANAGEMENT OF THE DEEP CARIOUS LESION

Indirect pulp capping

The objective of this technique is to protect the pulp from bacterial contamination via a pulpal exposure. A pulpal exposure is recognized by pulpal haemorrhage. It must be noted that a microexposure may be present. Therefore the classic bleeding exposure is a relatively severe pulpal wound. Deep cavities should be managed under *rubber dam* to decrease bacterial contamination of microexposures, pulpal exposures or carious exposures (p. 174).

Technique

> Indirect pulp capping should be used for all cavities where it is considered there may be a microexposure or where removing further remnants of caries is likely to cause classic pulpal exposure. A layer of calcium hydroxide (setting) is placed over the dentine closest to the microexposure. This is reinforced by a structural lining.

Direct pulp capping

An exposed vital pulp may be pulp capped. Less successful than indirect pulp capping.

Direct pulp capping is most likely to succeed when: • pulpal exposure is small (<1–2 mm) • pulp is free of salivary contamination • carious exposure is not present (pulp already likely to be chronically inflamed) • tooth was symptom free prior to cavity preparation (less initial pulpal inflammation) • patient is young (better pulpal blood supply).

Technique
Haemorrhage is arrested with a sterile paper point or cotton-wool ball. Cavity cleaned with sterile saline. Calcium hydroxide flowed over exposure and allowed to set. Structural lining placed.

Mode of action of calcium hydroxide in pulp capping Calcium hydroxide has several actions in pulp capping:

Antibacterial action Demineralization and staining precedes bacterial invasion of dentine. Calcium hydroxide can render this demineralized dentine sterile via its inherent antibacterial activity due to its high pH, although quickly neutralized.

Remineralization Calcium hydroxide may be involved in the remineralization of carious dentine. This is not fully understood.

Reparative dentine formation In the pulpal tissue adjacent to calcium hydroxide there is a zone of necrosis followed by repair, by formation of intertubular or intratubular mineralization of dentine, or by the formation of atubular dentine.

An alternative option gaining popularity is mineral trioxide aggregate (MTA) as this seems to be particularly biocompatible.

CARIOUS EXPOSURES

A carious exposure means that the exposed pulp is contaminated with bacteria and essentially undergoing a chronic inflammatory process. The treatment of choice for a carious exposure is removal of the pulp and conventional root canal treatment.

Use of corticosteroid–antibiotic preparations in management of the deep carious lesion Corticosteroid–antibiotic pastes have been used for many years to relieve acute pain associated with deep carious lesions.

Mode of action: *anti-inflammatory* (from the steroid) and *antibacterial* (from the antibiotic). Useful when there is a hyperaemic pulp and failure of local anaesthesia; most commonly when there is an irreversible pulpitis and/or carious exposure. Use of these pastes may cause relief of symptoms, decreased inflammation with ability to successfully anaesthetize the tooth on the next occasion.

> ⚠ It is imperative to realize that once these pastes have been used, conventional root canal treatment should be performed on the tooth. Use of these materials as a long-term indirect or direct pulp cap is not advised.

ALTERNATIVE CAVITY PREPARATION TECHNIQUES

Alternative methods of cavity preparation have recently been introduced in the form of *sonic* and *air abrasion* techniques.

Sonic preparation

Technique uses the vibration of a series of diamond-coated sonic tips to remove tooth tissue. Some tips are coated on one side to allow preparation of approximal cavities without damaging the adjacent tooth.

Air abrasion

Tooth preparation is undertaken using aluminium oxide particles (20–50 μm) delivered via a small-diameter nozzle at 240–960 kPa (40–140 psi). Useful for the preparation of pits and fissures, as this technique produces saucer-shaped cavities that are ideal for restoration with composite resin and other adhesive materials. Preparation needs to be carried out under rubber dam and using high-volume suction to minimize the spread of the aluminium oxide dust.

CROWNS

> A crown is a restoration that encompasses coronal tooth tissue, covering remaining tooth substance and restorations. When insufficient tooth tissue remains, the root canal can be used to aid retention – a post crown.

Types of crowns

Full coverage • Full-veneer crowns (usually made of gold for posterior teeth) • porcelain jacket crowns (anterior teeth) • metal ceramic crowns.
Post crowns • Cast gold core • prefabricated core.
Partial coverage • Three-quarter crowns and reverse three-quarter crowns.

Assessment of teeth for crowns

Case selection is important. In order to plan treatment appropriately, when considering crowns, assess: • tooth vitality • periodontal support and gingival condition • oral hygiene • caries control • occlusion • radiographic appearance • aesthetics (including patient's expectations) • adjacent teeth.

In some cases study casts, clinical photographs and a diagnostic wax-up of anticipated appearance may be useful.

CLINICAL STAGES IN MAKING CROWNS
1. Preparation

Crown preparation involves removal of enough tooth substance allowing sufficient thickness of material (from which the crown is to be made) to provide strength and aesthetics. Preparation must not damage the pulp. Preparation must provide sufficient retention for the crown. This can be achieved by taper of 5–20° (especially in cervical third of preparation), and inclusion of retention grooves or slots is useful in teeth of reduced occlusogingival height. Preparation should involve minimal gingival trauma. Preparation should have smooth curves, not right angles or sharp edges. Finishing lines depend on the material from which the crown is to be made. Options for finishing lines:

- *Butt joint*, e.g. porcelain jacket crown.
- *Chamfer*, e.g. palatal margin metal–ceramic crown.
- *Taper*, e.g. full-veneer gold crown.

Preparation is usually achieved by a selection of high-speed diamond burs.

2. Temporization

Prepared teeth require temporization for aesthetics, pulpal protection and prevention of overeruption or drifting of opposing or neighbouring teeth.

Types of temporary crowns

Anterior teeth • polycarbonate preformed crowns
• polyethylmethacrylate crowns fabricated using an alginate impression.
Posterior teeth • stainless steel • polycarbonate or polyethylmethacrylate.

Usually temporary crowns are cemented with temporary cement. Occasionally, a more permanent luting cement may be used when the temporary crowns are to be worn for a prolonged period or preparations are of reduced occlusogingival height. Heat-cured acrylic temporary crowns may be used if temporization is for a prolonged period.

3. Impression

An accurate impression of the preparation is *essential* if the crown is to fit. Materials used in crown impressions include polyvinylsiloxane, polyether, polysulphide (usually with an individual tray) (p. 131).

To ensure an accurate impression:

- Follow the manufacturer's instructions for the particular material selected.
- Good moisture control essential as all impression materials hydrophobic.

Obtain gingival retraction where a preparation is subgingival via use of appropriate thickness of retraction cord or occasionally using electrosurgery.

- Examine the set impression critically, paying particular attention to air blows, voids, tears and shiny surfaces (lack of flow of impression), and if necessary repeat.
- In difficult cases use of impression copings or proceeding to a trial of a casting may ensure a satisfactory end result.
- An impression of the opposing arch in irreversible hydrocolloid is required.
- Jaw registration is essential and is usually achieved by 'best fit' when sufficient teeth are present. Wax, reinforced wax or silicone rubber can be used as an alternative.
- Use of a facebow for mounting models on a semi-adjustable articulator is often desirable.

4. Prescription of technicians

The dentist should communicate information about crown shape, shade, irregularities and design (e.g. type of margin, type of material, rest seats/undercuts/guide planes) clearly to the technician.

5. Cementing a crown

On receipt of a crown from the laboratory check that: • the cast has been trimmed correctly; compare impression margin and cast margin • the neighbouring teeth on the cast have not been abraded • the crown fits the cast • the correct design features are present • the occlusion is correct • the shade looks broadly correct.

The temporary crown should be removed from the mouth and any adherent temporary cement removed (often this requires local anaesthetic).

The permanent crown is tried in. The following should be carefully checked:

- Marginal fit
- Contact point with neighbouring teeth. This should be such that interdental cleaning is possible.
- Gingival emergence angle
- Occlusion in all mandibular movements.

When the dentist is satisfied, the patient should be shown the crown aesthetics and modifications made if required. When both dentist and patient are satisfied, the preparation is degreased (with alcohol), dried and the crown cemented with a permanent luting cement. If there is any doubt, it is prudent to use a temporary luting cement and review the situation. Excess cement must be removed from around the crown margin. The patient should be given oral hygiene instruction regarding the crown.

COMMON FAULTS WITH CROWNS

Despite careful attention to detail the following faults with crowns occur commonly:

Overhanging margin • Usually due to poor impression or poor technical work. • Can in some cases be corrected by trimming with a bur, but often requires a remake. • If uncorrected leads to plaque accumulation, gingival inflammation or recurrent caries.

Negative margin • Usually due to poor finishing line delineation, over-trimming of die or over-vigorous polishing of crown margins. • Patient often feels sensitivity. • Risks recurrent caries or poor aesthetics.

Poor gingival emergence angle • Usually due to lack of communication between dentist and technician. • Overbulking of material at the gingival margin leads to plaque accumulation.

Poor contact point • Usually due to under-preparation of mesial and distal walls or overbulking of interdental area by technician. • Hinders interdental cleaning.

Poor aesthetics • Can be due to incorrect shade, shape or under-preparation leading to insufficient space for material. • Occasionally patients have unrealistic expectations.

Persistent debonding • Often due to inadequate retention on preparation • May be due to occlusal interference (esp. lateral excursion) • In post crowns may be due to poor post design or longitudinal root fracture.

ANTERIOR CROWNS

Indications • Protection of heavily restored teeth • aesthetics • bridge retainer • tooth wear.

Types of anterior crowns

Metal–ceramic crown • Used when limited occlusal space and high functional loads. • Relies on ability of porcelain to bond to metal oxide. • Modern metal–ceramic crowns have excellent aesthetics. • Can have metal (when very limited occlusal space) or porcelain palatal surface. • Often have butt joint labially (1.5 mm shoulder to

...v adequate metal and porcelain for aesthetics) and chamfer
...gin palatally.
    A typical metal–ceramic crown preparation for an anterior
...oth is shown in Figure 11.3.

Porcelain jacket crown • Used when aesthetics of prime concern.
• Problem in high-load situation as porcelain in thin section and
liable to fracture. Not usually suitable for posterior teeth.• Usually
butt joint around whole preparation (minimum 1 mm shoulder to
allow adequate porcelain for aesthetics).• Need 1.5 mm thickness of
porcelain incisally.• A typical porcelain jacket crown preparation
for an anterior tooth is shown in Figure 11.4.

Other anterior crowns Porcelain crowns with superior aesthetics
and with higher tensile strength than conventional porcelain jacket
crowns are finding increasing use – employ sintered alumina cores
or injection moulding of ceramic. Require even reduction;
preparation similar to a conventional aluminous porcelain jacket
crown. Use of dentine-bonded crowns and reverse three-quarter
crowns involve significantly less tooth destruction.

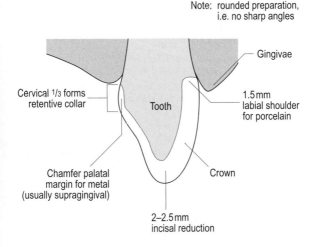

Note: rounded preparation,
i.e. no sharp angles

Gingivae

Cervical 1/3 forms
retentive collar

1.5 mm
labial shoulder
for porcelain

Tooth

Chamfer palatal
margin for metal
(usually supragingival)

Crown

2–2.5 mm
incisal reduction

Lateral view

Figure 11.3 Metal–ceramic crown preparation of upper anterior tooth.

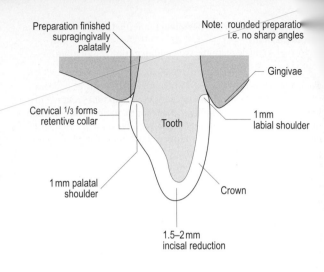

Preparation finished
supragingivally
palatally

Note: rounded preparatio
i.e. no sharp angles

Gingivae

Cervical ¹/₃ forms
retentive collar

Tooth

1 mm
labial shoulder

1 mm palatal
shoulder

Crown

1.5–2 mm
incisal reduction

Lateral view

Figure 11.4 Porcelain jacket crown preparation of upper anterior tooth.

POST RETAINED CROWNS

Indications When there is insufficient coronal dentine to withstand
occlusal forces or retain a crown. Root dentine is used and loads
transmitted via a post to the root dentine. The post retains the
crown. Usually root-filled teeth (but not every root-filled tooth
requires a post crown).

Assessment of teeth for post crowns Careful assessment of
individual teeth is required before considering a post crown.

Root length A long post is favourable for crown retention and a
post extending to within 5–6 mm of the root apex is ideal. Root
length may vary due to apicectomy, resorption, fracture.

Root width A wide post is often desirable; however, teeth such as
first premolars or lower incisors are often extremely narrow and
a wide post would leave such a tooth very weak.

Root alignment Curves and dilacerations complicate post design.

Root canal filling In general a sound root canal filling must be
present (leave 4 mm) with no apical pathology evident before
post placement.

Problems with post crowns

Failed post crowns are a common occurrence. Problems include:

Root perforation Occurs after failing to judge root alignment. More common with engine-driven instruments.

Root fracture Occurs particularly with wide posts (in high occlusal load situations) where root dentine is excessively weakened.

Post debonding Occurs especially with short, tapered posts. Likely with high occlusal load or root fracture.

Fractured post Thin cast posts are susceptible to fracture due to occlusal loads or trauma. Removed with a trephine system.

Corrosion Can be a problem if core and post are made of dissimilar metals.

Types of post crowns

A multitude of post crown systems exist. There is no single post core system that is suitable for all situations.

Basic types • Cast post core systems • prefabricated post core systems. Within these systems, posts may be parallel sided, tapered, threaded, serrated or parallel pins.

Cast post core systems Usually made of cast gold, sometimes wrought gold post and cast gold core. Problems involve casting porosity. Used successfully for many years. Tooth preparation should preserve as much coronal dentine as possible. Resist rotational forces by means of anti-rotational grooves or parallel pins. Post hole preparation should ideally be achieved with hand instruments to avoid risk of perforation.

Impression techniques may be indirect or direct indirect:

Indirect Involves use of wire or preformed plastic in the canal and an impression in an elastomeric impression material. An opposing arch impression and jaw registration is taken and the post core waxed up in the laboratory, invested and cast. Can sometimes make post core and final crown using single impression.

Direct indirect Involves use of a plastic post and either inlay wax or self-cured acrylic, modelled at chairside to gain an impression of the post hole and core shape. This is then invested and cast in the laboratory. Advantage – clinician has control over core shape.

Prefabricated post core systems These may be subdivided into:
• post and integral core • post (core built in plastic restorative material). Wide range of materials are in use – stainless steel, brass, titanium, nickel–chromium, ceramic, carbon-fibre.

Advantages • Can be placed directly, so avoiding laboratory stage • material properties often superior to cast gold • easy to use • cheap.

Disadvantages • Increased clinical time • preparation often involves mechanical instruments so increased risk of root perforation or fracture • often designed for 'average' teeth so do not meet needs of teeth with wide or narrow root canals • failure of core (if made in plastic restorative material).

When using prefabricated post systems, the dentist should bear in mind the individual manufacturer's recommendations, the limitations of the particular system and the core material to be employed.

Core materials Amalgam, resin composite, glass ionomer, glass cermet or resin-modified glass ionomer. Use of autocured or dual-cured materials is important so that restorative material is properly set (p. 119).

Clinical tips

The 'first bite of the cherry' principle Post crowns are most successful the first time they are constructed on a particular tooth. Treating failures is difficult as the preparation is already compromised. If fortunate to have the 'first bite of the cherry' in post crown treatment ensure: • as much coronal dentine as possible is maintained • post of adequate length and width to enhance retention but not compromise root strength or apical seal of root canal filling • there is adequate resistance to rotational forces in the preparation • post crown system most appropriate to clinical situation is chosen • final crown design is known at the outset in order that core can be designed properly • if using an indirect cast post system, instructions on design are clearly communicated to technician.

Cementation Luting failures are common. The tooth should be dried. A spiral paste filler should be used to transport luting cement into the canal and to coat the walls; further luting cement is placed on the post and the post core firmly seated.

Variations

Posterior teeth In molars and some premolars, roots are often narrow and at differing angulations leading to an increased risk of perforation or fracture by use of posts. Therefore use only posts essential for core retention. Consideration should be given to the use of dentine pins or packing of plastic restorative materials into root canal orifices to enhance core retention (so-called amalgam 'post'/Nayaar core).

Diaphragm Where there is subgingival root fracture, use of a cast post core and diaphragm may be appropriate.

Angulated teeth Minor tooth angulation problems, e.g. retroclined individual tooth, may be corrected by altering core angulation within the confines of occlusal harmony.

Apicected teeth Often have fairly short roots; thus post retention may be particularly difficult. Consideration should be given to making the final restoration non-functional.

POSTERIOR CROWNS

Indications • Aesthetics (some posterior teeth only) • bridge retainer • tooth wear • protection of heavily restored teeth • partial denture abutments.

Types of posterior crowns

Metal–ceramic crown Used when insufficient occlusal space, high functional loads, or aesthetics important. Metal (when limited occlusal space) or porcelain occlusal surface. Junction of metal and porcelain should not be in area of high occlusal stress. Can have metal or porcelain (superior aesthetics) labial margin. Often have *butt joint* labially (1.5 mm shoulder to allow adequate metal and porcelain for aesthetics) and chamfer margin palatally or lingually. Functional cusps (in Class I occlusion upper palatal cusps and lower buccal cusps) need additional tooth reduction (extra 0.5 mm) by means of a functional cusp bevel. A typical metal–ceramic crown preparation for a posterior tooth is shown in Figure 11.5.

Full-veneer crown Used when aesthetics of minimal concern (usually second or third molars). Usually made of cast gold. Tooth preparation should be as conservative as possible with the following features: • buccolingually and approximally, a 5° taper is ideal; chamfer margin removing all undercut areas. • Should finish supragingivally – not always possible as preparation should extend more gingivally than existing restorations so that preparation finishes on sound dentine. • Require minimum of 1 mm reduction occlusally to allow for gold to cover preparation. • Functional cusp bevel is needed to allow more occlusal clearance (1.5 mm) over functional cusps. • A typical full-veneer crown preparation for a posterior tooth is shown in Figure 11.6.

Other posterior crowns Cast gold partial-veneer crowns such as three-quarter crowns are occasionally useful to preserve a single

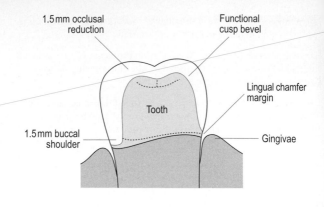

Distal view

Figure 11.5 Metal–ceramic crown preparation on lower molar with porcelain labial shoulder and metal lingual shoulder.

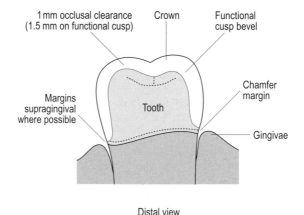

Distal view

Figure 11.6 Full-veneer crown preparation on lower molar.

intact cusp (usually mesiobuccal cusp of upper first molar). Porcelain crowns using sintered alumina cores or injection moulding of ceramic are finding increasing use in posterior crown situations.

VENEERS

> A veneer is a facing placed on either the labial or palatal surface of a tooth.

Types of veneers
• Labial veneers • palatal veneers • adhesive/dentine-bonded crowns.

LABIAL VENEERS

Uses • Aesthetic improvement of discoloured teeth • closure of diastemas • reshaping of hypoplastic teeth (e.g. peg laterals) • aesthetic masking of minor tooth position problems (e.g. slightly in-standing tooth) • trauma to anterior teeth • very rarely, as a bridge retainer in low occlusal stress situations.

Materials • Porcelain laminate veneers • direct composite veneers • indirect composite veneers.

In modern fixed prosthodontics, the porcelain laminate veneer is most commonly used as a labial veneer. Occasionally composite veneers may be used following trauma (usually in children until gingival margin stabilizes at around 18 years).

Case selection Existing caries, periodontal disease, occlusion and endodontic status should be assessed. Often porcelain laminate veneers are provided for aesthetic reasons so patient expectations should be determined. Teeth with large mesial or distal plastic restorations are usually not suitable for veneers due to increased risk of recurrent caries. Tooth wear and parafunctional habits should be assessed; veneers are often ill advised in such situations. Smile lines should be determined to identify which teeth require veneers.

Types of laminate veneer preparation (Figure 11.7)
Intra-enamel A localized area within the labial surface of a tooth. Often requires minimal preparation.

Feathered incisal This preparation involves 0.5–1 mm reduction on labial surface with chamfer margins approximally, incisally and at gingival margin. There is no incisal overlap.

Overlapping incisal As for feathered incisal, except that there is 1 mm of incisal reduction and the incisal edge is overlapped.

No preparation Sometimes (often interim measure in children) there is no preparation. This, however, leaves an overbulked tooth.

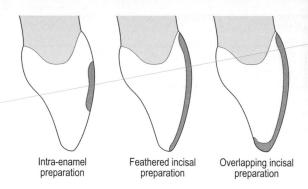

Intra-enamel
preparation

Feathered incisal
preparation

Overlapping incisal
preparation

Lateral view maxillary incisors

Figure 11.7 Porcelain laminate veneer preparations.

CLINICAL STAGES
1. Preparation
- The appropriate type of preparation is chosen and undertaken with an air turbine and a selection of fine grit diamond burs.
- Usually in enamel only and so local anaesthesia is not required.
- With the improved performance of dentine bonding agents, veneers are being used on teeth with exposed dentine so increasingly veneer preparations extend into dentine.

2. Impressions
Usually performed in an elastomeric material with alginate impression of the opposing arch.

3. Temporization
Temporary veneers are usually not required. Patients should be warned of some postoperative sensitivity and poor aesthetics.

4. Cementation
The finished veneer should be tried in and checked for occlusion, fit and aesthetics.

- Isolate tooth.
- Try in veneer with water-based try-in paste and assess appearance, fit and occlusion.
- When happy, clean fitting surface of veneer.
- Apply silane coupling agent to fitting surface of veneer.

- Place matrix strip mesially and distally.
- Enamel is etched with 37% phosphoric acid.
- Composite luting cement is placed on veneer and veneer seated. Use dual cure cement if veneer is very thick.
- Remove excess material with a brush and light-cure.
- Remove any remaining cement flash and check interdental contacts.

Note: Where there is dentine present labially, a suitable *dentine bonding agent* should be used.

Life span: 10 years plus; 5% prone to chipping around incisal edge.

Alternative

Direct placement composite veneer Usually used as medium-term restoration in adolescents until level of gingival margin stabilizes at around 18 years of age.

Preparation: either no preparation or as for ceramic veneer.

Acid etch and place directly using plastic matrix strips to protect adjacent teeth.

Life span: 3–5 years; more prone to chipping and discoloration.

PALATAL VENEERS

Facings on the palatal surfaces of upper anterior teeth only.

Uses • Tooth wear (in particular acid erosion) • decrease dentine sensitivity • restore aesthetics • protect pulp. Can extend onto worn incisal edge to improve appearance.

Types

Direct composite veneers Primary treatment method in tooth wear cases. Easy to place, adjust and repair. Can be extended onto worn incisal edge to improve appearance. Can be placed 'high' in occlusion using Dahl approach and posterior teeth allowed to erupt back into contact (approx. 3 months). Commonly used as they are easy to repair.

Gold palatal veneers Oxidized fit surface (400°C for 3–5 min) provide copper oxide layer that bonds with Panavia. Can be very thin. Poor if translucent incisal edge present as metal shines through (but better aesthetically than nickel–chromium). May have a role in deep overbite cases.

Nickel–chromium backings Can be very thin. Poor if translucent incisal edge is present as metal shines through. Better mechanical properties than gold. Useful if attrition is the main cause of tooth wear.

Ceramic palatal veneers Should be about 1 mm thick. Rarely used due to concerns about long-term wear effects on opposing lower incisors.

ADHESIVE/DENTINE-BONDED CROWN

Has features of both a porcelain laminate veneer and a porcelain jacket crown. This restoration involves enamel reduction labially, approximally and incisally and from the incisal quarter of palatal or lingual surfaces. All finishing lines are a heavy chamfer to enable a butt joint with porcelain (Figure 11.8).

Uses • Fractured incisal edges • closure of diastemas • discoloured teeth • labial caries • alternative to conventional crowns in lower anterior teeth.

Advantages

Advantages over porcelain laminate veneer • Greater strength • larger area for retention • less overbulking gingivally • potentially improved aesthetics • more accessible approximal margins.

Advantages over porcelain jacket crown • More conservative of tooth tissue • decreased gingival problems • less abrasion of opposing tooth • some exposed dental tissue available for future vitality testing.

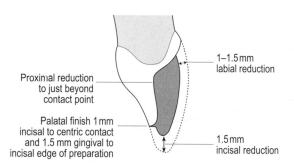

Proximal reduction to just beyond contact point

Palatal finish 1 mm incisal to centric contact and 1.5 mm gingival to incisal edge of preparation

1–1.5 mm labial reduction

1.5 mm incisal reduction

Lateral view maxillary incisor

Figure 11.8 Adhesive/dentine-bonded crown.

Disadvantages Adhesive crowns may fracture under high occlusal load, e.g. parafunctional habits or canine teeth.

Common problems with veneers include • Poor gingival emergence angle • fracture in function • fracture on cementation • poor interdental contact • aesthetics not ideal (especially if need translucent incisal tip) • lack of positive seating on cementation so cemented incorrectly.

INLAYS AND ONLAYS

INLAYS

> Inlays are intracoronal restorations which are manufactured in the laboratory and cemented into place.

Types • Gold inlays • composite inlays • porcelain inlays.

Uses Main use is in Class II cavities. Historically gold inlays have had limited use in Class III and Class IV cavities.

Advantages • Offer an alternative to amalgam as an intracoronal restoration • protects weakened cusps • more aesthetic than amalgam (composite and porcelain have superior aesthetics).

Disadvantages • Require two clinical stages and one laboratory stage • increased tooth tissue destruction • microleakage and recurrent caries can be a problem • luting cement flash causing gingival irritation (worst with porcelain inlays) • gold inlays may result in galvanic reaction if amalgam in opposing or adjacent teeth • radiographic marginal diagnosis not easy with composite or porcelain inlays as they are less radio-opaque than metal.

Clinical techniques In all inlays the usual features of cavity design should be followed; that is, caries removal, retention and resistance form. Linings and structural linings should be placed as they would be for a plastic restoration.

GOLD INLAYS
1. Preparation
Cavity must ensure a path of insertion and removal of inlay (5° ideal taper). Margins usually a fine taper or chamfer. Often need to cusp protect, i.e. cover functional cusps. If retention is poor, additional retention by means of parallel pins (pinlays) may be incorporated.

2. Impressions

Indirect Involves an impression in an elastomeric impression material. An opposing arch impression and jaw registration is taken and the inlay waxed up in the laboratory, invested and cast.

Direct indirect Involves use of either inlay wax or self-cured acrylic. The dentist models self-cure acrylic or inlay wax to gain an impression of the inlay cavity and models the inlay shape. This is then invested and cast in the laboratory.

3. Temporization

Inlay temporization is difficult, particularly if fine chamfer margins exist. The usual temporary crown materials (p. 254) are used but are not ideal. In some cases a temporary restorative material such as zinc oxide–eugenol may be used.

4. Inlay insertion

Once fit, occlusion and contact points have been checked, the inlay is adjusted and polished; it may be cemented with a conventional luting cement, e.g. polycarboxylate. With the advent of improved bonding systems, sandblasting and tin plating the inlay, and cementing with dual or autocured resin composite, is becoming popular.

COMPOSITE INLAYS

1. Preparation

Cavity taper wider than gold (15–20°). Cuspal coverage not usually required. Chamfer margins not required. Where possible, margins should be supragingival and based on enamel to reduce microleakage.

2. Impressions

An indirect technique as for gold inlays is used. In the laboratory, inlays are heat-, pressure- or light-cured (or a combination of these methods) depending on individual manufacturer's recommendations.

3. Temporization

Similar to gold inlays.

4. Cementation

a. Enamel etched.
b. On dentine, a suitable *dentine bonding* agent should be used and light-cured (follow manufacturer's recommendations).
c. Unfilled resin is placed on enamel, excess blown off with air and light-cured.

d. Unfilled resin is placed on inlay, excess blown off with air and light-cured.

e. Filled *dual-cured* resin is placed on inlay and inlay seated.

f. Optional seating using ultrasonic scaler for 30 seconds (special tips); gives improved seating.

g. Excess flash removed before light curing.

h. Any remaining flash is removed and interdental contacts checked.

PORCELAIN INLAYS

1. Preparation
Similar to composite inlays except that a *butt joint* is required; therefore greater destruction of tooth tissue.

2. Impressions
An indirect technique as for gold inlays is used. In the laboratory, inlays are waxed up and injection moulded ceramic can be used. There is increasing manufacture of inlays by both CAD-CAM technology and using sintered alumina cores.

3. Temporization
Similar to gold inlays.

4. Cementation
Similar to composite inlays except that the fitting surface of the inlay is often silane coupled prior to application of unfilled resin.

ONLAYS

> Onlays are extracoronal restorations on the occlusal surface of a tooth.

Types • Gold onlays • composite onlays • porcelain onlays.

Uses In tooth wear cases they are a less destructive alternative to increasing vertical dimension of occlusion than crowns. (*Note*: In severe attrition cases may not withstand parafunctional forces.) Also used for arrested caries, fractured cusps.

Onlays often require minimal tooth preparation and are supragingival. The composite/porcelain onlay, however, requires a butt joint so often a shoulder of 0.5 mm or more is needed. Clinical techniques are similar to inlays.

FIXED BRIDGES

> A bridge is a dental prosthesis that replaces a missing tooth or teeth and is attached permanently to one or more natural teeth (or implants). It is not removable by the patient.

Definitions

> *Abutment* tooth A tooth which supports a bridge.
> *Retainer* Part of a bridge which is cemented to an abutment tooth.
> *Pontic* Each replacement tooth in a bridge.
> *Unit* Each part of a bridge, i.e. abutment or pontic, is referred to as a unit. Thus two abutments and one pontic constitutes a three-unit bridge.
> *Pier* Non-terminal abutment.

The components of a bridge are illustrated in Figure 11.9.

Indications for bridgework • Aesthetics • occlusal stability – prevention of drifting, tilting, overeruption • function – usually in posterior regions • periodontal – a bridge is tooth supported (and covers less tissue) so is often considered more favourable to the periodontium than a removable prosthesis • small bounded saddles – ideal for fixed bridgework.

Disadvantages of bridgework • Tooth tissue destruction • expensive • difficult to repair.

General considerations in bridgework

Patients Patients often consider a fixed prosthesis more favourable than a removable prosthesis. However, bridges are costly in terms of tooth tissue, time and money.

Saddle Small saddles are more favourable than large saddles; however, marked resorption is a problem as cannot replace alveolar tissue (so bridge may cause aesthetic or speech problems).

Abutment teeth Teeth of small occlusogingival height unfavourable – as are tilted teeth, teeth with caries, endodontic problems,

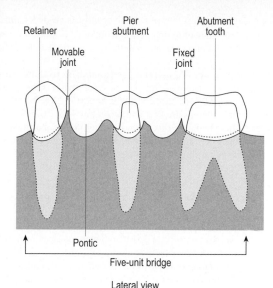

Figure 11.9 Bridge components.

perforations, periodontal disease. Require careful assessment as to suitability as an abutment.

Occlusion Deep overbites, evidence of severe bruxism and overeruption of opposing tooth into saddle are all unfavourable.

Support Bony support of abutment teeth and root morphology important.

Complications of bridgework

Short term • Traumatic periodontitis (occlusal imbalance) • pulpitis (following tooth preparation) • debonding (unretentive preparation) • 'sprung' retainer (bridge debonds from one abutment predisposing to caries under debonded retainer) • pain (irritant cement, pulpitis).

Long term • Loss of vitality of abutments • caries • periodontal disease • fracture of bridge component (e.g. porcelain facing) • 'sprung' retainer • persistent debonding • abutment mobility (excessive loading).

Care with case selection and attention to detail in clinical stages can reduce incidence of complications and failures.

Ante's Law

This law states: 'The combined pericemental area of the abutment teeth should be equal or greater than the pericemental area of the tooth or teeth to be replaced.'

In bridgework this is a useful 'rule of thumb' as to suitability of teeth as abutments. There is evidence, however, that it is the quality and not quantity of bone support that is important. Teeth with large pericemental areas are first and second molars, canines, premolars. These teeth are often good-quality bridge abutments. Teeth with small pericemental areas include upper lateral incisors, lower incisors; not optimal as abutment teeth for bridgework.

Pontic design

Pontic design is extremely important for good aesthetics and hygiene.

Broad principles of pontic design

Occlusal surfaces As narrow as possible to prevent excessive force on abutments (posterior teeth).

Buccal and palatal lingual surfaces Should be in same plane as surfaces of adjacent teeth to be in harmony with cleansing action of lips/cheeks/tongue.

Contact angle Angle of pontic to gingivae – contact should be as wide as possible to prevent food stagnation.

Contact area Where pontic joins mucosa should be as small as possible.

Mucosal contact Avoid concave contacts as patient cannot clean under them.

Interdental spaces (embrasures) Narrow spaces should be avoided. Space should be available for cleaning by an interdental brush or superfloss.

Material in contact with mucosa In a metal–ceramic bridge, mucosal contact should be with glazed porcelain.

A commonly used anterior pontic (*modified ridge lap*) is shown in Figure 11.10. An all-gold posterior pontic (sanitary pontic) is shown in Figure 11.11.

Retainers

Many types of retainers are used in bridgework. Factors influencing choice of retainer include: • retention required • occlusogingival height of abutment teeth • quality and quantity of dentine remaining after preparation • existing restorations in the tooth • the amount of metal that can be seen without compromising aesthetics • requirement for cusp or incisal protection.

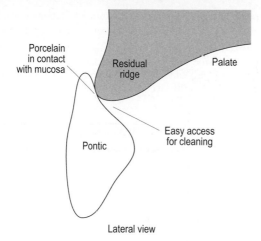

Figure 11.10 Anterior pontic design (modified ridge lap).

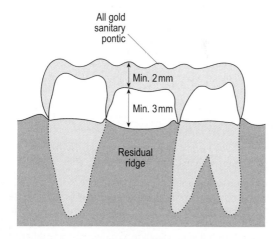

Figure 11.11 Posterior pontic design (sanitary pontic).

Usual retainers are • full-veneer gold crowns (posterior teeth)
• metal–ceramic crowns (anterior teeth).

Other retainers used include • three-quarter crowns (rarely)
• adhesive crowns/porcelain veneers/porcelain jacket crowns (for
all-porcelain bridges) • inlays/pinlays (in declining use) • telescopic
or milled crowns (for tilted teeth).

CONVENTIONAL FIXED–FIXED BRIDGE

> All joints are cast (or soldered) in one piece to connect
> abutment teeth rigidly.

Crown preparation has been discussed previously (p. 254). Only
difference in fixed–fixed bridge is the need to parallel the abutments
to achieve a common path of insertion of the bridge. This may
necessitate over-tapering of a tooth surface in teeth which are
slightly tilted in relation to each other.

Clinical procedures
1. *Abutment preparation* Tooth preparation should be undertaken
   after planning the prosthesis as the amount of preparation will
   vary according to design: • metal occlusal surface (less tooth
   reduction occlusally) • porcelain occlusal surface (more tooth
   reduction occlusally) • metal collar (chamfer margin buccally)
   • porcelain shoulder (wider buccal shoulder).
2. *Impressions* Elastomeric impression of abutments, often with
   the use of gingival retraction cord. In extensive bridgework,
   individual tray or reversible hydrocolloid may be needed.
   Subgingival preparations may need tissue management with
   electrosurgery before impression. Alginate or elastomeric
   impression of opposing arch is required.
3. *Occlusal registration* Recorded in either wax or
   polyvinylsiloxane; in extensive bridgework, mount casts on a
   semi-adjustable articulator using facebow registration.
4. *Shade taking* Individual teeth in a bridge may have different
   shades.
5. *Temporary bridge* Can be made at the chairside or in the
   laboratory. Laboratory-fabricated are more satisfactory as
   made in heat-cured acrylic and stronger.
6. *Try-in of casting* In extensive bridgework it is sometimes useful
   to try in the metal casting as it may need to be sectioned and
   relocated.

7. ***Checks prior to bridge cementation*** The following should be carefully checked: • marginal fit • occlusion • aesthetics • contact points • access for oral hygiene measures • speech.
8. ***Trial cementation*** In most cases it is advisable to cement the bridge temporarily for a short time (1–2 weeks). Thus if problems arise bridge can be removed and modified.
9. ***Final cementation*** Undertaken usually with conventional luting cement, e.g. glass ionomer, zinc polycarboxylate. Can sandblast, tin plate and use composite or chemically active resins with metal bonding components. A postcementation radiograph is useful as baseline data for further review.
10. ***Review*** At usual check-up times bridges should be carefully assessed for oral hygiene, carious margins, debonding from retainers, periodontal support. Periodic radiographs are useful for early detection of caries, endodontic or periodontal problems involving abutment teeth.

Life span: 10–15 years.

CANTILEVER BRIDGE

This type of bridge has a pontic connected to a retainer at one end only.

Indications • Low occlusal loads • replacement of lateral incisors with canine as abutment • replacement of one premolar (often pontic is merely an aesthetic facing) • can use twin abutments, e.g. first molar and second premolar as abutments to first premolar.
Advantages • One abutment does not require parallelism • more conservative of tooth tissue.
Disadvantage • Excess force on abutment.

FIXED–MOVABLE BRIDGES

A fixed–movable bridge has a joint allowing limited movement between pontic and retainer.

Uses
Malaligned abutment teeth Use of a joint allows for differing paths of insertion, e.g. mesially tilted lower molar.

Pier abutment In long-span bridgework where there are three abutments, the centre abutment acts as a fulcrum and is subjected to large occlusal forces. Addition of a joint reduces load on the pier abutment tooth.

Retrievability In long-span bridgework incorporation of a joint enables part of the bridge to be removed should one retainer fail, avoiding the need to replace the complete bridge.

Combination of materials e.g. mesial part of bridge metal–ceramic; distal gold. Allows combination of materials without solder joint.

Mobile teeth If one abutment is mobile, may help dissipate unfavourable forces.

Joints

Laboratory made Simplest is tube lock.

Precision attachments Can be intracoronal or extracoronal. A wide variety exist.

Fixed–movable bridges offer an alternative to fixed bridgework. The joint, however, builds in complexity and if a precision attachment is used, sufficient occlusogingival height is required.

These bridges are very successful but case selection is critical.

SPRING CANTILEVER BRIDGES

Support a pontic at some distance from the retainer. A gold bar which is in contact with palatal mucosa connects pontic to retainer. Rarely used.

Indications Replacing spaced anterior teeth.

Design Retainer usually one or two premolars or a single molar. Connector should be oval in shape for cleansing. Bridge should be rigid near retainer and flexible near pontic.

Careful case selection is important. This is not an ideal prosthesis as it results in an area of mucosa permanently covered by the bar.

ADHESIVE BRIDGES

Modern adhesive bridgework relies on the micromechanical bonding of composite resin or chemically active resin to etched enamel and etched or sandblasted metal.

Case selection

• Short span • Sound enamel available • Favourable occlusion (minimal or no overbite) • Small occlusal forces (no bruxism) • Intermediate restoration. • Missing lateral incisors. • Young patients with large pulps • 'Virgin' abutment teeth. • Splinting teeth.

Modern types of adhesive bridges

Unperforated framework Most commonly used. Relies on micromechanical bonding, e.g. Maryland bridge.

Perforated framework Relies on macromechanical retention, e.g. Rochette bridge.

Temporary Uses either natural tooth or acrylic or composite as a pontic.

Design of bridge

Most commonly, unperforated frameworks are used. Cover maximum area of available enamel – 180° wrap around. Currently debate over whether enamel needs preparation, particularly in young patients.

Using two abutments increases torquing forces on least mobile tooth so bridge may 'spring'. Therefore design is often cantilevered off single abutment tooth. There is currently great debate as to whether one or two abutments is the design of choice.

Anterior design Incorporate largest area of enamel without compromising aesthetics. Need 0.5 mm occlusal clearance, supragingival chamfer margin, guide planes mesially and distally, parallel grooves mesially and distally along path of insertion, cingulum rest.

Posterior design Similar to anterior design, except uses mesial and distal occlusal rests rather than cingulum rests. Maximize axial wall enamel incorporated in design.

Clinical tips

The bridge should be tried in and assessed for fit, aesthetics and occlusion prior to cementation. Do not extend preparation too far incisally as incisal edges will look grey. After cementation *do not* polish without water coolant as this reduces bond strength.

Preparation of metal surface For bonding to resin, the metal substructure of the adhesive bridge must be treated by one of the following methods:

Electrolytic or chemical etching Uses hydrofluoric acid in the laboratory. Bond may be severely compromised by salivary contamination so very technique sensitive.

Sandblasting Sandblasting with 50–150 µm aluminium oxide gives some degree of micromechanical retention; sandblasted surface is more robust than etched surface.

Cementation To ensure good moisture control this is best performed under rubber dam.

Types of cements available

Composite resins Low-viscosity microfilled composite resins (autopolymerizing or dual-cured with thin film thickness) can be used for cementation. Enamel should be etched with phosphoric acid and an unfilled resin used for bonding.

Chemically active resins Metal pretreatment with 4-META (4-methacryloxyethyl trimellilite anhydride) improves bonding. Chemically active resins typically have a monomer with a phosphate group and bond well to a sandblasted surface.

Recementing debonded adhesive bridges An assessment should be made as to why the bridge has debonded, check occlusion, look critically at the preparation, consider other treatment options – a conventional bridge may be more appropriate.

The tooth should be cleaned, the bridge ultrasonically cleaned and re-sandblasted before recementation.

Life span: Mean survival time 7.5 years. Unperforated framework more successful than perforated framework. Cantilever adhesive bridges also perform well.

TOOTH WEAR

Tooth wear is also known as tooth surface loss, non-carious tooth surface loss and non-bacterial tooth surface loss.

AETIOLOGY OF TOOTH WEAR

Tooth wear comprises *attrition, abrasion, erosion and abfraction.* These are often interrelated. Wear is much worse where more than one aspect is present simultaneously.

Tooth wear is increasing in prevalence and affects both adults and children. In the future, the effects of tooth wear will present many restorative challenges as individuals retain their teeth for longer.

> Attrition is the loss of tooth substance by wear due to mastication or contact between occluding surfaces.

Aetiology of attrition

- Bruxism (grinding, clenching).
- Lack of posterior support and occlusal collapse.
- Salivary flow and composition.
- Compromised tooth structure (amelogenesis/dentinogenesis imperfecta).

It is unknown why people brux. Several factors are involved, although the relative importance has not been established.

Factors involved in bruxism • psychogenic • genetic • local • systemic • occupational • instinctive (thegosis).

> Abrasion is the loss of tooth substance by wear due to factors other than tooth contact.

Aetiology of abrasion

• Aggressive oral hygiene techniques (toothbrush, toothpaste, interdental cleaning) • habitual chewing (pens/pencils, fingernails, nut shells) • occupational chewing (electrical wire, fishing line, ironmongery, etc.).

> Erosion is the progressive loss of hard dental tissues by a chemical process not involving bacterial action.

Bulk loss of surface enamel when pH < 4.5 (c.f. caries which is initially subsurface loss prior to cavitation).

Aetiology of erosion

• Acidic diet (carbonated drinks, fruit juices, citrus fruits, alcopops, white wine, cider, fruit teas, pickled foods, mouthwashes) • acid regurgitation (bulimia nervosa, gastrointestinal problems, chronic alcoholism, morning sickness) • industrial processes (armament production, battery workers) • medical problems (compulsive achievers, 'chewing the cud') • leisure activities (swimming) • tooth structure • salivary flow and salivary composition.

In over 30% of cases it will not be possible to elicit any significant aetiological factor in individuals displaying tooth wear.

Abfraction

Abfraction is loss of cervical hard tissue due to occlusal overloading. Possibly a form of stress corrosion involving interaction between occlusal loading and erosion.

DIAGNOSIS AND ASSESSMENT OF TOOTH WEAR

Case history A detailed case history should be taken to determine the nature of the problem, including: • patient's view of the nature of the problem • duration of the problem and whether or not in the patient's view the problem is ongoing • history and longevity of current restorations • assessment of aetiological factors (take diet history) • patient concerns over appearance, function or pain.

Clinical examination Clinical examination in cases of tooth wear should pay particular attention to the following: • occlusogingival height of worn teeth • lack of posterior support • overeruption of teeth • occlusal assessment • assessment of freeway space • craniomandibular disorders • state of existing restorations.

Additional information, particularly in assessment of the occlusion, is often required in complex tooth wear cases. Occlusal assessment involves: • study casts • use of mounted casts on a semi-adjustable articulator • diagnostic wax-ups of possible occlusal schemes • trial occlusal adjustments on mounted casts.

Assessment Once a detailed history and examination have taken place the following questions should be considered: • What are the immediate problems or concerns of the patient? • Can these be addressed? • Does the patient have unrealistic expectations? • What are the major aetiological factor(s)? • Can the aetiological factors be modified to give a long-term satisfactory outcome? • Is intervention desirable? • Is the patient capable of undergoing a complex restorative treatment plan or would a simple approach be better? • Is the scope of the problem within the clinician's capabilities?

Answering these questions will enable the clinician to decide upon a management strategy that may include appropriate monitoring, initial treatment, definitive treatment or referral.

Measurement of tooth wear Tooth wear is often measured subjectively. Various indices exist which are used primarily for research, e.g. Smith and Knight tooth wear index.

Prevention of tooth wear

A detailed wear history and establishment of a diagnosis is important in the prevention of tooth wear.

Practical aspects of tooth wear prevention

Dietary advice Patients should be advised to reduce carbonated drink intake (including 'diet/light' drinks); avoid excessive intake of citrus fruits, pure fruit juices and acidic dilutable drinks. Avoid chewing very abrasive foods. Remember not only is the frequency of consumption important, the pattern of consumption may result in prolonged exposure to acid, e.g. drinking a can of beverage very quickly or sipping it over a period of hours.

Oral hygiene Brushing within 30 minutes of exposure to erosive agents will remove more softened enamel/dentine. Advise patients to brush before meals rather than after (esp. breakfast).

Fluoride Daily use of a fluoride mouthwash encourages fluorapatite formation (p. 159).

Splint therapy Useful where attrition is the main aetiological factor. Splints may be *hard* or *soft* and can be made for *upper* or *lower* arches. It is unclear if the splint acts as a habit breaker for bruxism or is merely a damage limitation exercise as the splint wears in preference to tooth substance. Splints may be worn night-time, daytime, full time or during periods of the day when bruxism is known to occur (often stress/anxiety related).

Hypnotherapy Occasionally used to eliminate bruxism.

Tricyclic antidepressants Often useful, using their side effect of muscle relaxation, in the prevention of further bruxism; may also help with underlying psychological problems. Need to liaise with patient's General Medical Practitioner.

Monitoring tooth wear

Need to decide if tooth wear is excessive relative to patient's age. Monitoring of patients experiencing tooth wear is important to determine if the wear is progressive and in deciding the timing of treatment. Merely observing a patient's dentition periodically is insufficient to detect small changes in wear. Progression can be evaluated using serial study casts and clinical photography.

Management of tooth wear

Definitive management options are extremely varied. In general the following basic principles apply:

1. Control aetiological factors (avoid; use straw with carbonated drinks).
2. Modify oral health practices (brush before meals).
3. Pain and caries control.
4. Period of observation to determine if wear is progressing.
5. Provisional intervention:
   – provision of posterior support, e.g. partial dentures
   – increase in vertical dimension, e.g. splint, temporary denture.
6. Definitive rehabilitation:
   – direct composite palatal veneers, using Dahl approach if limited space
   – crown restorations
   – definitive dentures/overdentures.
7. Review.

Frequently an increase in the vertical dimension of occlusion is required. This should be provided in a reversible manner in the first instance.

Tooth wear failures

A small proportion of patients (particularly bruxists) fail to control aetiology despite rehabilitation. Over a period of years these patients present with a number of failures, including porcelain debonding from metal, root fracture, bent/fractured posts and cracked cusps.

Failure can be reduced by attention to detail when treatment planning. Where possible avoid multiple anterior post retained crowns in bruxists and use metal occlusal surfaces in crown restorations.

BLEACHING

Bleaching techniques aim to whiten darkened/discoloured teeth. Approach differs for vital and non-vital teeth.

CAUSES OF STAINING

- *Extrinsic* – tobacco, dietary tea and coffee, chlorhexidine.
- *Intrinsic* – trauma, hypocalcification, tetracycline, other systemic causes.
- *Age related* – secondary dentine formation.

Chemistry

Most products are based on either hydrogen peroxide or carbamide peroxide (also known as urea peroxide). Ten per cent carbamide peroxide will break down to 3.35% hydrogen peroxide and 6.65% urea. This means that for similar concentration products, hydrogen peroxide is the stronger bleaching agent.

Mechanisms of action

Bleaching agents diffuse through porous enamel.
Oxidation – larger chromogens broken down into smaller molecules that reflect less light.
Whitening/bleaching of tooth structure – especially of dentine.
Most teeth seem to bleach to a terminal point (often Vita shade B1).

CLINICAL TECHNIQUES

Techniques depend on whether tooth is vital or non-vital.

Vital teeth

This is potentially a huge growth area in dentistry. The options available are:

- Over-the-counter (OTC) products
- Professional home-use products.
- Professional surgery applied products.

Over-the-counter products

A variety of OTC products are available, including paint-on products and bleaching gel applied in 'boil and bite' bleaching trays. White strips (currently only available in USA) contain small amounts of hydrogen peroxide in a plastic strip or bandage that is wrapped over the upper or lower anterior teeth worn for 30 min twice a day. Usually effective in about 2 weeks.

Whitening toothpastes contain high levels of detergents, but will only remove extrinsic stains.

Professional home-use products

Also known as nightguard vital bleaching. Bleaching gel contains up to 15% peroxide together with thickening agents (carbopol), colourants and desensitizing agents (e.g. potassium nitrate).

Applied for 2–3 hours per day for 2–3 weeks using custom fabricated bleaching tray.

Technique

1. Preop assessment; shade guide/photos/check allergies/warn patient that composite restorations will need replacing.
2. Alginate impression.
3. Bleaching tray adapted to gingival margins constructed with labial reservoirs.
4. Check tray for fit and comfort; advise to use 2–3 hours per day; warn patient about possible transient sensitivity (affects up to 75% of patients); avoid chromogenic food/drink for 2 hours post-treatment.
5. Professional prophylaxis prior to first use.
6. Review weekly; usually takes 2–3 weeks to complete.

Notes

Technique totally reliant on patient compliance.

Need 2-week period post-bleaching before replacing composites (residual oxygen causes transient reduction in bond strength).

May need 'top-up' every 2–3 years.

Sensitivity management use desensitizing toothpaste applied topically, fluoride mouthwash, reduce time tray is worn, reduce frequency (bleach every other day).

Tetracycline staining is a special case; may need to bleach for up to 6 months depending on intensity of discoloration.

Professional surgery applied products

Also known as 'power bleaching'.

These techniques use much higher concentrations of hydrogen peroxide (up to 35%) in the surgery. Due to the higher concentrations, bleaching is much quicker (approx. 1 hour), but the soft tissues *must* be protected from the corrosive peroxide. Use either rubber dam or flowable composite applied to marginal gingivae.

Technique often includes application of light (visible light/xenon–halogen/blue laser light). Claimed that light will accelerate breakdown of peroxide and heat generated by light will enhance penetration and chemical reaction rate of peroxide. Little evidence to show that light has significant additional benefit.

Technique

1. Preop assessment; shade guide/photos/check allergies/warn patient that composite restorations will need replacing.
2. Prophylaxis with pumice and water.
3. Protect gingivae either with sealed rubber dam or paint on dam (flowable composite).
4. Activate hydrogen peroxide liquid and prepare fresh mix of bleaching gel.
5. Apply to teeth in smile zone 2–3 mm thick.
6. Activate with light, if using.
7. May need to repeat 2–3 times over 1 hour.

Notes

Sensitivity – use fluoride gel or potassium nitrate containing toothpaste applied topically.

May need to supply top-up home kit as shade regression is common.

Avoid chromogenic food/drink and warn about shade regression with time.

Avoid replacing composite restorations *for at least 2 weeks*.

Non-vital teeth

Options include:

- Chairside bleaching.
- Walking bleach technique.
- Inside–outside bleaching.

Preoperative assessment Regardless of technique, the status of the root filling needs to be assessed with a periapical radiograph. Replace if defective.

Chairside bleaching

1. Remove restoration obturating access cavity and any obvious grossly stained dentine.
2. Apply rubber dam and seal margins with varnish or unfilled resin (do *not* etch enamel).

3. Cut back coronal gutta-percha to just below gingival level (check with perio probe) and seal with thin layer of GIC/polycarboxylate.
4. Etch dentine with phosphoric acid gel for 30–60 s to remove smear layer and open up dentinal tubules. Wash and dry.
5. Load cotton wool pledget with 30% hydrogen peroxide and place in coronal pulp chamber.
6. Apply heat using flat plastic or similar.
7. Repeat 5 or 6 times.

Walking bleach technique

1. Remove palatal restoration, apply rubber dam and seal coronal access cavity as for chairside bleaching.
2. Combine 35% hydrogen peroxide with sodium perborate to give thick consistency.
3. Etch dentine with phosphoric acid gel for 30–60 s to remove smear layer and open up dentinal tubules. Wash and dry.
4. Apply peroxide/perborate mix to coronal dentine and seal in place using cotton wool pledget and GIC/polycarboxylate.
5. Review in 1 week; may need to repeat 3 or 4 times.
6. Restore with dentine-bonded composite.

Inside–outside bleaching

1. Provide patient with bleaching tray (see *Professional home-use products* above).
2. Remove restoration from palatal access cavity and seal coronal access cavity as for chairside bleaching.
3. Patient applies bleaching gel labially and to palatal access cavity for 2–3 hours per day.
4. Restore with dentine-bonded composite once desired colour change achieved.

MICROABRASION

Used for improving appearance of mottled enamel (usually due to fluorosis). Works best when mottled enamel is superficial and with yellow or light brown stains. Opaque white spots do not generally respond to microabrasion, but bleaching techniques (above) may help mask appearance.

Technique

1. Apply rubber dam.
2. Etch enamel with phosphoric acid for 60 s.
3. Carefully remove surface layer of enamel using abrasive discs (e.g. Soflex) or using a slurry of pumice and glycerine with a prophy brush.
4. Repeat as necessary taking care to avoid exposing dentine.
5. Apply topical fluoride.

ENDODONTICS

Endodontics involves treatment of the dental pulp.

Causes of pulpal damage
• Dental caries • trauma • periodontal disease • damage during operative procedures.

Diagnosis
Diagnosis of pulpal damage involves a comprehensive pain history (p. 232). In addition, special tests are often required to ascertain a correct diagnosis: • percussion testing of teeth • vitality testing of teeth (heat/cold/electric) • periapical radiographs.

CONVENTIONAL ROOT CANAL THERAPY

Conventional root canal therapy is undertaken for non-vital teeth, dying teeth, teeth where the pulps are so badly damaged that the pulp must be removed if the tooth is to remain in function and elective treatment where the root canal must be treated for the crown to be restored.

Aims of root canal treatment
• To cleanse the pulp cavity of infected debris, toxic materials and pulpal remnants. • To seal the pulp cavity apically, periodontally and coronally. • To maintain the tooth in function.

Instrumentation

There are many instruments in use in root canal treatment. Commonly used instruments include:

Files Used to widen the root canal, e.g. K flex files, K files and Hedström files (Figure 11.12). Files may be hand held or operated in a handpiece or ultrasonic handpiece.

Rotary files Used to widen the root canal, especially the coronal part, e.g. Rotary files of greater taper, safety Hedström files. Files should be used correctly in speed-reducing handpieces and not autoclaved too many times (leads to instrument fracture within canals).

Broaches These instruments, e.g. barbed broach, are used for vital tissue removal. Use with care – liable to fracture.

Side-cutting burs Used for preparation of the coronal two-thirds of the root canal.

Spiral paste fillers Used for placing sealer or intracanal dressings into the pulp cavity. Use with care – liable to fracture.

Spreaders and compactors Used in root canal obturation.

Instruments are usually standardized and colour coded (Table 11.3).

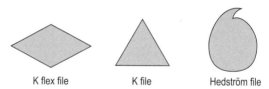

K flex file   K file   Hedström file

Figure 11.12 Cross-section of common file types.

TABLE 11.3 Dimensions and colour coding in endodontic instruments

Colour	Tip diameter (mm)	Size
White	0.15	015
Yellow	0.20	020
Red	0.25	025
Blue	0.30	030
Green	0.35	035
Black	0.40	040

Standardized files have a taper of 0.02 mm/mm and range in size from 008 to 140.

Rubber dam

 Rubber dam isolation is ESSENTIAL in modern root canal treatment.

See page 174.

Access cavity preparation

Knowledge of dental anatomy is essential for appropriate access cavity preparation.

Maxillary and mandibular canines and incisors Access cavity should permit straight-line access to within 1 mm of the apex. Ideally access cavity is close to incisal edge on the palatal or lingual surface of tooth. Triangular shape with broadest portion incisally. Mandibular incisors may need access through incisal edge. Access through Class III cavities results in sharp instrument bends and is not recommended.

Maxillary and mandibular premolars Access cavities should be ovoid buccolingually and through the occlusal surface.

Maxillary molars Access cavities should be through the occlusal surface, triangular in nature, with the base of the triangle buccally and the apex palatally.

Mandibular molars Access cavities should be through the occlusal surface, triangular in shape, with the base of the triangle mesially and the apex distally. Occasionally need to remove mesiobuccal cusp to access mesiobuccal canal.

Working length determination

Working length is usually determined by estimating a length from the preoperative radiograph. Length of a canal may be finalized by:

Working length radiograph Using files of known length to a stable reference point. Multiple radiographs of multirooted teeth may be required to show all roots.

Electronic apex locators Able to accurately assess working length in both wet and dry canals (e.g. Apit, Apex Finder AFA, Justy, Raypex, Root ZX). Need to be used in conjunction with working length radiograph.

During instrumentation of curved canals, working length must be reassessed as it may change as a canal straightens.

TECHNIQUES FOR CANAL PREPARATION

Options are:

- manual preparation with ISO instruments
- manual preparation with increased taper instruments
- rotary preparation.

Regardless of preparation technique, it is useful to initially open the canal system using size 15–35 K files then irrigate and check for patency.

Manual preparation with ISO instruments

Three common techniques are described:

- step back
- step down
- balanced force.

Step-back technique In this technique the working length to the apical constriction is determined and the canal filed to the apex using a master apical file (MAF). Further larger files are inserted in an incremental step back, 1 mm coronally in the canal each time, recapitulating to the working length with the MAF. Good technique for straight, simple canals. For example, if MAF is size 030 at 21 mm, file sequence will be 030 to 21 mm; 035 to 20 mm; 030 to 21 mm; 040 to 19 mm; 030 to 21 mm; 045 to 18 mm and so on.

Step-down technique Principles are: • coronal access • then radicular access • then apical instrumentation.

Technique Gain coronal access. Radicular access with 015–025 Hedström files with an up-and-down action (away from furca in multi-trooted teeth), together with side-cutting burs. Step-back technique at apex.

Advantages • Straighter access to apex • removal of dentinal interferences • bulk of coronal bacteria removed before apical instrumentation • working length less likely to change during apical instrumentation as canal curvature has already been reduced • allows deeper penetration of irrigating solutions • good for molars.

Balanced force technique Introduced by Roane in 1985.

Technique

1. K-file introduced into canal system using clockwise motion with no apical pressure.
2. File rotated anticlockwise with downward pressure (cutting stroke) – this balances force with which file wants to back out of canal. This is usually accompanied by a 'click' as dentine shears.
3. File turned quarter-turn clockwise with no pressure to remove debris.

Advantages • Circular preparation in centre of tooth • Little risk of ledging and transportation • Efficient cutting.

Manual preparation with increased taper instruments

This approach uses files of nickel–titanium (NiTi), which give:
• increased flexibility • can rotate in canals with reduced risk of fracture

NiTi Greater Taper (GT) files have:

● four different tapers; 0.12 (blue), 0.10 (red), 0.08 (yellow) and 0.06 (white)
● taper 3–6 times greater than standard ISO files
● size 20 non-cutting tip
● large pear-shaped handles to apply high rotational forces.

Technique

1. Initially open canal system using size 15–35 K files, then irrigate.
2. Use GT files in sequence 0.12 (blue), 0.10 (red), 0.08 (yellow) and 0.06 (white) using crown down approach. Files are used with clockwise balanced-force motion.
3. Once apical third is reached, stop instrumentation and determine working length.
4. Use standard NiTi instruments at working length to gauge canal diameter and complete apical preparation.

Rotary preparation

There are a number of rotatory NiTi systems available, including tapered systems (GT systems, K3, Hero 642 and ProTaper) and one taperless system (Lightspeed).

All these systems are slightly different and practitioners should become familiar with their chosen system in the laboratory before clinical use.

However, there are a number of points that are common to all:

- Access must be straight.
- Speed of rotation is critical and can be maintained with torque-controlled motors.
- Instruments should be fed into the canal system with low-amplitude up-down movements.
- No instrument should be in the canal for more than 5 s before being removed and inspected.
- Instruments should be kept constantly moving.

Root canal cleansing

Cleansing of a root canal is essential for successful root canal treatment. Cleansing disinfects the canal contents, flushes out debris, in some cases dissolves organic debris and softens dentine.

Cleansing is achieved by irrigating solutions into the root canal either endosonically or using a syringe with a 27 gauge needle and an endodontic tip (which has a side perforation to reduce risk of cleansing fluid being forced through the apex). Solutions which may be used are as follows:

Sodium hypochlorite solution Most commonly used cleanser, effective antibacterial action. Commonly used at 1–5% concentration.
Ethylenediamine tetra-acetic acid (EDTA) Removes smear layer.
EDTA and urea peroxide Releases nascent oxygen.
EDTA and sodium hypochlorite.
Saline.
Chlorhexidine.

Copious amounts of irrigant should be used for root canal cleansing.

Intracanal dressings

Inter-visit dressings are frequently required. After instrumentation, canals should be dried with paper points. Non-setting calcium hydroxide is the material of choice as an inter-visit intracanal dressing. Other materials in use include 35% solution of camphorated monochlorophenol and betamethasone (anti-inflammatory, antiseptic), 1% triamcinolone and 3% dimethylchlortetracycline paste (used for hyperaemic pulps). Coronally 3 mm of temporary dressing is required to obtain an adequate seal.

Root canal obtuation

Obturation of the root canal implies occlusion of the canal and accessory and lateral canals in order to prevent the movement into or out of the canal of tissue fluids, micro-organisms and toxins (hermetic seal).

Criteria for root canal obturation Canal must be dry and must usually be symptom free.

Materials used for root canal obturation Although many materials have been used for root canal obturation (e.g. silver points, absorbable pastes), root canals are most commonly obturated with gutta-percha and sealer.

Gutta-percha Available as cones (standardized or non-standardized), thermoplasticized.

Sealers Gutta-percha alone does not provide an adequate seal; therefore, sealers are required. Sealers may be based on calcium hydroxide, zinc oxide–eugenol, resin, glass ionomer or PVC.

Common obturation techniques

Laterally condensed cold gutta-percha Extension of single cone technique. Single cone fits only in apical 2 mm. Unfilled spaces are obturated around the master gutta-percha cone with accessory cones. Create space by using a spreader. Useful for ovoid canals. Time consuming.

Vertically condensed hot gutta-percha (Schilder's technique) Uses heat to plasticize gutta-perch, which is then vertically condensed to create a homogenous root canal filling of greater density, especially apically. A heat carrier (pointed root canal spreader) is heated until cherry red then plunged 3–4 mm into the gutta-percha and the softened material is condensed apically with a series of pluggers. Requires a wide preparation in the coronal third of the tooth, which may complicate subsequent tooth restoration.

Hybrid technique Combination of lateral and vertical condensation.
  Laterally condensed warm gutta-percha same as cold lateral condensation, except that a warmed spreader is used.

Thermomechanical compaction of gutta-percha Uses an Archimedean screw at 8000 rpm to provide frictional heat. Technically difficult procedure. Can be used only in straight portion of a canal. Generates lots of heat.

Thermoplasticized gutta-percha Uses alpha gutta-percha, which is tacky and flows better than normal (beta) gutta-percha. Uses inserts made of plastic, titanium or stainless steel. Requires slow-setting sealer.

Injection techniques with thermoplasticized gutta-percha Can be either high heat (>160°C) or low heat (<75°C). Marked shrinkage as cools. Problem with extruding gutta-percha through apex.

There is no ideal obturation technique for all situations. An appropriate technique should be chosen, depending on individual clinical situation.

Successful root canal treatment
For a root canal treatment to be deemed successful the tooth must be: • functional • symptom-free • of normal radiographic appearance with complete bony infill of radiolucencies • periodontium of normal radiographic appearance.

Restoration of the root canal treated tooth
Previous restoration and access cavity often leaves a root-filled tooth compromised. Coronal leakage is a major factor in failed root canal treatment so a sound coronal restoration is important.

The amount of tooth substance remaining and its ability to withstand occlusal loads should be assessed. In the absence of sufficient sound dentine, a post crown restoration should be considered.

Single-visit root canal treatment
Conventionally, root canal treatment is carried out over 2–3 visits. This is time consuming for the patient and often clinically unnecessary.

Indications for single-visit root canal treatment
• Elective root canal treatment • apical radiolucency but draining sinus present • patient requiring antibiotic cover for medical reasons • irreversible pulpitis.

Disadvantages Emergency treatment for drainage is complicated by presence of a root canal filling, appointment may be too protracted for patient (especially curved canals in molars).

Contraindications • Excessive exudates • symptom-free teeth with periapical radiolucencies and no sinus (these often cause acute symptoms after first visit).

Problems in conventional root canal therapy
Fractured instruments More likely with small-sized instruments, incorrect filing techniques (e.g. 'watchwinding'), old

work-hardened instruments, instruments autoclaved too many times, incorrect handpiece used for rotary instruments. Removal can be attempted with endosonics or further filing. Removal not always possible!

Perforation May occur due to over-instrumentation of apex, furcal perforation during access cavity preparation and perforation of concave surface of curved molar roots during filing. Can be repaired using mineral trioxide aggregate (MTA) using an intracanal approach. Alternatively, may be repaired by surgical endodontics. Perforation may be a cause of postappointment pain.

Zipping (or transportation) Occurs by using straight large files in curved canals. Minimized by instrument precurving and use of files with blunt tips.

Failures 95% of root canal treatments can be successful if appropriate techniques are chosen and followed. Common causes of root canal treatment failure include breakdown of coronal restoration, inadequate cleansing, shaping or obturation and root fracture.

Pulp therapy in deciduous teeth and permanent teeth with open apices is discussed on pages 180–184.

SURGICAL ENDODONTICS

PERIRADICULAR SURGERY (INCLUDING APICECTOMY)

> Apicectomy is the surgical removal of the root apex and surrounding tissue and is often combined with retrograde filling.

Surgical aspects of apicectomy are discussed on page 397.

Indications for apicectomy • Extreme canal curvature • sclerosed canal • inaccessible lateral canals • heavily restored tooth where root canal is occluded by a post which cannot be removed without risk to the tooth • fractured instrument in canal which cannot be removed by conventional means • root fracture of apical part of root • bay cyst • extruded root filling causing symptoms • open apex that cannot be sealed conventionally.

Apicectomy should be considered only for well-motivated patients with good oral hygiene and controlled caries. In addition the tooth to be apicected should be restorable after the procedure.

Retrograde root filling A good coronal seal is required so, before apicectomy, a sound orthograde root filling should be placed where possible. Sometimes a retrograde root filling is required. This involves preparation of a Class I cavity apically and restoration with reinforced zinc oxide–eugenol or MTA. Historically amalgam was used but this has fallen from favour.

Other types of procedures in surgical endodontics

Root amputation Used when one root is untreatable by conventional means. Root is sectioned and crown reshaped to be self-cleansing. Usually upper molars. May also be used if one root is periodontally involved.

Hemisection 'Premolarization', usually lower molars. Used when one root is untreatable conventionally. It is sectioned and extracted. May also be used if one root of a lower molar is periodontally involved.

Periapical curettage Similar to apicectomy, except leaves root apex intact.

'Through and through' root filling Combined orthograde root filling with periapical curettage; useful in lower incisors.

Reimplantation of teeth Replacement of tooth in socket after trauma. Light splinting is required for 1 week and conventional root treatment required. Complicated by root resorption.

Transplantation of teeth One tooth (immature) transplanted into a socket of another; fairly unsuccessful; often results in root resorption.

Incision and drainage of endodontically associated swellings Sound treatment for dental abscesses. Immediate relief of patient's symptoms.

Perforation repair Intracoronal repair using MTA is beginning to become treatment of choice for perforations and specific instruments are available to help place the MTA. Alternatively, this can be attempted surgically or by a combined approach; orthograde root filling through perforation then immediately trimming surgically.

RELATIONSHIPS WITHIN RESTORATIVE DENTISTRY

Total patient care often requires a combined approach between the disciplines of fixed prosthodontics, removable prosthodontics, periodontology and endodontics. Of particular importance in integrated treatment planning are:

Endo-perio lesions

Endo-perio problems involve pulpal inflammation or necrosis associated with periodontal bone loss around the same tooth.

Endo-perio lesions arise as: • primary endodontic lesions • primary endodontic lesions with secondary periodontal involvement • primary periodontal lesions with secondary endodontic involvement • true mixed lesions – aetiology a combination of both primary causes.

In general, root canal treatment should be attempted first. Prognosis is best for primary endodontic lesions (p. 287).

Crowns and partial dentures

It is frequently the case that crowns are made before partial denture construction. It is imperative that the partial denture design is decided before crown construction. This enables the crowns to be constructed with appropriate rest seats, undercuts and guide planes or crowns to be milled so that the partial denture has improved retention, support, function and aesthetics.

Surgical crown lengthening

Used to increase the height of the clinical crown prior to restoration where occlusogingival height is small.

Indications for this treatment include: • tooth wear cases • subgingival horizontal root fracture • subgingival caries or restoration margins.

Surgical technique involves bone removal and bone contouring of the alveolar crest.

Periodontal tissues need to heal for 3 months prior to definitive restorations.

CHAPTER 12

REMOVABLE PROSTHODONTICS

Treatment planning   300

Changes following
extraction of teeth   304

Complete dentures   304

Partial dentures   314

Precision attachments   321

Copy dentures   321

Overdentures   322

Immediate dentures   324

Other prosthetic
appliances   325

Repairs, relines and
additions   325

Craniomandibular
disorders   327

Implant borne
prostheses   330

Maxillofacial
prosthetics   336

The shortened dental
arch   337

Prescription to
technicians   338

Advice to patients   339

TREATMENT PLANNING

HISTORY TAKING

 Obtaining a comprehensive history is critical to the prescription of appropriate prosthodontic treatment.

Factors required in prosthodontic history

The general principles underlying taking a history apply (Chapter 2). The following are of particular relevance in relation to prosthodontics.

Patient complaints Appearance, function, problems with present or previous dentures, pain, retching, problems eating with prostheses, attitude to wearing a prosthesis.

Denture history Age of dentures? Are present dentures a matched set? When was first denture worn? How many sets of dentures worn? Material from which dentures constructed?

General dental history Presence of crowns, bridges, periodontal problems, orthodontic therapy, splints. Previous treatment tried for present complaint.

Medical history In particular look out for anxiety and depression, history of stroke, muscle disorders.

Social history Determine mobility, access for treatment.

EXAMINATION

Extraoral examination

In prosthodontics, extraoral examination may reveal many interesting features:

Signs of craniomandibular disorders such as joint clicking, masseteric hypertrophy, tenderness in joints or muscles of mastication.

Facial contours Loss of dental bulge, perioral wrinkles, angular cheilitis, vertical dimensions.

Overall aesthetics of dentures.

Intraoral examination

Mucosa Overall health of mucosa should be carefully checked. Features of particular relevance in prosthodontics include presence of xerostomia, denture-related candidal infection, ulceration, hyperplasia or lip/cheek chewing which may indicate active parafunction.

Periodontal health In partially dentate patients, oral hygiene, gingival condition, periodontal status, mobility and drifting of remaining teeth should be assessed.

Caries In partially dentate patients, teeth with active, recurrent or arrested caries should be identified.

Restorations The status of existing restorations should be assessed, and contour noted to determine suitability for retention or support.

Occlusion Particular attention should be paid to skeletal class, overerupted teeth, tilted teeth (buccal–lingual tilting as well as mesiodistal) and crowding or spacing.

Endodontic status Teeth should be confirmed as apically healthy or unhealthy, vital or non-vital prior to denture therapy.

Support of edentulous areas Determine the quality of support in saddle areas. The degree of resorption of bone should be noted. In addition anatomical features such as presence or absence of tori, tubercles, bony or flabby ridges or muscle attachments are important.

Denture examination

Present dentures (and in some cases previous dentures) should be examined both in and out of the mouth.

With existing dentures in situ consider • Is the freeway space appropriate? • Is the retruded contact position registered correctly? • Are the lips supported well? • Are both posterior and anterior occlusal planes in harmony? • Are the dentures retentive at rest? • Are the dentures stable in function? • Is there any pain on occlusion? • Does the patient like the appearance of the dentures? • Can the patient articulate properly with the dentures?

With existing dentures out of the mouth consider • Is the base extension appropriate? Dentures are frequently *underextended* in lingual pouches, retromolar pads and distally on the hard palate. Dentures are frequently *overextended* to the external oblique ridge of the mandible. • Is the tooth position appropriate? Common problems include excessive lingual positioning of posterior mandibular teeth and excessive labial positioning of anterior teeth. • Has the denture been altered since insertion? e.g. additions, relines, repairs or excessive adjusting. • Is there any sign of parafunction? e.g. wear in excess of denture age, wear facets.

Radiographic examination

Comprehensive radiographic examination, particularly of partially dentate patients, can reveal: • periodontal bone levels • caries

• apical pathology • retained roots and unerupted teeth • ridge contours • bone height and width • anatomical features such as nerve canals and foramina, maxillary sinus • temporomandibular joint anatomy.

Useful radiographs in prosthodontics are: periapicals, panoramics, occlusals, lateral cephalometric views and tomograms.

Additional features of prosthodontic examination

In some cases special tests are required. These are listed below:

Study casts Determine inter- and intra-arch relationships. Reveal overerupted or tilted teeth. Help in denture design. Can be used for individual tray construction. Outline difficult saddle areas.

Surveying Surveying of casts is useful in showing areas of undercut and determining potential paths of insertion, removal or displacement of prostheses. Useful in denture design.

Full occlusal assessment Determination of lateral jaw movements, etc., may be required using facebow mounting of a maxillary cast and the use of a semiadjustable articulator. Particularly useful in tooth wear and craniomandibular disorders.

Diagnostic wax-up May aid evaluation of alternatives. Can aid patient evaluation of options.

Digital photography Can help in assessment of aesthetic needs, planning and communication with technician.

DIAGNOSIS AND MANAGEMENT

A good history and thorough examination are crucial in making a sound diagnosis and effecting appropriate management of prosthodontic patients.

Diagnosis in edentulous patients

Patients fall into the following categories:

Good denture wearers whose dentures require replacement because they are worn, lost, broken, aesthetically poor or loose These patients usually have simple histories and present few prosthodontic problems.

Good denture wearers with poor dentures These patients have a good history but their present dentures often have a major fault, e.g. grossly excessive vertical dimension. Correction of the fault can often lead to success.

Poor denture wearers who, if provided with very well designed and constructed dentures, may tolerate their dentures These patients often have a history of many replacement dentures from different dentists, never being totally satisfied with dentures.

Poor denture wearers who do not tolerate dentures despite very well designed and constructed dentures These patients have complex histories and conventional prosthodontics can offer them little. Particularly in this group, look out for gross anatomical or support problems or a psychological problem. These patients require specialist care.

Diagnosis in partially dentate patients

Patients who are partially dentate differ in their response to dentures.

Important additional features of diagnosis in partially dentate patients include:

Design changes Changing a denture design may improve results, e.g. a cobalt-chrome denture rather than an acrylic denture; altering clasp positions.

Denture alternatives In partially dentate patients, fixed prosthodontics or implant-retained prosthodontics, or not wearing dentures at all, may in some cases solve denture problems.

Management

Preprosthetic management In general, caries, periodontal disease and major endodontic problems must be controlled prior to prosthesis construction. In some cases, temporary relines of existing dentures (when the mucosa is traumatized) or provision of occlusal pivots (for very worn dentures with collapsed occlusion) may be required to ensure ultimate success of a prosthesis. Preprosthetic and ongoing preventive advice is essential especially the reduction in sugary snacks and the use of topical fluoride.

> ⚠️ Remember – not treating is a sound option in prosthodontics. Just because there is a saddle does not mean there has to be a prosthesis, especially if there are no aesthetic or functional problems and the occlusion is stable or in harmony.

Management options in prosthodontics

Who? It must be decided who is the most appropriate person to make new dentures. Referral to a specialist for advice or treatment should be considered in difficult cases.

What? Take history, examination and diagnosis into account for decisions such as conventional or copy denture; acrylic or cobalt–chrome denture.

When? Sometimes delaying treatment is useful, e.g. to treat pre-existing mucosal infections; in craniomandibular disorders; whilst patient undergoes medical treatment; for patient personal commitments.

Where? Patient mobility must be assessed to determine whether a patient can be treated in a surgery or on a domiciliary basis.

How? Some cases are clinically and technically demanding, e.g. precision attachments. Dentists should ensure they and their technicians are familiar with protocols in individual cases.

CHANGES FOLLOWING EXTRACTION OF TEETH

Changes following extraction of teeth may be divided into three categories: facial, intraoral and psychological.

Facial changes • loss of the dental bulge • loss of lip support • 'witches chin' • lips fold inwards and look thinner.

Intraoral changes • loss of mandibular height – 9–10 mm over 25 years; 4 mm after 1 year • loss of maxillary height is one-quarter of loss of mandibular height • decreased masticatory performance • decreased proprioceptive ability • resorption of buccal bone width.

Psychological changes Some patients find edentulousness difficult to accept, perhaps as a sign of 'growing old'. Consequently some patients despise the thought of dentures and require careful management; indeed, some patients equate the effects of loss of their teeth to loss of a limb.

COMPLETE DENTURES

PRINCIPLES
Aims

Complete dentures should replace tissues and teeth in approximately the same quantities and positions from where the tissues and teeth have been lost. Complete dentures should fill the 'denture space'.

> **Denture space** is the space previously occupied by teeth and supporting tissues.

atures of complete dentures

hese comprise good retention, good support, good muscle balance, good occlusal balance and stability.

Retention

> **Retention** is the resistance to displacement of a denture away from the ridge.

Good retention gives psychological comfort. Retention requires intimate contact between denture and tissue. However, dentures can still be retained following resorptive changes, achieved by neuromuscular control. In the mandible the mobility of the floor of the mouth makes retention more difficult than in the maxilla.

Support

> **Support** is the resistance of vertical movement of a denture towards the ridge.

Support is the foundation on which a denture rests. Effective support requires: • the denture to cover the maximal surface area without moving or impinging on friable tissues • tissues most capable of resisting resorption to be selectively loaded during function • tissues most capable of resisting vertical displacement to be allowed to make firm contact with denture base during function • compensation to be made for different tissue resilience.

Primary and secondary support areas, areas to be relieved and non-compensatory support areas are shown in the maxilla (Figure 12.1) and the mandible (Figure 12.2). These may require modification in the presence of flabby ridges, prominent genial or mental tubercles, etc.

Muscle balance

> **Muscle balance** is achieved when the muscular forces of tongue, lips and cheeks do not dislodge a denture during functional movements of the mouth with the teeth out of contact.

Concave shapes of denture polished surfaces give a vertical seating force when buccinator contracts. A thinner denture flange

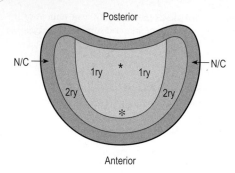

1ry = Primary support area (hard palate)
2ry = Secondary support area (ridge crest)
N/C = Non-contributing to support (denture border)
 * = Occasionally the midline suture and incisive papilla require relief

Figure 12.1 Support – complete maxillary denture.

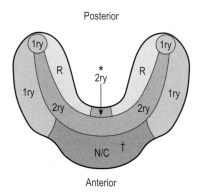

1ry = Primary support area (buccal shelf and pear-shaped pad)
2ry = Secondary support area (ridge crest and genial tubercles)
N/C = Non-contributing to support (labial ridge incline)
R = Relief area (lingual ridge incline and mylohyoid ridge)
 * = Requires relief in the presence of prominent genial tubercles
 † = May require relief in the presence of prominent mental tubercles

Figure 12.2 Support – complete mandibular denture.

. the premolar region results in more free movement of the
nodiolus (the site of muscle fibre decussation from buccinator and
orbicularis oris muscles).

Occlusal balance

> **Occlusal balance** is achieved when the forces of one denture
> on another do not dislodge either denture during functional
> jaw movements with the teeth in contact.

This can be achieved by a balanced articulation.

Stability

> **Stability** is the ability of a denture to resist displacement by
> functional stresses.

Stability gives physiological comfort.

DESIGN

Complete dentures in general should have the following design
features:

Maximal extension of denture base The complete denture should
cover the whole of the available denture-bearing area. In the
maxilla, extension posteriorly should lie just anterior to the line
of flexure of the soft palate. In the mandible, care should be
taken to extend the denture base into the retromolar pad and
posterior lingual sulci regions.

Peripheral seal This is an area of contact between mobile mucosa
and the denture surfaces and is determined at the master
impression stage. Good peripheral seal is important for retention
and stability.

Postdam A rounded smooth line at the junction of hard and soft
palate aids the peripheral seal of a maxillary denture.

Fraena An impression technique should be used to obtain fraenal
relief.

Relief areas Small tori, prominent mylohyoid ridges and prominent
mental nerve foramina often have to be relieved.

Retruded contact position Complete dentures should be registered
in the retruded contact position (the position of the mandible

when the condyles are in their most retruded position in the glenoid fossa) as this is the most reproducible position (p. 239).

Balanced articulation Complete dentures should aim to have balanced articulation, which is a continuous sliding contact of upper and lower cusps all around the dental arch during all closed grinding movements of the mandible.

Freeway space 2–4 mm of freeway space is a guide to restoration of the vertical dimension in complete denture patients although this varies depending on an individual's mandibular movements in speech.

Tooth position

Upper anterior Teeth should usually be set labial to the residual ridge. They should usually be 10 mm labial to the middle of the incisive papilla. About 2–3 mm of teeth should show when lips are apart and relaxed.

Lower anterior If there is little ridge resorption, teeth should be placed marginally in front of the ridge crest. In cases with lots of resorption, teeth should be placed over the buccal sulcus.

Upper posterior Teeth should be slightly buccal to the residual ridge and parallel to the ala–tragus line.

Lower posterior Teeth should be set directly over the ridge.

Aesthetics The dentist should establish individual needs of a patient and try to accommodate these without loss of important functional concepts.

These design features are merely a guide. In individual cases one feature may have to be compromised for the sake of another, depending on patient complaints and needs.

CLINICAL STAGES

Stages in complete denture construction are: examination, diagnosis and treatment plan, primary impressions, master impressions, jaw registration, trial of teeth (and if required retrial), insertion of prosthesis, review.

1. Examination, diagnosis and treatment (p. 300).

2. Primary impressions

Aims • To outline the denture-bearing area. • To construct an individual tray. • To show potential problems, e.g. prominent mylohyoid ridge.

Clinical technique An edentulous stock tray is selected and usually warm impression compound is used to take the impression. In the andible great care should be taken to place material into the lingual sulci. Then cool the impression and take a wash impression in irreversible hydrocolloid. The impression is disinfected and sent to the laboratory where it is cast in plaster. An individual tray is made. Both the individual tray and the cast should be returned to the dentist.

3. Master impressions

Aims • To accurately record the denture-bearing area. • To selectively load tissues capable of resisting load. • To relieve tissues that are friable.

Types of impressions
Mucocompressive An impression under load so that mucosa is reduced in volume equally and is evenly condensed.
Mucostatic An impression made without load application so that mucosa is neither compressed nor displaced.

Types of individual impression trays
Individual trays are usually made of self-cure acrylic. Trays are separated from the primary cast by wax spacers. Wax spacer thickness depends on impression material and technique chosen. Trays may be perforated and have localized relief areas or vents. May have handles or stops.

Clinical technique
Individual trays should be tried in the mouth prior to use. Gross overextension or infringements on muscle attachments should be corrected by trimming the tray.

Maxilla Warm tracing stick compound should be placed on the tray in the midline rugal area of the palate to act as a locating stop to correctly centre the tray. Tracing stick should also be applied in postdam areas and buccally to delineate the position of cheeks and lips.

Mandible The depth of the lingual flange is extremely important. This is checked by asking the patient to protrude his/her tongue gently. If the tray rises the flange is overextended. Warm tracing stick should be applied posteriorly to the retromolar area and on the lingual flange to define the lingual pouch

The master impressions should then be taken. Clinical techniques vary and are dependent on choice of material. The impression is disinfected and sent to the laboratory where it is cast in stone. A record block is made. Both the record block and the cast should be returned to the dentist.

Suitable materials for master impression
Maxilla Hydrocolloid; plaster; polysulphide, polyvinylsiloxane, polyether.

Mandible Zinc oxide–eugenol; plaster; polysulphide; polyvinylsiloxane, polyether.

4. Jaw registration

Aims • To register the jaw relationship in the retruded contact position. • To determine the vertical dimension of occlusion. • To determine lip support. • To determine anterior and posterior occlusal planes. • To record the midline correctly. • To select teeth of appropriate shade, shape, size and form.

Clinical aspects

- Wax record blocks are used to register the jaw relationships.
- These can be made more stable by addition of heat-cured acrylic or shellac baseplates.
- In jaw registration the labial contour is first restored by modifying the maxillary wax block to a 90° angle between the philtrum and columella.
- The anterior occlusal plane is registered usually 2–3 mm below the relaxed level of the upper lip parallel to a line between the pupils.
- Posteriorly the upper block is trimmed by continuing the anterior occlusal plane level posteriorly in a line parallel to the ala–tragus line.
- The midline is marked on the block; this is usually in the centre of the philtrum but varies in cases of facial asymmetry.
- The lower block is then placed in the mouth and trimmed until the rims contact evenly.
- Vertical dimension is then checked by a Willis bite gauge or calipers, with dots on the nose and chin, or by assessing the closest speaking space of 1 mm. Use of more than one method will give a better guide. If incorrect, wax is either added or removed from the block.
- Once satisfied with the registration, check notches are marked on both sides between rims and final registration taken using a bite registration paste.
- In difficult cases, use of a facebow to record the relationship of the upper cast to the skull is useful so that a case may be set up on a semiadjustable articulator and an accurate balanced articulation achieved.
- Teeth are selected for the dentures. This is often difficult. As a general rule, teeth should harmonize with the dominant colours of the complexion. In addition, tooth shape should harmonize with face shape. Patients often wish to be actively involved in tooth selection.

The record blocks (registered) will be sent to the technician with information about shades and moulds for setting up a trial of teeth.

5. Trial of teeth

Aims • To check the vertical dimension of occlusion is correct. • To check the horizontal jaw relationship has been registered correctly. • To check the anterior and posterior occlusal planes are correct. • To check the aesthetics are appropriate and that the patient is satisfied with aesthetics.

Clinical aspects

- The trial dentures should be examined critically prior to insertion – is tooth position correct, e.g. lower posteriors over the ridge?
- Trial dentures are inserted and all design features carefully assessed. If incorrect, chairside adjustments or re-registration and retrial may be required.
- The patient must be permitted to see the trial and an opportunity given to discuss and, if necessary, alter aesthetics, e.g. tooth shape, position, shade and colour.
- When both dentist and the patient are satisfied, the trial dentures may be sent to the technician for flasking, packing and processing into heat-cured acrylic.

6. Insertion of prosthesis

Aims • To deliver completed dentures to patient. • To check there have been no processing errors. • To instruct the patient on denture wear.

Clinical aspects

- The completed prostheses ideally should be presented on holding casts with an articulator. Thus the occlusion can be checked prior to patient's arrival.
- The fitting surface of the denture should be closely inspected and any 'blebs' or gross undercuts removed.
- The dentures should be inserted and occlusal balance and muscle balance checked. If occlusal balance is incorrect, can be identified using articulation paper and modified by selective grinding. If a larger error is present it may be necessary to re-register and remount the dentures in the laboratory and grind them to an appropriate occlusion. If there are muscle balance problems, grinding of the denture periphery may be required.
- Obvious gross overextension should be corrected, speech checked and the patient allowed to comment on the appearance.

● Before leaving, the patient should be instructed about
expectations of new dentures (p. 339).

7. Review

Aims • To assess how the patient is coping with new dentures. • To
relieve discomfort. • To motivate patient.

Clinical aspects

● Patient complaints should be carefully noted. This will help
determine how the patient is coping with new dentures.
● The occlusion should be reassessed, retention and stability
checked.
● The mucosa and support areas should be closely examined for
signs of ulceration or redness and the dentures adjusted.
● If major faults exist, these may require further laboratory stages.

OTHER CLINICAL ASPECTS OF COMPLETE DENTURES

Special impression techniques

Denture space technique Uses an acrylic base with upstanding
flanges; denture space is formed by moulding impression
compound. Useful for delineating the polished surface of a denture
and setting up teeth within the confines of the denture space.

Upper displaceable ridge Primary impression in mucostatic material
then composition impression of the resulting cast. In the mouth
composition is reheated and moulded over firm but not flabby areas.
Final wash impression. This technique compresses soft supporting
tissues without distortion so utilizes these areas for support.

Lower unemployed ridge Masticatory loads are borne by peripheral
tissues and not the ridge, where the ridge offers poor-quality
support. Primary impression in mucostatic material. An individual
tray is made with perforations over ridge crest. Then a composition
impression of primary cast is taken. Composition is removed from
over the ridge crest and a wash impression taken.

Occlusal pivots

With old, worn dentures the perioral muscle activity may become
deranged. Prior to construction of new dentures, masticatory
muscle activity may need to be retrained to ease the transition to
new dentures. Temporary acrylic pivots on existing dentures may be
placed in the premolar region of the lower denture to effect these
changes.

OMMON DENTURE PROBLEMS

Inadequate support • pain on digital pressure on support areas • discomfort under denture as day goes on • burning sensation in denture-bearing area with no redness or ulceration.

Try and redistribute support to areas most suited. Relief by trimming of poor support areas. In some cases the support is so poor there is little that can be done.

Inadequate retention • patient complains of denture looseness at all times (including at rest) • denture can be removed from mouth with no resistance • denture drops down after being firmly seated in the mouth.

Attempt to improve peripheral seal by self-cure acrylic. Relining may be required.

Muscle balance problem • dentures loose only when patient eats or speaks • dentures feel too large • cheek biting • lower denture rises on tongue protrusion.

Careful trimming of denture areas encroaching on muscles often solves the problem.

Occlusal balance problem • patient wears dentures well except at mealtimes where there is pain or looseness • dentures move when teeth ground together.

Selective grinding, laboratory remount and resetting of teeth help these problems.

Appearance problems Often fall into the following categories: • shade of tooth wrong • shape of tooth wrong • too much or too little tooth shows • lips look odd • face looks asymmetrical • patient unhappy with appearance but uncertain about precise nature of problem.

Often management of appearance problems involves resetting of different teeth. In some cases they may be due to incorrect recording of vertical or horizontal components of occlusion.

 Occasionally some patients have totally unrealistic expectations of dentures.

Speech problems • Often problem is lisping 'f' and 'v' sounds or hissing 's' sounds. • May be due to problem with tooth position or vertical dimension of occlusion. • Notoriously difficult problems to solve.

Retching • This is a protective reflex. • In some patients simple examination is difficult and impression taking almost impossible. • In some patients there is a psychiatric element to retching. • Treatment options include progressive adaptation to dentures by constructing baseplates first. Hypnotherapy or desensitizing therapy may help.

Acrylic allergy In rare cases where there is proven acrylic allergy an alternative material should be considered. Nylon or polycarbonate are useful as alternative base materials. Porcelain teeth are an alternative to acrylic teeth.

Irritant reactions to free monomer in new dentures (corrected by recuring) should be differentiated from genuine acrylic allergy.

PARTIAL DENTURES

> A partial denture is a prosthesis which replaces one or more, but less than all, of the natural teeth and is removable by the patient.

PRINCIPLES
Aims
There are many similarities in complete and partial denture prosthetics. Partial dentures should replace lost teeth and tissues and fill the denture space. Partial dentures should not damage adjacent teeth or restorations. Partial dentures should be designed with periodontal health in mind and should restore function and aesthetics.

The problems in failure to restore lost natural teeth If missing natural teeth are not replaced the following problems may occur: • drifting and tilting of teeth • overeruption of teeth • decreased masticatory function • craniomandibular disorders • overloading of remaining teeth or mucosa • tooth wear • poor oral hygiene • speech problems • aesthetic problems.

The negative effect of partial dentures Whilst partial dentures provide many benefits, they have a number of potential drawbacks: • increased plaque accumulation • caries • gingivitis and periodontitis • gingival stripping • overloading of abutment teeth.

Partial dentures must be designed to reduce the risk of these negative sequelae. Careful patient selection is required and motivation, improved oral hygiene and elimination of dental pathology in remaining teeth should be achieved prior to prosthesis construction.

Design (Table 12.1)

 A systematic approach to partial denture design must be followed for each case.

One such systematic approach is as follows:

Stage 1: Classification of support for each saddle
A saddle may be either mucosa borne, tooth borne or tooth and mucosa borne.

Typical examples are • mucosa borne – bilateral free end saddle • tooth borne – small bounded saddle.

> **Saddle** describes that part of the alveolus from which teeth are missing.

Stage 2: Connect saddles together
Saddles should be connected to produce a rigid unit.

Types of connectors in the maxilla
Anterior palatal bar Used for an anterior saddle only or as indirect retention in a bilateral free end saddle.
Midpalatal bar Connects two posterior bounded saddles.
Posterior palatal bar Has its posterior border on the vibrating line. Only indicated as a rigid strut for the distal ends of free end saddles.

TABLE 12.1 Kennedy classification of edentulous spaces	
Class I	Bilateral free end saddle
Class II	Unilateral free end saddle
Class III	Unilateral bounded saddle
Class IV	Anterior (across the midline)

Palatal horseshoe connector For anterior saddles.
Full-coverage palatal plate Used when very few natural teeth present.

Types of connectors in the mandible
Lingual bar Needs to be 4 mm deep, 3 mm thick, 1.5 mm away from
the gingival margin and 1.5 mm above the highest level of floor
of mouth.
Lingual plate Used when insufficient room for lingual bar.
Lingual bar and continuous clasp Provides more indirect retention
than lingual bar alone but has many sharp edges.
Buccal bar Indications are few.
Sublingual bar Lies very low in floor of mouth.

Stage 3: Choose the path of insertion and delineate undercuts
The partial denture must be easily inserted and removed from the
mouth; therefore the denture requires a path of insertion. A study
cast is required for this and a *surveyor* is used. Ideally a slight distal
tilt of the cast is required to ensure a simple path of insertion for
the patient. Suitable undercuts are surveyed and marked in pencil
on the cast by the surveyor pencil.

Stage 4: Resistance of movement away from the teeth
Retainers are usually placed on abutment teeth. Retention is
usually achieved by a clasp, which is a flexible arm, the tip of which
lies in an undercut. If there are fewer than four quadrilaterally
opposed retainers there is a tendency for rotation.

Stage 5: Indirect retention
If the direct retainers do not provide sufficient resistance then
indirect retention must be considered.

> **Indirect retention** occurs where the direct retainers act
> indirectly to resist movement of a saddle that can only be
> directly retained at one end.

Example of indirect retention – free end saddle If the saddle lifts, it
does so by rotation around a fulcrum on a line through the clasp
tips on the abutment teeth. If the framework is extended on the
other side of the fulcrum line (away from the free end saddle) as far
as possible from the fulcrum, the clasps will indirectly resist
movement as the saddle rises (Figure 12.3).

Stage 6: Resistance of movement towards the teeth and tissues
A partial denture requires support, usually provided by an *occlusal
rest*. Without good occlusal support there may be tissue damage.

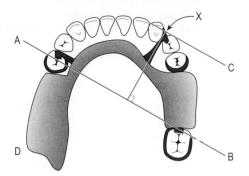

The incisal rest 'X' transfers fulcrum line A–B to A–C. As D rises on new fulcrum, clasps act indirectly to resist this movement. The further C is away from A–B the more effective the indirect retention.

Figure 12.3 Indirect retention.

Occlusal rests should transfer load to the teeth parallel to the long axis of the tooth. Where possible, a quadrilateral distribution of rests is required to minimize rotational axes. In a distal extension saddle, the most distal occlusal rest should be placed mesially on the abutment tooth to prevent torque on this tooth.

Stage 7: Resistance to horizontal movement
Some parts already added to the denture will resist horizontal movement, e.g. clasp arms, contours of palate, etc.

Resistance to forward movement Only a problem in a large anterior bounded saddle. Movement forward prevented by contours of tissue and framework around abutment teeth.

Resistance to backward movement A problem in free end saddles. Prevented by addition of spurs on the mesial side of the mesial abutment.

Resistance to lateral movement Bracing arms to clasps and the contour of the palate/lingual sulcus resist this movement.

Stage 8: Simplification
The denture design should be critically appraised and any excessive or unwanted aspects removed.

Clasp design
There are many designs of clasps and only general principles are described.

Undercuts The deeper the undercut, the greater the retention. However, clasp deformation must not stress the clasp beyond its elastic limit. Therefore, for different undercut depths, different materials are appropriate: • cast cobalt–chromium useful for 0.25 mm undercut • wrought gold useful for 0.5 mm undercut • wrought stainless steel useful for 0.75 mm undercut.

Clasp flexibility A long clasp arm produces a more flexible clasp, e.g. gingivally approaching clasp is more flexible than occlusally approaching clasp. A thick clasp is less flexible than a thin clasp.

Aesthetics Particularly in anterior region, clasps may be very noticeable. Consideration should be given to placing tips in distal undercuts, gold plating the clasps or using tooth-coloured clasps.

Bracing A clasp consists of a *retentive arm* (which engages an undercut) and a *reciprocal (or bracing) arm* (which ensures retentive arm does not act like an orthodontic appliance).

Minor connectors When considering clasp position it is important to remember the clasp must be connected to the main denture framework by a minor connector. This is particularly important where there is little interocclusal space.

Common types of clasp include • occlusally approaching clasp • gingivally approaching clasp • I bar clasp (Figure 12.4).

Rests

Rests provide tooth support. Common types of rests include:

Occlusal rests Are placed mesially or distally on occlusal surfaces of molar or premolar teeth. Sometimes tooth preparation is required. Must not interfere with occlusion.

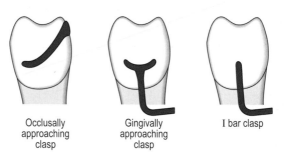

| Occlusally approaching clasp | Gingivally approaching clasp | I bar clasp |

Lateral view

Figure 12.4 Partial denture clasps.

Cingulum rests Placed on the cingulae of incisor and canine teeth. May require tooth preparation.

Guide planes

Surveying frequently reveals unfavourable tilting of teeth. To obtain a favourable path of insertion, it is sometimes necessary to cut guide planes on the tooth to correspond with the path of insertion of the denture. In some instances tooth cutting is so extensive that a *milled crown* must be made for a tooth to obtain a satisfactory guide plane.

Choice of material

Partial dentures are usually made of *cobalt–chromium* or *acrylic.*

Reasons for choosing acrylic • cheap • transitional or immediate partial dentures • mucosa borne denture • previous history of long-term successful acrylic denture wear • resistance of patient to anterior clasping.

Reasons for choosing cobalt–chromium • definitive dentures • tooth, or tooth and mucosa borne denture • easier to keep clean • less palatal coverage • temperature discrimination.

Bilateral free end saddle dentures

Bilateral free end saddle dentures have particular problems. The 500 μm resilience of the residual ridge and 20 μm resilience of the teeth provide a huge support discrepancy. This may manifest itself in excess loading on the distal abutment teeth. To overcome this several design concepts have been proposed for the design of this type of denture:

Flexible denture base Stress-breaker designs – result in trauma distal to the last abutment tooth.

Floating denture base A mucostatically recorded denture base is related to the abutment teeth under pressure.

Mucofunctional impression An impression technique is used to record the tissue surfaces in the shape that the residual ridges take under functional loads. This requires the use of an *altered cast impression technique.*

Particular partial denture designs

More complex designs may provide alternatives in difficult cases. They are, however, clinically and technically complex and may require the patient to have some degree of manual dexterity.

Two part This type of denture is designed to engage alveolar or approximal undercuts on individual paths of insertion. The two parts are locked together to retain the prosthesis.

Hinged flange This denture engages alveolar or approximal undercuts by closing into them from the buccal side once the denture base is seated.

Disjunct A tooth borne element splints the natural teeth and retains a mucosal borne element which replaces the missing teeth. Useful in Kennedy Class I and II cases.

Swinglock This denture has a flange which locks after the denture is seated, engaging undercuts gingival to interdental contact points. Useful for retention but also as a mask for unsightly gingival recession. Has a splinting action. A high standard of oral hygiene is required for this design.

CLINICAL STAGES

The clinical stages in partial dentures fabrication are similar to those in complete dentures, namely: planning, primary impressions, master impressions, jaw registration, trial, insertion and review.

Some important differences

Planning stages The status of the remaining natural teeth should be looked at carefully prior to partial denture construction. Unsatisfactory restorations should be replaced, endodontics undertaken, caries treated and crowns constructed prior to beginning other stages of partial denture construction.

Primary impressions Casts are often mounted and surveyed and used for denture design. Occasionally diagnostic wax-up of tooth position is performed.

Master impressions At this stage tooth preparation may take place, e.g. guide planes, rest seat preparations.

Jaw registration Often record blocks are not required and maxillary and mandibular casts may be related by use of wax or silicone rubber.

Trial In the case of metal-based dentures, in addition to a trial of teeth, a trial of the casting must be undertaken.

Insertion Instructions to patients should include modifications to oral hygiene measures affecting natural teeth.

Review The effect of the dentures on the abutment teeth should be assessed.

PRECISION ATTACHMENTS

Precision attachments are used in removable prosthetics to provide additional retention.

Uses • overdentures • implant-retained dentures • bounded saddles • flexible denture base (stress breaker) in free end saddles • in conjunction with fixed prosthodontics.

Types
Extracoronal Studs, bars, magnets.
Intracoronal Often in conjunction with fixed prosthodontics.
  A huge number of individual designs exist.

Advantages of precision attachments • retentive • aesthetics (decrease need for anterior clasping) • enable use of tilted teeth for retention and support.

Disadvantages of precision attachments • expensive • require large occlusogingival and inter-ridge height • technically and clinically complex • long-term maintenance a problem as parts may wear and need to be replaced • fracture of acrylic in saddles as it is in thin section to accommodate attachment • oral hygiene often more difficult.

Case selection for precision attachment designs is critical. Consider only in well-motivated patients with good oral hygiene and controlled caries.

COPY DENTURES

Copy dentures (also known as replica dentures) are a method of producing replacement dentures which are similar in shape and dimension to the patient's existing dentures.

Indications • elderly patients • patients with old, worn or loose dentures which were otherwise successful • where patient is extremely satisfied with an aesthetic result and wishes this reproduced • poor patient cooperation, e.g. dementia.

Advantages • enhances neuromuscular adaptation to new denture as they are basically of similar shape • one less clinical stage • registration of jaw relationship is often simple • gives technician much more of a guide to tooth position and moulds, etc.

Disadvantages • large errors are difficult to correct • only used in complete denture prosthetics.

Clinical stages

1. Modification of existing dentures, e.g. underextension of lingual pouches modified by tracing stick to lower denture.
2. Putty impression of fitting and polished/occlusal surfaces of modified existing dentures and relocated together as a mould.
3. In laboratory putty moulds are poured into copy dentures with either wax (sometimes with shellac baseplate) or pour-cure acrylic.
4. Replicas used for master impressions (usually in polyvinylsiloxane) and jaw registration at the same clinical visit.
5 Set up, trial of teeth and insertion as for a conventional complete denture.

OVERDENTURES

An overdenture is a prosthesis that gains support from one or more abutment teeth by enclosing them beneath its fitting surface.

Advantages of overdentures • maintains alveolar bone • maintains proprioceptive feedback, which controls masticatory force and monitors mandibular position in function and discriminates size and texture of foods • decreases psychological trauma of tooth loss • decreases mobility of mobile teeth • eases the progression to edentulousness • may increase denture retention.

Disadvantages of overdentures • caries on abutment teeth • periodontal disease on abutment teeth • cost • more complex clinically • more maintenance required • often abutments require root treatment.

Indications for overdentures • complete denture in one arch • cleft palates and surgical or traumatic defects • hypodontia • tooth wear • overerupted teeth • doubtful conventional partial denture abutments.

Clinical aspects

Motivated patients should be selected who can demonstrate good oral hygiene and whose caries rate is controlled.

Abutment selection Potential overdenture abutment teeth should in general fulfil the following criteria: • sufficient coronal tooth substance to maintain integrity • capable of (or not requiring) endodontic therapy • periodontal status favourable • no gross bony undercuts (unless no flange required) • sometimes ability to have positive retention on abutments is desirable • ideally, overdenture abutments should be spaced around the dental arch • adequate inter-ridge space.

Abutment teeth can be prepared – *dome* or *thimble shaped*.

Attachments Attachments to abutment teeth can be used to increase the retention of the overdenture. However these have certain disadvantages: • increased cost • complex maintenance • increased bulk may weaken denture base • higher load onto abutment • more difficult to clean abutment.

Types of attachments to overdentures commonly used are: studs, bars, magnets, hollow posts. These are either prefabricated or placed on top of gold post and diaphragms.

Impression technique for overdentures As the abutment tooth and mucosa are of varying compressibility a close-fitting individual tray, perforated over the abutment teeth, is often made. Sometimes when using prefabricated attachments there will be impression 'dummies' and individualized impression techniques depending on the type of attachment used. In such cases close attention should be paid to manufacturers' instructions. Frequently, immediate overdentures are made with preparation of abutment teeth at the insertion stage. This requires immediate modification of the surface over the abutment teeth by use of self-cure acrylic with vent holes to the polished surface of the denture.

Care of abutments Following insertion of an overdenture the following procedures are desirable for maintenance: • toothbrushing of abutments with a fluoride-containing toothpaste • denture hygiene, including removal of prosthesis at night • self-application of topical fluoride to the abutments by the patient • dietary advice regarding reduction of sugar in diet • frequent recall visits to check status of abutment teeth.

IMMEDIATE DENTURES

An immediate denture is a prosthesis used to replace one or more teeth and inserted on the day of extraction of the tooth or teeth.

General features Immediate dentures may be used for complete or partial dentures. They should be considered as *transitional* and are therefore usually made of *acrylic*. Patients should be advised preoperatively of their shortcomings, i.e. retention problems, aesthetic problems, necessity for relines, initial pain and discomfort.

Treatment planning When many teeth are to be extracted consideration should be given to either staging of extractions or post-immediate dentures (let sockets heal then make prosthesis).

Reasons for immediate dentures • aesthetics • psychological • improved masticatory function • stabilization of wound.

Problems with immediate dentures • lots of aftercare required, e.g.: temporary linings and relines • frequent adjustments • often do not equate to patient's perceived expectations both functionally and aesthetically • sometimes considerable postextraction discomfort, especially if dry sockets or difficult/multiple extractions involved.

Clinical aspects
Removing teeth from cast The correct method of trimming a tooth to be extracted from a cast prior to immediate denture construction is to cut across from one gingival papilla to another following ridge contour. Socketing of teeth is not desirable as this limits clot size and decreases fibrous tissue deposited.

Aesthetics Digital photography pre-extraction gives a baseline position which can aid the selection of appropriate tooth position, shape and shade of denture teeth. Good aesthetics will enhance patient acceptance of immediate dentures.

Flanges If possible, immediate dentures should have full flanges rather than be gum fitted. This ensures peripheral seal although may involve undercut trimming at insertion.

Follow-up At the time of immediate denture insertion, some checks are not possible as the patient may be locally anaesthetized or swollen. Ideally the patient should be seen the following day for occlusal and other checks to be made.

OTHER PROSTHETIC APPLIANCES

Gingival veneers Useful to mask recession following periodontal disease.

Palatal lift appliances Used with or without existing dentures to improve speech. Especially useful in motor-neuron disease and most successful when there is joint management with a speech therapist.

Gumshields An essential feature of trauma protection in contact sports; individual custom-made soft vinyl splints can be made in a wide variety of colours; cheap and easy to make and should be actively promoted by dentists.

Anti-snoring appliances (e.g. mandibular advancement) May be useful in reducing snoring and in sleep apnoea.

Mouthpieces for diving and wind instrument playing Highly specialized appliances but essential for these occupations.

Bleaching splints Thin flexible splints with spacers for use in dentist-controlled vital home bleaching.

REPAIRS, RELINES AND ADDITIONS

REPAIRS

Denture fracture is fairly common.

Common types of fracture • midline fracture of complete dentures • tooth detaching from denture • piece of flange lost • clasp fracture • anterior maxillary saddle area fracture • acrylic saddle detaching from cobalt–chromium baseplate.

Reasons for fracture • impact, i.e. patient drops denture • work hardening, e.g. clasp fracture • thin sections of acrylic undergoing normal forces • parafunctional forces • odd habits, e.g. nail biting • close bite, e.g. anterior maxillary saddle • dentures with soft linings (very difficult to repair accurately) • original denture processing problem, e.g. porosity in denture base, incorrect bonding of denture teeth to denture base.

Repair protocols

Simple If there is a simple fracture and the broken pieces of the prosthesis can be located easily together, send to laboratory without impression where the pieces can be located together, a cast poured, the fractured area removed and new acrylic processed, e.g. midline complete denture fracture.

Lost part of prosthesis An impression is taken with the prosthesis in the mouth. A cast is poured and the new part added, e.g. lost flange or broken clasp.

Unrepairable Some fractures, e.g. denture smashed into many pieces, are not repairable.

Acrylic–cobalt–chromium Use of 4-META or silicoating of cobalt–chromium may improve retention of an acrylic saddle to a cobalt–chromium baseplate.

Temporary repairs May be effected with cyanoacrylate glues or cold-cure acrylic.

 If persistent denture fracture occurs, re-evaluate the treatment plan. Often a replacement denture of a different design is required.

RELINES

A reline of a denture involves placing new material on the fitting surface.

Types of reline

Temporary This usually involves a soft material and is useful for tissue conditioning of grossly ill-fitting dentures prior to new denture construction. Other uses include following insertion of immediate dentures.

Soft Often uses molloplast or silicone-based materials. Useful as a cushion in patients with parafunctional habits or irregular ridges. Unfortunately plasticizer leaches, so soft linings may become hard and need fairly frequent replacement. Bacteria may colonize lining so it is often unhygienic and in addition there is some doubt over the clinical efficacy of soft linings.

Permanent Hard acrylic reline. Useful in: • gross peripheral seal problems • correction of errors which occurred at master impression stage • prolonging the life span of old dentures • immediate and post-immediate dentures.

Clinical aspects • Some relining materials are available for use in the mouth and are self-cured. • Usual method involves an impression of the fitting surface. • The denture must be prepared prior to impression by removing overextended flanges and undercuts.

• Tracing stick reforms peripheral seal. Holes need to be drilled through areas, e.g. palate, to relieve pressure and an impression taken with impression paste or low-viscosity polyvinylsiloxane. Occlusion is checked during the impression procedure. • The denture is processed in the laboratory and returned to the patient. Occlusion must be carefully checked as registration error is common after relines.

Relines are most frequently used in complete denture prosthetics. Sectional relines of partial denture saddles are occasionally useful, especially following immediate partial dentures.

ADDITIONS

> Describes the placing of an additional tooth or part of a denture to an existing prosthesis.

Indications

Immediate addition Where a tooth is lost subsequent to denture construction and a tooth added on the day of extraction.

Post-immediate addition Where a tooth is lost subsequent to denture construction and at a later date a replacement tooth added.

Retention Where retention of a denture is poor, a clasp may be added to improve retention.

Clinical aspects Additions usually involve an impression of the arch with the denture in the mouth. Occasionally it is possible to perform a chairside addition using self-cure acrylic, although this is often temporary in nature.

CRANIOMANDIBULAR DISORDERS

Craniomandibular disorders (CMD) (see also p. 471) are a range of musculoskeletal disorders affecting the temporomandibular joint (TMJ) complex (including the muscles of mastication), which may be transient and self-limiting, often resolving without serious long-term effects but causing much morbidity when they are present.

Alternative names CMD is known by several other names, some of which are not entirely synonymous: • TMJ dysfunction syndrome • myofascial pain dysfunction syndrome.

DIAGNOSIS

If craniomandibular disorders are suspected a thorough pain history must be taken to exclude other non-CMD causes such as dental pain, pharyngeal or parotid neoplasia.

Differential diagnosis • jaw muscle disorders, e.g. muscle spasm • TMJ derangement • trauma • degenerative joint disease • inflammatory joint disease • chronic hypomobility, e.g. ankylosis • growth disorders.

History Pain history is most important. Features often include pain on waking, pain radiating to temporal region of head. May be some craniocervical pain. Pain is often chronic and recurrent but rarely constant.

Symptoms and signs • Pain on function • limited jaw opening • audible joint click • signs of tooth wear or denture wear.

Examination

Joint examination The TMJ should be assessed in static and dynamic positions.

Static examination • Tenderness may be assessed by palpation • TMJ morphology can be assessed by tomography or arthroscopy.

Dynamic examination
   Mobility The range and limitations of TMJ movement should be recorded.
   Sounds Palpation and auscultation may aid diagnosis.

Muscle examination The range, limitation of movement and pain on movement should be assessed in all functional mandibular positions. Muscle pain may also be assessed by direct palpation of masseter and temporalis muscles.

Occlusal examination Study casts and facebow registration of casts for mounting on a semiadjustable articulator may prove useful in occlusal assessment and as a diagnostic aid to management possibilities.

MANAGEMENT

Management goals in CMD • Decreased pain • decreased adverse loading • restored function • restored daily activities.

Management options

Patient education and palliative home care This involves: • patient reassurance • avoidance of heavy mastication, yawning, sighing, singing, object biting • home physiotherapeutic exercises

• application of heat or cold by patient to muscles. About 60% of patients are relieved by these simple methods alone.

Behaviour modification This attempts to change persistent habits, e.g. parafunction by methods such as progressive relaxation, hypnosis, lifestyle counselling and biofeedback.

Drug therapy This may relieve symptoms of CMD by reducing pain, inflammation, muscle hyperactivity, anxiety and depression. The following drugs may be useful: • analgesics • non-steroidal anti-inflammatory drugs • corticosteroids (short-term systemic or local injection) • muscle relaxants • benzodiazepines (useful in acute trismus) • tricyclic antidepressants.

Exercise therapy The following exercises of the TMJ may be useful:
   Repetitive exercises Establish coordinated muscle function.
   Isotonic exercises Increase range of TMJ motion.
   Isometric exercises Increase muscle strength.

Mobilization Repeated joint manipulation is useful in TMJ articular disc displacement.

Physical agents Aim to produce analgesia, heat and cold, muscle relaxation and increased joint mobility. Electrotherapy (TENS), ultrasound, vapocoolants, local anaesthetic injections and acupuncture are occasionally useful.

Splint therapy Interocclusal splints are in common use in the treatment of CMD.

   Splints aim to: • alter occlusal relationships and redistribute occlusal forces • prevent tooth wear • decrease bruxism and parafunction • treat masticatory muscle pain and dysfunction • modify relationships and forces within the TMJ.

   It is well documented that painful symptoms often decrease after splint insertion.

Types of splints

Stabilization splints Flat plane or muscle relaxation splints. Work by altering mandibular posture to a more relaxed position. Made in hard acrylic. Usually worn at night time. Often initial positive response in 3–4 weeks.

Repositioning splints Mandibular orthopaedic repositioning appliances (MORA). Used in disc displacement to decrease joint pain, sounds and secondary muscle pain. Work by decreasing adverse load in joint and altering condyle to disc relationship. Mandible is positioned into a protrusive position. Made in hard acrylic. May cause a posterior open bite. Poor success at maintaining joint structural changes.

Provisional splints Often used as a short-term measure. Include soft resilient splint, anterior bite plane and occlusal pivots.

Occlusal therapy Some clinicians advocate altering occlusal loads as a treatment of CMD. This is rarely required and should only be considered and undertaken by a specialist practitioner. However, provision of posterior support in the form of partial dentures is often useful.

Other therapy Other forms of therapy include acupuncture, orthodontics, orthognathic surgery and joint surgery (useful for articular disorders but of limited value in CMD).

> ⚠ With the vast range of potential management options available, CMD can appear most confusing. In addition, many workers have specific treatment regimes that are often anecdotal and 'work for them'. In general, patient education and home care is a useful start, with perhaps progression to stabilization splints. In cases that do not respond to these treatment modalities, specialist help should be sought.

IMPLANT BORNE PROSTHESES

Types of implants • subperiosteal • osseointegrated • transmandibular. Osseointegrated titanium implants are most common.

Uses of implants • complete overdentures • full arch fixed bridges • partial fixed bridges • partial overdentures • single tooth replacement • natural tooth–implant bridges • orbital, nasal, auricular and hearing aid prostheses.

OSSEOINTEGRATED IMPLANTS

> *Osseointegration* A direct structural and functional connection between ordered, living bone and the surface of a load-carrying implant.

To achieve optimal osseointegration requires:

1. Material biocompatibility – usually commercially pure titanium.
2. Adequate implant design – large surface area; shape that permits stabilization during healing; surface irregularities better than smooth
3. Bone – adequate bone height, width and quality is required.

4. Surgical technique – bone tissue damage occurs at temperatures over 47°C so atraumatic surgery imperative.
5. Loading conditions – do not overload implants.

There are many proprietary systems. Basically two forms:
Transmucosal (use one-stage surgery).
Submucosal (use two-stage surgery).
Typical mechanical components of an osseointegrated implant are shown in Figure 12.5 and tooth replacement solutions for osseointegrated implants in Figure 12.6.

Dentists who undertake implant treatment should be appropriately trained and competent to deal with any and all complications.

Case selection

Planning of implant procedures is extremely important. This involves teamwork between oral surgeon and prosthodontist.

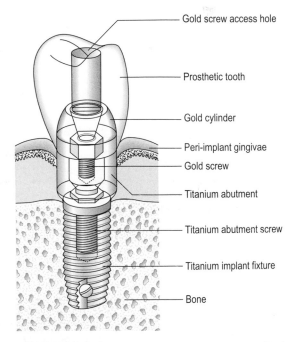

Gold screw access hole
Prosthetic tooth
Gold cylinder
Peri-implant gingivae
Gold screw
Titanium abutment
Titanium abutment screw
Titanium implant fixture
Bone

Figure 12.5 Typical mechanical components of an osseointegrated implant.

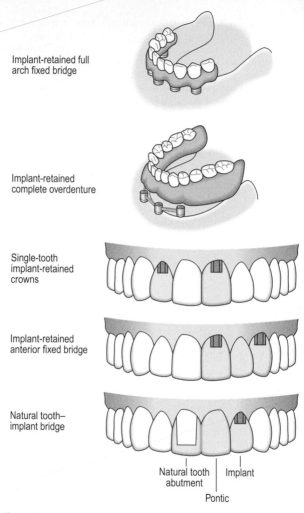

Implant-retained full arch fixed bridge

Implant-retained complete overdenture

Single-tooth implant-retained crowns

Implant-retained anterior fixed bridge

Natural tooth–implant bridge

Natural tooth abutment   Implant

Pontic

Figure 12.6 Some tooth replacement solutions for osseointegrated implants.

General considerations • Patients must be medically fit to undergo surgery and complex prosthodontic treatment over multiple visits. (Caution in patients with uncontrolled diabetes, irradiated bone, coagulation problems, smokers have much higher failure rate, patients on high-dose steroids.) • The bony implant site must have bone of sufficient height, width and quality for implant placement. • The implant site must not impinge on key anatomical features, e.g. mental nerve foramen. • Implants must be placed in such a manner that the teeth and tissues to be restored may be placed in appropriate functional and aesthetic positions. • Implants should ideally be placed into two cortical bone layers. • The patient must be fully informed of complications and the nature of implant treatment.

Dental considerations • Patients should be capable of good oral hygiene. • Pre-existing periodontal disease and caries should be controlled. • There should be enough inter-ridge space for implant superstructures and prosthesis (minimum 7 mm). • There should be enough space between existing teeth for implant placement without tooth damage (minimum 7 mm). • Implant therapy is sometimes a more appropriate solution than conventional prosthetic treatment to a patient's difficulties. Therefore, the patient should be allowed to make an informed choice as to whether or not to undergo implant treatment.

Planning

Planning should be meticulously undertaken. Occasionally, specialist help from a prosthodontist or oral surgeon is required. The role of the prosthodontist is: • to determine if the patient's symptoms would benefit from implant treatment • to decide provisionally what method of retention to the fixtures should be employed • to estimate likely tooth positions • to assess occlusal possibilities • to counsel the patient • to make surgical guides and radiographic templates.

Radiographs

Maxilla: panoramic, periapicals are usually required; sometimes lateral cephalogram, serial tomograms and computed tomography (CT) scans are required.

Mandible: panoramic and lateral cephalogram required; occasionally periapicals or, in the posterior mandible, CT scans or serial tomograms. Specialized software programs may act as an adjunct to radiographic planning.

Radiographic templates These are useful, particularly in edentulous patients. Usually the denture in the arch to be considered for implants is copied in clear acrylic. Gutta-percha or ball-bearing inserts are placed at selected areas and radiographs taken with this in the mouth. This helps localize specific bony areas so that potential implant sites may be found.

Surgical templates Made in clear acrylic to help the surgeon decide on probable implant sites (p. 421).

Diagnostic wax-up Useful for tooth positioning and assessing potential problem areas.

Digital photography Assessment of likely tooth position.

Temporization
Following implant surgery, ridge and gingival contours may change. Existing prostheses may not fit well and so temporary soft linings or gross reduction of acrylic or the construction of temporary prosthesis may be needed. This is particularly important in immediate and early loading cases.

Prosthodontic treatment
Although components of different systems vary, the prosthodontic phase of implant treatment is similar to the stages in other methods of prosthetic treatment. However, individual tray design may be different and a specialized impression technique used, depending on system employed.

Maintenance
Regular follow-up, particularly of implant-retained overdentures, is required. The role of the dental hygienist in motivation and oral hygiene instruction is highly important for maintenance of peri-implant health.

Complications of implant treatment
Some common complications of implant treatment are: • failure of osseointegration • failure to seat abutment properly • screw fracture • implant fracture • denture fracture • peri-implantitis • gingival hyperplasia.

Current developments in implant treatment
Immediate loading of implants This is now accepted as a useful treatment option where bone conditions and occlusal factors are favourable and there is good primary implant stability. Best sites are anterior mandible and posterior mandible. Posterior maxilla less good. Use of resonance frequency analysis is helpful for case selection.

Socket implants Placement of implants into extraction sockets is now more commonplace. Advantages are less traumatic surgery, good implant position as follow line of root, in limited bone cases the bone has not resorbed at time of extraction. Disadvantages are bone resorption unpredictable so difficult to determine crestal height of implant, cannot be used where acute infection, if loss of buccal bony plates may need grafting of bone or use of guided bone regeneration membranes. Best cases are where there is a large block of mature bone beyond the extraction socket. In such cases the socket implant may be able to be immediately loaded.

Implants of differing shapes Development of wide and narrow implants, tapered and straight implants enable more cases to be treated with the implants in better positions. For example: narrow implants useful for lower incisors • tapered implants useful in sockets • wide implants useful in molar regions.

Natural teeth to implant bridges In the early days of implant treatment, a pontic supported by both a tooth and an implant was considered by some as inappropriate due to different loading characteristics. This is now an accepted treatment modality.

Scanned frameworks and prostheses Use of scanning technology can enable highly accurate prosthetic substructures to be made from solid blocks of titanium. Similarly, all ceramic crowns for implants can be made using scanning technology.

Soft tissue surgery Conservation of existing tissue is helpful in gingival recontouring around implants to improve aesthetics. Particularly useful in high smile line cases for implants in the anterior maxilla.

Insufficient bone Whilst bone grafting has a place in implant treatment (p. 421) smaller bony insufficiencies can be corrected by: harvesting of bone chips from implant placement • scraping of bone under the flap; use of inert material like coral • changing the angle of an implant (which can be corrected later by an angled abutment) • guided bone regeneration membranes • use of implants of different widths.

> ⚠️ **Osseointegrated implants are *not* a panacea. They are a well-recognized form of prosthetic rehabilitation which is of great benefit in individuals with poor neuromuscular control and retention difficulties. Implants are costly and complex, and good case selection is absolutely critical to success. It is particularly important for dentists undertaking implant treatment that they undertake continuing professional development with respect to implant treatment given the rapid changes taking place in this area of dentistry.**

MAXILLOFACIAL PROSTHETICS

Types of defects
Extraoral e.g. missing eyes, ears, nose.
Intraoral • acquired (mouth cancer, trauma) • congenital (cleft palate).

Maxillectomy

Commonly, patients with mouth/maxillary antral cancer. Defects may be hard palate, soft palate, both hard and soft palate, pharyngeal. Must be seen preoperatively to determine prosthetic rehabilitation.

Initial treatment Surgical obturator made, often a three-part Conroy obturator; may be screwed in with champy plates; sectional gutta-percha into defect with a temporary soft lining. In dentate patients Adams clasps on remaining teeth are used for retention. At surgery, impression should be taken for interim obturator.

Interim treatment For 6 months, straightforward acrylic prosthesis made from impression at surgery then relined.

Definitive treatment After about 6 months, final obturator design and replacement of interim obturator.

Types of obturators • One-piece hollow box • two-piece hollow box • detachable silicone or molloplast obturator • hollow box and detachable silicone or molloplast part • collapsible obturator.

Choice of obturator depends on size of defect, undercuts and success or failure of interim prosthesis. In dentate patients cobalt–chromium baseplates may be used with clasping for retention.

 Do not use hydrocolloid impression materials in maxillary defects as poor tear strength may leave them stuck in nasal conchae or tissue undercuts.

Cleft palate

In the Western world, most congenital cleft palates are repaired. Occasionally, small fistulae are left, leaving an oronasal communication. Many repaired cleft patients have missing teeth, Class III occlusion and often require partial prostheses. Prevention of caries and periodontal disease is extremely important in such patients as tooth loss leaves poor support for denture retention.

Unrepaired congenital clefts Mainly an elderly population. Same principles apply as for definitive dentures in maxillectomy patients, although defect is usually symmetrical.

Mandibular defects

Types superior marginal, inferior marginal, segmental.

Mandibular rehabilitation depends on: • extent of remaining mandible • degree of deviation • quality of remaining alveolar ridge • number and condition of remaining teeth.

Basic prosthetic principles apply but are complicated by prominent position of surgical fixators, e.g. champy plates, titanium mesh, wire. Soft tissues are also altered (e.g. glossectomy) and there may be anaesthesia or paraesthesia so neuromuscular control of prosthesis is limited. Sometimes use of a guide-flange prosthesis postoperation is useful to limit mandibular deviation from scarring. Osseointegrated implants have a valuable role in definitive rehabilitation of mandibular defects.

Craniofacial prostheses

Types auricular, orbital, nasal, other.

Most are made from silicones. Sunlight leads to degeneration and so often require yearly replacement. Osseointegrated implants have an increasing role in retention of these prostheses. Ocular (eye) prostheses need an ocular technician to achieve good lens colouring. Spectacles and hairlines are useful in masking border between prosthesis and skin. This is a highly specialized form of prosthetics and is usually only carried out in specialist centres.

THE SHORTENED DENTAL ARCH

Describes an arch consisting of anterior teeth and premolars.

Advantages • No partial dentures are worn so potential risks of partial denture wear, e.g. caries, decreased. • Most people can function adequately with a shortened dental arch. • Most people have no aesthetic problems with a shortened dental arch. • Simplifies dentition so oral hygiene regimes often easier. • Number and complexity of restorations reduced.

Disadvantages • No partial denture wearing experience so often poor transition to denture wear if a denture is required later in life.

• Tooth wear may be increased due to lack of posterior support.
• Caution should be exercised in patients with craniomandibular disorders. • Overloading of premolar teeth. • In patients who are severely compromised periodontally, increased mobility and drifting of teeth may result. • Extraction of four premolars is a common orthodontic therapy and in such patients a shortened dental arch is extremely short. • Patients with a high smile line may find a shortened dental arch aesthetically poor.

The shortened dental arch is becoming a more prominent concept as an increasing proportion of the population retain teeth into old age.

PRESCRIPTION TO TECHNICIANS

Communication with dental technicians is important to the success of a prosthesis. A good working relationship will benefit patient, dentist and technician.

General aspects • Treat technicians with respect; they are highly skilled individuals and essential members of the dental team.
• Write instructions clearly and legibly. • Ensure there is a mechanism for discussing difficult cases or problems. • In complex cases or cases using precision attachments ensure good communication and that the technician has access to materials and equipment needed. • Use of digital photography is useful for denture design and shade-matching purposes. • Ensure pick-up and delivery times suit the needs of dentist, patients and technician.
• Allow the technician sufficient time to complete a specific task.
• The dentist should know the capabilities of the technician. • If problems occur, look at the clinical side and ensure it is not the dentist who has made an error. • Always disinfect work to be sent to a laboratory.

Specific instructions

Casts The technician requires to know what material a cast should be poured in, the purpose of the cast, whether it should be surveyed or not.

Individual trays The technician should be informed of tray material, design, handles, spacers, vents, etc.

Record blocks The technician should be told of baseplate design for record blocks, e.g. wire, shellac, heat-cured (clear or pink) acrylic.

Trial setting of teeth Detailed information should be given to the technician regarding shade, shape, mould and setting of teeth.

Processing of denture Information regarding gingival stippling, use of coloured acrylics (e.g. for pigmented gingivae) and minute staining of teeth (for improved aesthetics) must be given to the technician at this stage.

Partial denture design This is the responsibility of the dentist. It must be communicated clearly, via design sheets or on casts, to the technician.

ADVICE TO PATIENTS

Patients require advice on what to expect from denture wear. This should certainly be reiterated on insertion of a denture. It is prudent however to give advice before and during denture construction so that the patient is fully informed and has the opportunity to discuss aspects of denture wear he or she is unsure of with the dentist.

Patients should usually be informed of the following:

Coping with new dentures Wearing new dentures can be extremely difficult and will take time and perseverance. To get used to new dentures they should be worn as much as possible. Dentures should not be worn overnight. Patients should not expect too much too soon from dentures.

Eating with new dentures Initially food should be cut into small pieces and only food that requires little chewing eaten. Gradually the patient should diversify and be more ambitious with foods eaten. Food often goes under the denture at first. The patient should attempt to chew on both sides at the same time.

Speaking with new dentures Speech is often a little difficult for the first few days. This usually improves relatively quickly.

Discomfort with new dentures It is quite normal to experience some discomfort after dentures are fitted. If the discomfort is minor, the patient should persevere with it until he/she sees the dentist again. If discomfort is severe the new dentures should be removed and the patient should revert to a previous prosthesis (if there is one) for a few days. Two days prior to the next visit to the dentist, the patient should recommence wear of the new dentures. This will help the dentist find the source of the discomfort. In addition the patient should be able to contact the dentist to discuss problems prior to the next visit.

Looseness of new dentures Initially dentures can feel a little loose until the patient adapts to the new shape. In most patients looseness improves with time.

Cleaning of new dentures Dentures may accumulate food debris, stain, plaque and calculus, so keeping them clean is important.

Dentures should be cleaned regularly after each meal using a *soft brush* and *soap*. Dentures should be immersed overnight in lukewarm water containing a tablet (or powder) of an *alkaline peroxide denture cleaner*.

Specific advice for patients with immediate dentures In addition to the above advice, immediate denture patients should be informed that in the weeks and months after extractions their denture may become loose and require multiple adjustments, relines or even replacement.

CHAPTER 13

ORTHODONTICS

Introduction   342

Risk/benefit considerations in orthodontic treatment   345

Classification and occlusal indices in orthodontics   348

Patient assessment/ examination   352

Cephalometrics   355

Principles of treatment planning   356

Management of the developing dentition   358

Class I malocclusion   361

Class II division 1 malocclusion   363

Class II division 2 malocclusion   365

Class III malocclusion   366

Removable appliances   368

Fixed appliances   374

Functional appliances   376

Orthodontic management of cleft lip and palate   377

Orthodontic aspects of orthognathic surgery   379

INTRODUCTION

WHAT IS ORTHODONTICS?

> Orthodontics is the branch of dentistry concerned with the growth of the face, development of the occlusion and the prevention and correction of occlusal anomalies.

WHAT IS MALOCCLUSION?

> Malocclusion is an irregularity in the occlusion beyond the accepted range of normal.

Not all malocclusions need treatment! Some malocclusions are only mildly unaesthetic and not detrimental to the health of the teeth or their supporting structures. In such cases there is likely to be little gain from treatment.

> *Ideal occlusion* Hypothetical concept based on the anatomy of the teeth.
> *Normal occlusion* An occlusion within the accepted deviation from the ideal.

PREVALENCE OF MALOCCLUSION

Based on morphology The UK population can be classified as:

Class I	50–55%
Class II div. 1	25–33%
Class II div. 2	10%
Class III	3%

using the British Standards Institute's Incisor Classification (p. 348).

Based on need for treatment Assessment of 12-year-old children using the Index of Orthodontic Treatment Need – Dental Health Component (p. 350): • one-third of children have a malocclusion showing a need for treatment • one-third have malocclusions which have borderline need for treatment • one-third have a malocclusion with little or no need for treatment.

WHO PROVIDES ORTHODONTIC CARE?

All dentists must be 'orthodontically aware'. Orthodontic appliance treatment is increasingly provided by specialists but the general dental practitioner (GDP) has a vital role to play. Good dental health is an essential prerequisite for future orthodontic treatment. The GDP is the gatekeeper to orthodontic care and should be competent in appropriate monitoring and recognition of malocclusion, as timely referral or treatment can alleviate orthodontic problems. The role of the GDP in orthodontics includes continuing preventive care, 'orthodontically appropriate' operative treatment such as management of primary molar problems, appropriate assessment of first permanent molars, monitoring of the developing occlusion, simple treatment skills – often in conjunction with advice from a specialist, extended treatment skills; further training via longitudinal part-time clinical attachments is available in some areas and can increase the range of malocclusions that can be treated by the GDP.

 The GDP will often wish to refer patients for advice or treatment. If in doubt, refer sooner rather than later, and before carrying out any intervention. The most difficult orthodontic problems are often those that have been referred too late, or have had previous unsuccessful or inappropriate orthodontic treatment.

Distribution of, and access to, specialist orthodontic practitioners is variable. At present, in many areas, demand for orthodontic treatment outstrips available resources. As a result, resources must be directed to those most likely to gain benefit from treatment. This excludes individuals with mild malocclusions, questionable dental health and poor oral hygiene. Orthodontic specialists undergo formal extensive postgraduate training. The GDP may refer patients to specialists working in a number of different environments: consultant orthodontic services based in regional hospitals or dental schools; specialist orthodontic practitioners; and orthodontists working in the community dental service.

Not all patients with a malocclusion require orthodontic treatment.

TIMING OF ORTHODONTIC INTERVENTION

When should orthodontic treatment be carried out? This is related to stage of dentition.

Deciduous dentition Treatment rarely indicated. Possible exceptions include malpositioned tooth causing marked mandibular displacement, supernumerary teeth, severe skeletal discrepancy or asymmetry.

Early mixed dentition Occasionally involves extraction of deciduous teeth, or interceptive procedures such as moving a tooth over the bite.

Late mixed/early permanent dentition Most treatment is carried out at this stage.

Later treatment Many forms of treatment are feasible in later life. Treatment involving orthognathic surgery is usually delayed until late teens.

Why do orthodontic treatment?

For many, orthodontic treatment is optional rather than essential. Benefits in terms of health gain are often limited and yet orthodontic treatment may cause iatrogenic damage. The risks associated with treatment are likely to be equally high in the management of a mild malocclusion or severe malocclusion. All potential patients must be aware of the benefits and risks of orthodontic treatment. The GDP must also be aware of these to give appropriate advice and guidance.

SCOPE OF ORTHODONTIC TREATMENT

Orthodontic treatment can be considered under the following headings: • monitoring and assessment of the developing dentition • management of problems of intra-arch alignment, e.g. anomalies in position of erupted teeth, transposition, ectopic teeth, crowding, spacing • inter-arch variation, e.g. anterior/posterior incisor relationships, overbite problems, centreline discrepancy, transverse buccal segment arrangement • management of skeletal discrepancies – in severe cases this may require a combination of orthodontics and orthognathic surgery • adjunctive orthodontic treatment, i.e. treatment designed to facilitate other areas of dentistry, e.g. uprighting teeth prior to bridgework, management of hypodontia.

RISK/BENEFIT CONSIDERATIONS IN ORTHODONTIC TREATMENT

POTENTIAL BENEFITS OF ORTHODONTIC TREATMENT

Can be categorized as: • improved dental health/function
• improved appearance.

Improved dental health/function

> The aim of orthodontic treatment is to produce improved
> function by the correction of irregularities and so to create
> not only greater resistance to disease, but also to improve
> personal appearance, which will later contribute to the
> mental as well as physical well-being of the individual.
> Memorandum on Orthodontics, BDA, 1954.

Despite this statement, there is limited scientific evidence
regarding the long-term effect of the various irregularities on
dental health. A variety of factors have, however, been discussed in
terms of improved health/function as a result of orthodontic
treatment.

Masticatory function Malocclusion has little to do with masticatory
efficiency. Even extreme states have little or no effect on
digestion or nutrition. Some occlusal problems, such as anterior
open bite, may however make incision of food awkward and
cause social embarrassment.

Dental caries Evidence is conflicting but suggests little relationship
between crowding and dental caries. However, grossly displaced
teeth may cause significant problems in cleaning and therefore be
prone to decay.

Periodontal disease Evidence is again conflicting. Recent research,
looking at specific crowded sites, shows a statistically significant
link between tooth alignment and plaque accumulation.
Improvements in toothbrushing are likely to have a greater effect
than orthodontic alignment of teeth in preventing periodontal
disease. As with caries, it would seem reasonable that extreme
malposition of teeth may predispose to problems. A suggested
benefit of orthodontic treatment is the opportunity for oral
hygiene instruction to be repeated and reinforced over a period
of time.

Overjet There is evidence that anterior teeth with an increased
overjet (>6 mm) are considerably more likely to suffer trauma.
Peak incidence is before age 10 and unfortunately treatment is
not commonly provided by this age. A slight increase in plaque

accumulation on teeth having either an increased or reverse overjet has also been shown.

Craniomandibular disorders (p. 327) These have a multifactorial aetiology. There is little evidence to suggest that malocclusion has any significant effect, or that orthodontic treatment brings any lasting benefit.

Tooth impaction Orthodontic treatment may be used to prevent tooth impaction.

Overbite Increased overbite may cause soft tissue damage to the palatal or lower labial mucosa.

Anterior crossbite Accelerated gingival recession may occur around lower incisors related to upper incisors in linguo-occlusion.

Conclusion The threat posed to dental health by malocclusion is generally modest. However, in some specific malocclusion traits there is the potential for significant damage.

Improved appearance

Malocclusion affecting appearance may also affect an individual's self-esteem, elicit an unfavourable social response or provoke negative stereotyping.

Self-esteem Only limited information is available but most suggests no link between level of malocclusion and self-esteem. However, there is great variation between individuals' perception of their appearance.

Social response Teasing may affect personality development.

Stereotyping It has been shown that faces evoke a more favourable response when there is normal anterior dental alignment, but that the level of background facial attractiveness is of greater importance.

Conclusion This is a difficult topic to investigate; intuitively it would seem that the chances of evoking an unfavourable social response are greater with more conspicuous dental defects.

POTENTIAL RISKS OF ORTHODONTIC TREATMENT

Can be categorized as: • tissue damage during treatment • increased susceptibility to dental disease • effects of treatment failure.

Tissue damage during treatment

Dental caries Especially likely around fixed appliances if poor plaque and dietary sugar control. Caries is entirely preventable – all potential orthodontic patients must have excellent oral hygiene, caries controlled and should use a fluoride mouthwash daily. This must be monitored closely throughout treatment.

Periodontal disease Mild gingivitis in patients wearing appliances is common. This is reversible, but requires careful control. Permanent loss of attachment can occur in some cases, particularly if teeth are moved outwith the arch or excessively tipped.

Root resorption Exceedingly common but usually insignificant in amount. Can be a significant problem in some cases and is more likely with fixed than removable appliances. History of trauma is a predisposing factor.

Pulp damage Occurs rarely, associated with excessive application of force. Minor circulatory changes occur and discomfort during orthodontic treatment is common. There is marked individual variation in response.

Ulceration Commonly arises from appliance components.

Enamel damage at debond There is the potential for enamel damage at debond as brackets are removed.

Headgear injury Dislodged headgear can cause facial and ocular injury. Headgear must be of an appropriate contemporary safety design, correctly fitted by an experienced operator and should be monitored carefully at each visit.

Increased susceptibility to dental disease

Craniomandibular disorders (p. 327) These have has been suggested as an effect of orthodontic treatment. Long-term studies seem to disprove this theory.

Periodontal disease Long-term follow-up of fixed appliance cases suggests this is not generally a significant problem.

Treatment failure

Can be due to a variety of factors: • poor patient cooperation • underlying skeletal constraints • inappropriate treatment technique. The effects of treatment failure will vary between individual patients.

Conclusion The effect of malocclusion on dental health in many cases is modest and it is vital that while seeking to improve appearance there is no iatrogenic damage. Active orthodontic treatment should be considered only in patients who have controlled dental health, excellent oral hygiene, and who have a significant degree of malocclusion that can be corrected with a reasonable degree of stability. The appropriate appliance should be used by an operator with appropriate training and experience. The patient must be fully informed of the scope of treatment, inconveniences involved and the likely long-term success.

Orthodontic treatment does, however, in appropriate circumstances, offer the opportunity to dramatically improve the appearance of the dentition.

CLASSIFICATION AND OCCLUSAL INDICES IN ORTHODONTICS

> An occlusal index is a rating or categorizing system that assigns a numeric or alphanumeric label to an individual's occlusion.

CLASSIFICATION

Numerous types of index have been developed. Whilst some are used to classify malocclusion for *diagnostic purposes*, e.g. British Standards Institute's Incisor Classification (Figure 13.1) and Skeletal Classification (Figure 13.2), other indices are designed to measure *treatment need*, e.g. Index of Orthodontic Treatment Need (IOTN) or *treatment outcome*, e.g. Peer Assessment Rating Index

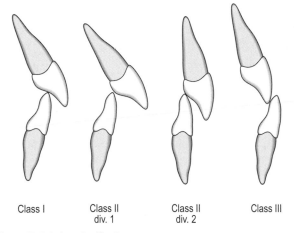

| Class I | Class II div. 1 | Class II div. 2 | Class III |

Figure 13.1 Incisor classification.

(PAR). There is also an Index of Complexity, Outcome and Need (ICON).

Incisor classification

Simpler and more relevant than Angle's classification. Now uses the British Standards Institute's (1983) classification of malocclusion based upon the relationship of the lower incisor edges and the cingulum plateau of the upper central incisors (see Figure 13.1).

Class I The lower incisor edges occlude with or lie immediately below the cingulum plateau of the upper central incisors.

Class II The lower incisor edges lie posterior to the cingulum plateau of the upper central incisors.

Class II div. 1 The upper central incisors are proclined or of average inclination and there is an increased overjet.

Class II div. 2 The upper central incisors are retroclined; the overjet is usually minimal but may be increased.

Class III The lower incisor edges lie anterior to the cingulum plateau of the upper central incisors; the overjet is reduced or reversed.

Skeletal classification

See Figure 13.2.

Class 1 skeletal pattern The lower dental base is normally related to the upper dental base. Point B lies a few millimetres behind point A (see Figure 13.3).

Class 2 skeletal pattern The lower dental base is retruded relative to the upper.

Class 3 skeletal pattern The lower dental base is protruded relative to the upper.

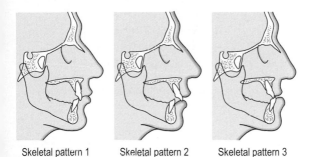

Skeletal pattern 1   Skeletal pattern 2   Skeletal pattern 3

Figure 13.2 Skeletal patterns.

INDEX OF ORTHODONTIC TREATMENT NEED (IOTN)

The IOTN has two components: • aesthetic component • dental health component. Both components can be applied to study models or clinically.

Aesthetic component of IOTN

The aesthetic component scores the need for treatment on the grounds of aesthetic impairment of the anterior teeth. The patient's teeth are compared with 10 photographs ranked in order of attractiveness, 1 being the most attractive and 10 the least aesthetically pleasing. The scale has been validated as follows:

Grades 1, 2, 3, 4   No/slight need
Grades 5, 6, 7   Borderline need
Grades 8, 9, 10   Need

Dental health component (DHC) of IOTN

The DHC records the various aspects of malocclusion using the MOCDO convention, where:

M =   Missing teeth
O =   Overjet
C =   Crossbite
D =   Displacement of contact points
O =   Overbite

This provides a reliable and rapid method of assessing the occlusion. A specifically designed measuring ruler is used and a grade awarded on the basis of the single most severe feature of the malocclusion. The index has been validated as follows:

Grades 1, 2   No/slight need
Grade 3   Borderline need
Grades 4, 5   Need

Limitations Aesthetic component cannot be used accurately in mixed dentition. There is a shortage of scientific information regarding the long-term effects of malocclusion. Nonetheless the DHC of IOTN provides a structured method for assessment of malocclusion.

Potential uses of IOTN

Resource allocation Enables identification of those most in need of treatment.

Outcome measure Both components of IOTN can be applied to treated cases to give an indication of the change resulting from treatment.

Uniformity of assessment Offers an objective structured assessment of malocclusion and the need for intervention.

Screening Can be used by GDPs for screening purposes.

Patient advice May be used to provide objective advice to a potential patient. The aesthetic component in particular can be used as a scale to advise patients who may have unrealistic concerns about the appearance of their teeth and similarly unrealistic expectations of orthodontic treatment.

PEER ASSESSMENT RATING INDEX (PAR)

Used to determine orthodontic treatment outcome. Assesses the outcome of treatment in terms of dento-occlusal change. Following a list of criteria and using a specially designed measuring ruler, this index is applied to the pre- and post-treatment study models. It measures the following features of the malocclusion: • overjet • overbite • centreline relationship • buccal segment relationship • upper and lower anterior alignment.

Limitations PAR is based solely on study models and does not account for changes in facial profile, iatrogenic damage, tooth inclination, arch width or posterior spacing, and is not appropriate for assessment of mixed dentition treatment.

PATIENT ASSESSMENT/EXAMINATION

The features of taking a history and examining a patient outlined in Chapter 2 apply. However, the following features are specifically relevant to an examination for orthodontic purposes.

The aims of orthodontic assessment are to document and evaluate facial, occlusal and functional characteristics, to decide if there is a problem and, if so, what action is required.

Notably important times for orthodontic examination are: • early mixed dentition • early permanent dentition.

As always, a logical structured approach must be followed to gather all the information efficiently and to ensure important features are not overlooked.

The following sequence should be employed.

PATIENT BACKGROUND

Note: • age • relevant medical history • relevant dental history, e.g. attendance record, oral hygiene, caries rate, trauma • social history: is there a complaint from the patient? Does the patient appreciate what orthodontic treatment involves? Level of parental support? Any friends/siblings having treatment?

CLINICAL EXAMINATION

Extraoral examination

Need to consider hard and soft tissues.

Hard tissues

Assessment is aimed at noting any disproportion or asymmetry. The skeletal pattern has an important effect on the dental arch relationship. The patient sits unsupported, with the head in the free postural position. Usually determined in profile. Assess in three dimensions.

Anterior–posterior Significant discrepancies between the two skeletal bases will be readily apparent. Retraction of the soft tissues provides easier visualization.

Vertical Need to assess the Frankfort–mandibular plane angle (normal, reduced, increased) and the lower facial height. The distance from a point between the eyebrows (glabella) to the base of the nose (subnasale) should be equal to that from subnasale to the underside of the chin (soft tissue menton).

Lateral (view from the front) Is there any significant asymmetry? Asymmetry in the lower part of the face can be due to a true skeletal asymmetry, a displacement on closure or a combination of both. Any significant lateral skeletal base discrepancy is usually apparent from the transverse arch relationship intraorally.

Soft tissues

Lips *Lip contour* Normal, everted, vertical? *Lip line* Where is the top of the lower lip relative to the incisors? Should cover about a third to a half of the upper central incisor. *Lip seal* Are the lips competent with mandible in the rest position? An attempt should be made to assess lip activity during swallowing.

Beware of cases with marked lip incompetence.

Tongue This is difficult to examine without interfering. Some positions of tongue activity can be inferred from the occlusion. With incompetent lips the tongue will tend to come forward to help maintain the anterior oral seal (adaptive tongue thrust).

By the end of the extraoral examination, a reasonable idea of what occlusal characteristics to expect should have been obtained. If they differ from the expected, why?

Intraoral examination

Look at the general features of dental health such as oral hygiene, caries experience, gingival condition, tooth number and form. Then examine each arch in isolation, followed by the two arches in occlusion.

Lower arch

Labial segment Count the teeth, assess alignment and angulation of the incisors.

Buccal segment Observe alignment problems (potential and present) and inclination of the canines.

Upper arch

Labial segment As for lower arch.

Buccal segment Determine inclination of the canines, note alignment problems; if the permanent canine is unerupted, is it palpable?

In occlusion As the teeth are brought together check path of closure. Is there a premature contact and associated displacement?

Incisor relationship Classify this according to British Standards Institute's Incisor Classification (p. 348).

Overjet Measure to the nearest millimetre.

> **Overjet** Relationship between incisors in the horizontal plane.

Overbite Is it average, increased or reduced; complete or incomplete?

> **Overbite** Relationship between incisors in the vertical plane.

Centrelines Check the relation of each dental midline to the facial midline and also to each other.

Arch anterior/posterior relationship Check the canine and buccal segment intercuspation.

Arch buccolingual relationship Check for any crossbites. If there is a posterior crossbite, is it bilateral or unilateral, and is there an associated displacement?

TMJ assessment An assessment should be made of any TMJ and myofascial symptoms or signs.

DIAGNOSTIC RECORDS

The following diagnostic records will aid assessment of the patient's orthodontic status:

Study models

Allow a more accurate assessment of some aspects of the occlusion and facilitate measurement. Models provide a good baseline record and help explanation of any problem to both the patient and parent. Diagnostic set-ups may be helpful.

Radiographs

Radiographs, if justified, should only be taken after a clinical examination has been carried out. A panoramic-type view is often appropriate, although this may need to be supplemented by other views where indicated, e.g. history of incisor trauma, localization of unerupted teeth. A lateral cephalogram may be required in certain cases. As with the clinical examination, radiographs should be examined in a standard, structured manner and reported upon (see Chapter 4).

Having completed the examination, a precise summary of the patient's condition should be recorded in the case notes.

CEPHALOMETRICS

> *Cephalometrics* The study of facial form as revealed in the analysis of lateral skull radiographs.

A lateral cephalogram is taken under standardized conditions in order that measurements can be compared between patients and between films of the same patient taken on different occasions. The head is held in a cephalostat so that there is a fixed constant relationship between the head, film and X-ray source.

In addition to clinical examination, analysis of a lateral cephalogram permits a more detailed evaluation of facial and dentoskeletal structures to aid diagnosis and treatment planning, especially in cases with a skeletal discrepancy. Also provides baseline measurements to monitor the effects of growth and treatment.

> **A lateral cephalogram is not needed, or justified, for all orthodontic assessments.**

ANALYSIS OF A LATERAL CEPHALOGRAM

An outline should be traced as in Figure 13.3. The following definitions are important:

- Sella (S) – midpoint of sella turcica
- Nasion (N) – most anterior point on the frontonasal suture
- 'A' point (A) – deepest point on maxillary profile between the anterior nasal spine and the alveolar crest
- 'B' point (B) – deepest point on the concavity of the mandibular profile between the alveolar crest and the point of the chin
- Posterior nasal spine (PNS) – tip of the posterior nasal spine

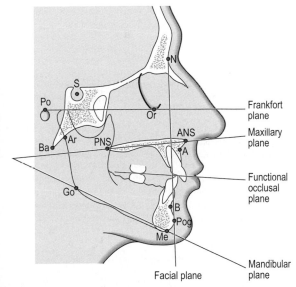

Figure 13.3 Cephalometric points and planes.

- Anterior nasal spine (ANS) – point of the bony nasal spine
- Gonion (Go) – most posterior, inferior point on the angle of the mandible
- Menton (Me) – lowermost point of the mandibular symphysis
- Pogonion (Pog) – most anterior point on the bony chin
- Porion (Po) – highest point on the bony external acoustic meatus
- Orbitale (Or) – most inferior point on the margin of the orbit
- Articulare (Ar) – point of intersection of the projection of the surface of the condylar neck and the inferior surface of the basiocciput
- Basion (Ba) – most posterior inferior point in the midline on the basiocciput.

From these points a number of planes can be described:

Frankfort plane Po–Or. It was once believed this plane was horizontal when the head was held in a free postural position. Now not so as there is individual variation.

Facial plane N–Pog. Indicates the general orientation of the facial profile.

Maxillary plane ANS–PNS. Indicates the orientation of the palate.

Mandibular plane Go–Me. Indicates the orientation of the mandible.

Occlusal plane Variety of definitions used. Functional occlusal plane (FOP) is a line following the occlusion of the molar and premolar teeth.

Interpret cephalometric measurements with caution and do not be overly concerned with minor variations in values.

Cephalometric analysis tends to utilize angular values which change little with either sex or age. A vast array of measurements have been suggested; the more common are listed in Table 13.1.

The anterior/posterior skeletal discrepancy is determined using angle ANB (Table 13.2). The vertical skeletal discrepancy is evaluated using the Max/Man plane angle. As the discrepancy in either increases, so do the difficulties in dealing with the problem.

A cephalogram can be used to determine incisor inclination. This permits judgements to be made as to the potential for tipping to correct incisor position, the need for bodily movement, or the skeletal pattern precluding either option.

PRINCIPLES OF TREATMENT PLANNING

Treatment planning is affected by many factors. In most instances the GDP should obtain a specialist opinion.

TABLE 13.1 Mean cephalometric values (Caucasian norms)

	Mean	Range (+ or −)
SNA	81°	3
SNB	79°	3
ANB	3°	3
Maxillary plane/mandibular plane	27°	4
Upper incisor/maxillary plane	108°	6
Lower incisor/mandibular plane	92°	6
Upper incisor/lower incisor	133°	10
Lower incisor/A–Pog	0 mm	2
Upper lip/aesthetic plane	0 mm	
Lower lip/aesthetic plane	0 mm	

TABLE 13.2 Relationship of ANB angle to skeletal pattern

Angle ANB (degrees)	Skeletal pattern
2–4	1
>4	2
<2	3

AIMS OF TREATMENT

The aim of treatment is to produce an occlusion that is stable, functional and acceptable in appearance. Must determine if treatment is indicated. If so, what are the goals of treatment – ideal or compromise result? The aims must be appropriate to the particular individual and must take account of likely compliance with treatment.

CONSIDERATIONS

Space requirements It is usual to plan around the lower arch. The form of the lower arch is usually accepted and the position of the lower labial segment labiolingually is altered only in specific circumstances. If the lower labial segment is crowded the lower canines need to be repositioned and extractions may be needed to facilitate this. Next, the upper arch should be planned around the lower arch and the upper canine placed in a Class I relationship with the lower.

Tooth movement Must decide on nature of tooth movement
required as this influences the type of appliance indicated.

Anchorage demands Anchorage requirements must be assessed. It is
best to err on the side of caution, as it is easier to lose than to
regain space in the later stages of treatment. Anchorage
demands involve an interaction of space needs, tooth movement
and the buccal occlusion goals.

Anchorage: The source of resistance to the reaction from the active
components of an appliance.

Retention This is vital and must be included in the initial treatment
plan. Each case will have specific retention requirements and it is
important that the patient understands these at the outset of
treatment.

TREATMENT OPTIONS

No appliance It may be that, following the provision of space,
spontaneous tooth movement will occur, e.g. extraction of first
premolars will allow mesially inclined canines to tip distally and
give some relief of crowding in the labial segment.

Removable appliances These can be used only if simple tooth
tipping alone is required.

Fixed appliances Indicated where bodily tooth movement is needed.

Functional appliances A functional approach will be indicated in
certain situations, most commonly early intervention in a Class
II division 1 malocclusion.

Orthognathic surgery If there is a significant skeletal discrepancy,
successful treatment may be outwith the scope of orthodontic
treatment alone and require a combined orthodontic/surgical
approach. This type of treatment is not usually undertaken until
late teens, when growth has reduced to adult levels.

> ⚠️ **The prospective patient must be fully aware of the
> treatment plan, goals and necessary implications for
> him/her in terms of extractions, appliances and cooperation.**

MANAGEMENT OF THE DEVELOPING DENTITION

The development of the dentition is discussed on page 172, and the
timing of tooth formation and eruption is detailed in Appendix C.
Awareness of the normal developmental pattern and sequence of
eruption is vital. This is more important than chronological

eruption guidelines, e.g. if an upper lateral incisor erupts before the upper central incisor further investigation is needed.

As part of the routine examination of children, the dentition should be assessed using the MOCDO convention as per the DHC of the IOTN described on page 350. This will permit referral of appropriate cases for orthodontic treatment/advice.

DECIDUOUS DENTITION

Natal teeth Are present at or shortly after birth. Rare; often in the lower incisor region – extract only if causing problems (e.g. with feeding).

Lack of space between anterior deciduous teeth just before they are shed is indicative of crowding in the permanent dentition.

The tendency is not to interfere in deciduous dentition other than to maintain good oral hygiene and dental health. Rarely, treatment for problems of a skeletal nature may be provided at this time.

Early loss of deciduous teeth Varying opinion on management of enforced extractions. Effect of loss of a deciduous tooth depends upon the age at which lost, the tooth lost and the degree of inherent crowding. May result in mesial migration of posterior teeth and spreading out of any crowded anterior teeth. Specifically:

Early loss of deciduous incisors Usually causes no problem; don't balance or compensate.

Early loss of deciduous canines Rarely lost through caries but may be pushed out by permanent lateral incisor if crowded. Consider a balancing extraction of early loss of deciduous canines to minimize any centreline shift that would complicate later treatment. Extraction of deciduous canines often allows some relief in anterior crowding; however, may result in exacerbation of the crowding, with mesial movement of the posterior teeth.

Early loss of deciduous molars Space loss may occur due to extraction or unrestored cavities or poor restoration. The earlier the extraction the greater the space loss.

Early loss of first deciduous molars Unilateral loss may cause a centreline shift. First permanent molar and second deciduous molars will drift forwards without rotation.

Early loss of second deciduous molars If lost before the first permanent molar erupts, will often result in considerable space loss. Space loss tends to be greater in the upper arch.

Space maintenance, balancing and compensatory extractions

The natural tooth is the ideal space maintainer. In cases with generalized crowding, space maintenance will rarely be appropriate. Further, children with high caries experience are seldom suitable candidates for long-term appliance wear. If only one tooth is a significant problem then consider pulp therapy.

Consideration should be given to compensating or balancing extractions.

Balancing extraction (same arch, opposite side), to maintain symmetry and centreline relationships.
Compensating extraction (same side, opposite arch) to maintain inter-arch relationship.

It is crucial that, before extracting teeth for orthodontic purposes, radiographs are taken to determine the presence/absence of suspected unerupted or missing teeth.

MIXED DENTITION

A variety of problems may present. Abnormalities of tooth number, form, position and structure may affect how the dentition develops. These are discussed on pages 190–193. Other factors affecting development of the dentition include:

Sucking habits Possible effects include: • upper incisor proclination • lower incisor retroclination • narrowing of upper arch, which may lead to mandibular displacement and a crossbite • anterior open bite (often asymmetric).

Such habits often stop spontaneously. The sooner the habit is stopped, the better the chance of spontaneous improvement of any associated problems. In some situations a habit deterrent appliance may be indicated.

Traumatic loss of upper central incisor If reimplantation is not feasible, initially space maintenance should be carried out and then plan long-term management.

Incisors in linguo-occlusion If corrected as early as possible and any associated displacement eliminated, the risk of gingival damage and of tooth wear is reduced. Often the upper incisor is tipped palatally and the tooth movement needed is suitable for a removable appliance incorporating posterior bite capping to free the occlusion. Once 'over the bite' the correction is often retained by the overbite.

Treatment of posterior crossbite Generally, a posterior unilateral crossbite with a displacement on closure should be corrected in the mixed dentition. Often, a simple removable appliance can be used.

Skeletal problems Any patient with a severe skeletal discrepancy should be sent for an early specialist assessment. Some forms of discrepancy will respond better than others to early treatment and the benefits, or otherwise, should be determined.

First permanent molars of poor prognosis The prognosis for first permanent molars should be assessed at age 8–9 and if there is doubt about the long-term outlook, a specialist opinion should be sought. Often the tooth condition and dental motivation will outweigh all other factors. For the best spontaneous improvement, timing is critical in the lower arch and loss of first molars is usually best when the furcation of the second permanent molar is just calcifying. If crowding is present, this will also help spontaneous space closure. Early loss of an upper first permanent molar can lead to rapid space loss.

CLASS I MALOCCLUSION

> Lower incisor edge occludes with or lies below the middle palatal third of the upper central incisor.

Problems encountered in Class I occlusions include crowding, spacing (much less commonly), crossbite, openbite and bimaxillary proclination.

Crowding
Cause Disproportion between tooth and arch size.
Dental health threat/appearance Threat to dental health is not as great as once thought. In general it is easier and more worth while to improve toothbrushing than to align the teeth to facilitate this. Aesthetics related to severity.
Stability Influenced by method of correction.
Treatment options: • Arch expansion – achieved by increasing the arch width or by proclination of the labial segments. Often unstable. • Extraction of teeth – particularly in severe cases. • Distal movement of teeth.

Increase in lower incisor crowding in the mid to late teens is common. Rarely poses any threat to long-term dental health and careful thought should be given before undertaking treatment as it will often involve fixed appliances and stability is not guaranteed.

Spacing

Cause Often due to missing teeth or a tooth/tissue ratio problem. Can be small teeth in average arches or normal teeth in large arches. In adults, spacing may occur secondary to loss of periodontal support and tooth drifting.

Dental health threat/appearance Usually there is no threat to dental health; aesthetics depends on severity.

Stability Frequently poor; requires permanent retention as great tendency to relapse.

Transverse problems – crossbites

Crossbite Deviation from the normal buccolingual relationship. Can be local or segmental.

Local crossbites Usually caused by crowding, e.g. lower second premolar forced to erupt lingually.

Segmental crossbites Involve most teeth in the buccal segment. From the dental health standpoint, of greater importance is whether or not there is an associated displacement on closure. There are three commonly presenting patterns of crossbite:

Unilateral crossbite with associated displacement
Cause Often due to mismatch in the arch widths and displacement into a position of maximum intercuspation. Displacement results in crossbite. Can be related to a thumb-sucking habit.

Threat to health/appearance Displacement on closure can be associated with TMJ problems, faceting and development of the dentition in a displaced position. Consider interceptive treatment using an upper removable appliance for midline expansion, incorporating posterior bite capping to eliminate the displacement.

Unilateral crossbite with no displacement
Cause Often a skeletal asymmetry.

Threat to health/appearance Often none, treatment seldom indicated.

Bilateral crossbite
Cause Skeletal base problem (both anterior/posterior and transverse).

Threat to health/appearance Usually there is no displacement and is unlikely to affect appearance. Often accept as treatment stability doubtful. Some advocate rapid maxillary expansion.

Vertical problems – openbite

Anterior open bite

In occlusion, incisors fail to contact and do not overlap in the vertical plane. May be due to digit-sucking habits, tongue thrust or skeletal pattern. Frequently there is an associated tongue thrust which is usually secondary and adaptive. If associated with a digit habit it will improve once the habit has ceased, although this is slow and may not be complete.

Posterior open bite

Rare. Aetiology unclear and treatment stability often poor.

Correction of an open bite due to skeletal discrepancy almost always requires a combination of orthodontics and orthognathic surgery.

Bimaxillary proclination

If this is present in a Class I relationship, the upper incisors cannot be retracted without first retracting the lower incisors. Long-term stability influenced by soft tissue equilibrium.

CLASS II DIVISION 1 MALOCCLUSION

> Lower incisor edges lie posterior to the cingulum plateau of the upper central incisors, overjet is increased, upper incisors may be proclined or of average inclination.

Occlusal features

Overjet Upper incisors are often proclined (digit habit, lip activity, developmental position). Where upper incisors are more upright, the increased overjet is associated with a skeletal pattern 2 or retroclined lower incisors (due to lower lip activity, habit, trapped behind vertical part of palate).

Overbite Variable, often deep and complete.

Buccal segments Often Class II (related to the skeletal pattern).

Alignment Crowding, spacing, etc., are all possible on top of arch malrelationship.

Skeletal features

Anterior/posterior Usually Class 2 skeletal pattern – the primary aetiological feature. As the severity of skeletal pattern increases, so does treatment difficulty.

Vertical Overbite will often reflect this and is variable. A high angle
pattern is often associated with an unfavourable facial profile.
Transverse Nil characteristic.

Soft tissues
Lips are often incompetent. For reasons of stability, lip competence
post-treatment must be aimed for.

Mandibular position/path of closure
May tend to posture the mandible to improve profile and lip
coverage – true displacement is rare.

Why treat?
If increased overjet is present, the incisors are at greater risk of
trauma. Incompetent lips may worsen gingivitis. Aesthetic reasons.
Occasionally may have an overbite problem.

Treatment options
Management of the overjet is the key factor in treatment planning.

No treatment May be acceptable, especially if mild.
Extractions only Rarely an option. May relieve crowding but no
beneficial effect on the incisor relationship.
Removable appliances A common approach historically but now
rarely appropriate.
Single-arch fixed appliance Only consider if no overbite problem or
would be unable to fully reduce the overjet due to the vertical
impedance of the lower labial segment.
Two-arch fixed appliances Frequently the most appropriate treatment
option. Gives the ability to deal with overjet, overbite and arch
relationship. Required when canines are unfavourable for tipping
distally or the upper incisors are unfavourable for tipping,
rotations are present, or controlled space closure is needed.
Functional appliance An option if considering early treatment.
Often needs a second phase of treatment with fixed appliances to
complete treatment. If successful, functional appliance
treatment may reduce the complexity/difficulty of second-phase
fixed treatment.
Orthognathic surgery With a severe skeletal pattern, orthodontic
treatment can only produce a dentoalveolar camouflage. A
combination of orthodontics and surgery allows the skeletal
pattern to be changed (p. 379).
Key factors in treatment planning Severity of skeletal pattern: can
the malocclusion be treated by dental camouflage or would this
have an adverse effect on the facial profile?

Post-treatment stability

 Control of the upper incisors by the lower lip is of paramount importance.

CLASS II DIVISION 2 MALOCCLUSION

The lower incisor edges lie posterior to the cingulum plateau of the upper central incisors. The upper central incisors are retroclined, the overjet is usually reduced but can be increased. The overbite is increased.

Occlusal features

Overjet Typically minimal but can be increased. Upper central incisors are retroclined. Upper lateral incisors are often proclined, mesially inclined and mesiolabially rotated. Lower incisors are often retroclined, contributing to lower incisor crowding, increased overbite and a poor interincisal angulation.

Overbite Usually increased and can be sufficiently severe to produce traumatic bite.

Buccal segments May present with a scissors bite.

Alignment Variable, there is often a typical arrangement of upper lateral incisors and the incisor retroclination may be associated with crowding.

Skeletal features

Anterior/posterior Often skeletal pattern 1 or mild 2. Tendency to bimaxillary retroclination.

Vertical Usually reduced or average. May have a closing growth rotation.

Transverse If severe, results in scissors bite.

Scissors bite Lingual crossbite of the lower posterior teeth.

Soft tissues

Lip line often high; accentuated labiomental fold, flattening of the upper lip profile with an obtuse nasolabial angle.

Mandibular position/path of closure

Usually a simple hinge closure but in severe cases a habitual downwards and forwards posture may be seen.

Why treat?
Possibility of overbite trauma; aesthetics.

Treatment options
No treatment Especially in a mild case this is often a very sensible option.

Extractions only Rarely an acceptable option.

Removable appliance Rarely appropriate because of the inter-incisor relationship. May, however, use a removable appliance in conjunction with fixed appliance treatment to help overbite reduction by taking advantage of the bite plane effect.

Single-arch fixed Limited application and really only in cases with a mild problem and no extremes of overbite or retroclination.

Two-arch fixed The vast majority of cases in this group, if treated, need upper and lower fixed appliances. This allows overbite control and, more particularly, control of the incisor inclinations – essential for long-term stability. If the incisors are retroclined it may be that the crowding can be dealt with by proclining the labial segments. This facilitates relief of crowding, overbite reduction, correction of the interincisal angulation, improves the profile and may help stability.

Functional appliances An option, but must first convert relationship to a Class II division 1. Has added advantage of dealing with the overbite using the bite plane effect. Likely to need fixed appliance to complete.

Orthognathic surgery May need to consider in an adult with a significant anterior/posterior discrepancy or very reduced lower facial height. As for functional treatment convert firstly to a Class II division 1. Indicated if profile poor.

Post-treatment stability
The rotated lateral incisors have a strong tendency to relapse. Overbite reduction stability is related to the interincisal angle achieved at end of treatment.

CLASS III MALOCCLUSION

Lower incisor edges lie anterior to the cingulum plateau of the upper central incisors. Overjet is reduced or reversed.

Occlusal features

Overjet Often see dentoalveolar compensation of the incisors. Upper incisors are often crowded and proclined. Lower incisors frequently retroclined (to compensate for the skeletal pattern). There may be an anterior displacement on closure.

Overbite Varies considerably.

Buccal segments Upper arch is often crowded, especially if there has been early loss of deciduous molars. Lower arch is often spaced. Crossbites are common due to a discrepancy in arch width and the lower arch being positioned relatively more anterior in a class III malocclusion.

Alignment Upper often crowded. Lower often spaced.

Skeletal features

Anterior/posterior Often the most important factor in producing a Class III. As the skeletal pattern gets more adverse so does the Class III malocclusion and the scope for successful orthodontic treatment alone. Skeletal pattern is associated with a variety of causes, e.g. large mandible, retrognathic maxilla, forward position of glenoid fossa, short anterior cranial base. Usually results from a combination of these factors.

Vertical Wide variation. Anterior height of the intermaxillary space may be large and associated with an anterior open bite.

Transverse In many cases the maxillary base is narrow and the mandibular base wide. This is further aggravated by the anterior/posterior discrepancy.

Soft tissues

Increased anterior intermaxillary height may result in incompetent lips.

Mandibular position/path of closure

Usually a simple hinge closure but an anterior displacement is often seen. Occasionally overclosure is evident.

In a Class III malocclusion growth is often a problem. It is unpredictable and it is best to assume that it is going to be unfavourable. By the time the patient enters the pubertal growth spurt, incisor compensation is often at its maximum.

Why treat?

Concerns about appearance. Modest link between mandibular displacements and craniomandibular disorders.

Treatment

Need to establish the true occlusal position in absence of any displacements. Do not rush into extractions – need to consider the longer-term effects of growth.

Key factors in treatment planning. Concerns of patient (profile or teeth), skeletal pattern severity (as is and possible future changes). Can the patient achieve edge-to-edge incisor contact? Is there an overbite which will help to retain the correction, amount of dentoalveolar compensation?

No treatment If crowding is minimal or there are no displacements may wish to accept and review at later date.

Extractions only Upper arch extractions would only provide relief of crowding.

Removable appliance May use as an interceptive measure in the mixed dentition but requires an adequate overbite to maintain the correction.

Single-arch fixed Could align the upper arch and accept the Class III incisor relationship.

Two-arch fixed Will allow dentoalveolar correction of the malocclusion. Requires careful consideration of the effects of unfavourable growth. May wish to delay treatment in view of this. Best results are obtained where skeletal discrepancy is mild and susceptible to dentoalveolar camouflage.

Functional appliances Less popular in Class III cases due to the undesirable effects of continuing growth. Protraction headgear may be appropriate in certain circumstances.

Orthognathic surgery An option for the severe Class III malocclusion. A phase of presurgical orthodontics will be needed to decompensate and align the arches before surgery in late teens.

Post-treatment stability

Dependent upon the overbite and long-term facial growth.

REMOVABLE APPLIANCES

An orthodontic device which can be removed from the mouth by the patient for cleaning. May be either passive or active:
Active Designed to achieve tooth movement (tipping) by means of active components such as wire springs and screws.
Passive Appliances designed to maintain teeth in their present position, e.g. space maintainers, retainers.

This section deals with the conventional type of removable appliance used when simple tooth tipping is indicated. Most functional appliances are also classified as removable appliances.

INDICATIONS

Use of removable appliances requires careful case selection. They should not be used in circumstances where fixed appliance therapy would be more appropriate. May be used as an adjunct to fixed appliance treatment.

Treatment options with removable appliances

Simple tipping movement of teeth A force applied to the crown of a tooth by a spring will cause tipping about a fulcrum roughly one-third to one-half of the way from the apex. As the crown tips in one direction the root apex will tip in the opposite. If the use of a removable appliance to tip a tooth is being considered, assess the angulation of the tooth, its desired position and decide if it is feasible to achieve this movement with simple tooth tipping. For example, correction of an anterior crossbite.

Overbite reduction In cases with a deep overbite, the use of a flat anterior bite plane may help overbite reduction by holding the posterior teeth out of occlusion and allowing continued vertical development.

Elimination of occlusal interferences and crossbite correction Posterior bite planes can be used to prop the occlusion and facilitate crossbite correction by freeing the occlusion and eliminating any displacement on closure.

Extrusion of teeth (if used with a fixed appliance component) A spring can be used to apply an extrusive force if a bracket is placed to allow force delivery. The acrylic coverage of the palate provides vertical anchorage to resist the effect of this extrusive force.

Space maintainer A removable appliance can be used to control the position of groups of teeth while awaiting further eruption.

Retainer Removable retainers are often used after active appliance treatment.

Habit deterrent A simple removable appliance may be used, where appropriate, to help discourage a finger-sucking habit.

Contraindications

Removable appliances are not indicated if simple tooth tipping is inappropriate, e.g. where multiple rotations or bodily tooth movement is required. The range of malocclusions that can be treated to a high standard with removable appliances alone is limited.

COMPONENTS OF REMOVABLE APPLIANCES

These can be described as: • fixation components • active components • baseplate.

Fixation components

Fixation is the method by which the appliance resists displacement from the mouth. Good fixation will help patient compliance, anchorage and tooth movement.

Typical fixation components are:

Adams' clasp Posterior teeth – 0.7 mm hard stainless steel wire.
Southend clasp Anterior teeth – 0.7 mm hard stainless steel wire.

Fixation is gained by engaging the undercuts of teeth. In appliance design the principle of three-point fixation should be adhered to.

Active components

Provide the force which moves the teeth. A variety of different methods are used, e.g. wire springs and bows, screws, elastics.

Springs Springs are activated in the intended direction of movement and when the appliance is seated the spring is displaced. The spring then attempts to return to its original position and applies force to the tooth. The force applied (F) is affected by the deflection of the wire (d), radius of the wire (r) and length of the wire (l), This is expressed in the equation:

$$F \propto \frac{dr^4}{l^3}$$

Examples: palatal finger spring, buccal canine retractor, Z-spring.

Points to remember • Stability ratio – ideally a spring should be flexible in the desired direction of action but not in others. • As light a force as possible for a given deflection is desired. • Coils are incorporated to increase the length within the confines of the oral cavity. The coil should unwind as the force is dissipated. Although simple in design, to be used to maximum effect careful attention to detail is needed. If poorly designed or adjusted they can cause tooth movement in the wrong direction. • The force applied to a single-rooted tooth should be about 0.3 N, which, for a 0.5 mm palatal finger spring, will be about 2–3 mm of activation. • A palatal finger spring should be boxed and guarded.

Bows Mechanically more complex than springs. Supported bows such as a Roberts' retractor have good flexibility and a good stability ratio.

Screws Can act either directly on a tooth or through the baseplate. Typical activation (one turn once or twice a week) is 0.2 mm and thus a large force is applied intermittently over a small distance.

Elastics Historically used as an alternative to a labial bow to improve the appearance, but may slide up teeth and traumatize the soft tissues. Furthermore, they tend to flatten the arch.

Baseplate
Removable appliances have an acrylic baseplate. It should fit well around the teeth that are not to move and is trimmed away from those required to move. The functions of the baseplate are: • to support and protect other components • to prevent unwanted drift of teeth • to contribute to anchorage. May be extended into bite planes.

Flat anterior bite plane Often used to free the occlusion or to encourage overbite reduction. At design stage, the height and length of the bite plane must be specified.

Posterior bite plane Can be helpful in eliminating a displacement and to free the occlusion sufficiently to push a tooth over the bite. Keep to minimal thickness.

The baseplate also has an important role in anchorage (p. 358). Anchorage can be:

Intramaxillary from within the same arch.
Intermaxillary from the opposing arch.
Extraoral from outwith the mouth (headgear, facemask).

With a removable appliance anchorage is aided by: • baseplate contact with teeth not being moved • baseplate contact with the palate • applying simple tipping forces • applying light tooth-moving forces • applying force to only a small number of teeth at any one time.

Anchorage can be reinforced by use of extraoral or intermaxillary anchorage.

DESIGNING A REMOVABLE APPLIANCE

When designing a removable appliance remember: • design for a specific task • design at chairside with patient still in chair • draw and describe the design on laboratory prescription sheet • use a systematic approach: – fixation – activation – baseplate and any baseplate modifications • *do not* attempt to put too many active components on one appliance.

APPLIANCE FITTING

When fitting a removable appliance:
1. Check the appliance provided complies with design.
2. Try the appliance in the mouth.
3. Ensure it is comfortable.
4. Adjust the appliance.
5. Take relevant measurements to assess progress.
6. Give patient instructions on:
   a. insertion, removal and care
   b. when to wear
   c. what to expect
   d. what to do if problems occur.
7. Arrange next visit – usually 4 weeks later.

APPLIANCE CHECK VISITS

At each visit assess: • tooth movement • anchorage • cooperation.

A standard approach is essential at each visit to allow this information to be gathered quickly and efficiently.

1. Ask the patient how he/she is coping. This will identify any specific problems and allows an assessment of speech.
2. Examine the patient with the appliance in situ. Does it fit? Are the active components seating correctly? Are the teeth still free to move?
3. Ask the patient to remove the appliance. How does the patient handle the appliance? Does it look worn?
4. Check measurements – progress of tooth movement and anchorage.

5. Adjust appliance:
   - fixation
   - active components
   - baseplate.
6. Check insertion and removal.
7. Revise instructions to patient.
8. Review in 4 weeks.

PROBLEMS WITH REMOVABLE APPLIANCE TREATMENT

Potential problems are: • no tooth movement • incorrect tooth movement • anchorage loss.

 If treatment progress is slow, identify a cause as soon as possible.

No tooth movement

Check at each visit – if teeth fail to move as expected check:

Is the tooth free to move? • Baseplate trimmed correctly • occlusal locking • retained root/other anatomical limitation.

Active components adjusted correctly? • Check screw turns • check springs correctly in place • springs activated at last visit.

Lack of wear? Signs of non-wear are: • broken appointments • broken appliances • poor speech with appliance in situ • poor fit • still active at each visit • no signs of wear on appliance/soft tissue • difficulty inserting or removing appliance.

Incorrect tooth movement

Check: • appliance design • position of coils • contact of active component with tooth.

Anchorage loss

Signs (if retracting a tooth) • An increasing overjet • developing crossbite in buccal segments • deterioration in buccal segment relationship.

Action • Reduce active component force • check appliance fit, design and wear • seek further advice from a specialist orthodontist.

ADVANTAGES OF REMOVABLE APPLIANCES

• Tip teeth efficiently • good for overbite reduction • bite planes can eliminate displacements/occlusal interference • tooth movements usually few and simple • less chairside time needed than with fixed appliances • fewer inventory problems than with fixed appliances • can remove for cleaning • good source of anchorage from baseplate.

DISADVANTAGES OF REMOVABLE APPLIANCES

• Limited tooth movement available • limited scope in lower arch • affect speech • removable by the patient!

FIXED APPLIANCES

> An orthodontic device in which attachments are fixed to the teeth and forces are applied by archwires or auxiliaries via these attachments.

COMPONENTS

Classified as attachments, archwires and auxiliaries.

Attachments

Act as a 'handle' to allow the application of forces to the teeth in three dimensions. Two types:

Brackets Fixed to the tooth by bonding and are used on most teeth.

Bands Cemented to the teeth; used on molars and teeth with persistent bracket failures.

The most commonly used type of fixed appliance is the preadjusted edge-wise appliance.

Archwires

The archwire is tied to the attachments. In the early stages of treatment (aligning and levelling) the archwire is active. At engagement, the wire is deflected and pulls the teeth with it as it returns to its original shape. In the later stages of treatment the archwire is passive and the teeth are moved along the archwire by auxiliary forces.

Auxiliaries

Springs or elastics Used to apply force to the teeth.

INDICATIONS FOR FIXED APPLIANCES

Fixed appliances are indicated where multiple tooth movement is required, e.g. derotation, bodily movement, controlled space closure at extraction sites. They require a suitably trained operator and suitably motivated patient – excellent oral hygiene, caries controlled, wishes treatment and understands the implications, i.e. 18–24 months duration, visits 4–8-weekly, brush teeth after every meal, fluoride mouthwash daily, modify diet, wear elastics/headgear if required, some discomfort, retainers at end of treatment. Even then, relapse may sometimes occur.

To achieve the highest standard of care, fixed appliances are usually indicated. They are, however, demanding of patient cooperation. Treatment should be undertaken only when the patient fully understands the implications.

If in doubt, delay and do not treat – choosing a simple compromise option may preclude full correction at a later date.

CONTRAINDICATIONS FOR FIXED APPLIANCES

• Poorly motivated patient • poor dental health • operator without appropriate training in use of fixed appliances • some malocclusions may not be amenable to fixed appliance treatment, i.e. outwith the scope of orthodontics alone.

ADVANTAGES OF FIXED APPLIANCES

• Precise tooth control possible • multiple tooth movements can be made concurrently.

DISADVANTAGES OF FIXED APPLIANCES

• Aesthetics • oral hygiene requirements • demanding in terms of materials and operator time • anchorage control/treatment monitoring more difficult.

FUNCTIONAL APPLIANCES

> The term functional appliance describes those appliances
> which engage both arches and act principally by holding the
> mandible away from its normal resting position, and utilize
> the forces of the circumoral musculature.

CLASSIFICATION

There is no universally accepted method of classification. Most are
named after their originator, e.g. Andresen, Bionator, Harvold,
Frankel appliances, Twin–Block.

MODE OF ACTION

Most functional appliances act by utilizing one or more of the
following: • a forced mandibular posture, which transmits forces to
the teeth and jaws • a screening effect, which can either use or
relieve direct forces on the teeth from the circumoral soft tissues
• bite planes which produce differential eruption.

CASE SELECTION

Can be used for different types of malocclusion but most effective
in Class II division 1. For success, virtually full-time wear is needed.
It is important to review progress carefully after 6 months and if
treatment is not proceeding satisfactorily, an alternative approach
should be considered.

Functional appliances may be used for definitive treatment or
as Phase 1 of two-phase treatment: e.g. Phase 1 to reduce the
overjet, overbite and correct the sagittal jaw relationship; Phase 2 to
complete alignment using fixed appliances.

ADVANTAGES OF FUNCTIONAL APPLIANCES

• May utilize growth potential • can start treatment in the mixed
dentition • effective vertical control of increased overbite • chairside
adjustment time is minimal.

DISADVANTAGES OF FUNCTIONAL APPLIANCE

• Precise tooth movement not possible • very dependent on p[...] cooperation • often need Phase 2 treatment to complete • tre[...] duration is often prolonged.

ORTHODONTIC MANAGEMENT OF CLEFT[...] AND PALATE

Cleft lip and palate (CLP) is the most common cong[...] deformity in the craniofacial region. There is a wid[...] presentation ranging from bifid uvula to a comple[...] of lip and palate.

Incidence (UK)

Approximately 1 in 700 live births. Some raci[...] Caucasians: • CLP is more common in male[...] occur more often on the left side • isolated [...] common in females.

Classification

Patients with cleft lip and palate can b[...] groups.

Cleft lip ± cleft palate Those with cl[...] CP), or those with *cleft lip alone*[...]
Cleft palate Those with *cleft pala*[...]

Aetiology

Not fully understood. Certain[...] Genetic predisposition may [...] factor. May occur in isolati[...]

Cleft lip and palate

Main problems in ortho[...] malalignment, esp[...] into, and the e[...]

Dental
T[...]

Majority of occlusal problems occur secondary to
pair of the defect. Postoperative scarring impedes
of the maxilla in all three planes of space. A Class
nship is often seen with posterior crossbites also

is usually a skeletal 3 dental base
of surgical scarring and maxillary
Palate repair has a more serious effect
one. Differences are most

h varying degrees of

of the normal

variation. In

range

bilate

unilateral cle

left palate is more

divided into two distinc

ft lip and cleft palate (CL +
(CL).
alone.

cleft types show family history.
e triggered by an environmental

associated problems

dontic management are tooth
at cleft site, lack of bone to move

ial growth.

e cleft side may be ab
, hypoplastic, or d
, more comm

3. *Mid-mixed dentition* If an alveolar cleft is evident, secondary alveolar bone graft is routinely performed at age 9–10 years. Cancellous bone from the iliac crest is placed in the alveolar cleft and will: • facilitate eruption of the permanent canine • allow alignment of teeth adjacent to the cleft • promote orthodontic rather than prosthodontic repair • help stabilize the maxillary segments • assist closure of fistulae • improve vestibular anatomy.

4. *Early permanent dentition* Treatment indicated is dictated by the concerns of the patient and severity of the skeletal discrepancy. If skeletal discrepancy is not severe then conventional fixed appliance treatment can be carried out. A significant proportion of cleft cases will have a severe skeletal pattern 3, the full correction of which requires combined orthodontics/orthognathic surgery in the late teens.

5. *Late teens* If orthognathic surgery is indicated, the Class III incisor relationship is corrected by fixed appliance treatment to decompensate and coordinate the dental arches prior to surgery such as a Le Fort I osteotomy and a mandibular set-back osteotomy. A genioplasty may also be indicated (p. 432).

ORTHODONTIC ASPECTS OF ORTHOGNATHIC SURGERY

Orthognathic surgery is used to correct malocclusions outwith the scope of orthodontics alone, i.e. when there is a significant skeletal discrepancy. This approach to treatment is not usually carried out until growth has reduced to adult levels in the late teens.

Candidates for combined orthodontic/surgical treatment must be fully assessed at a combined clinic by an orthodontist and oral surgeon. Treatment is highly demanding of patient cooperation, and careful preoperative explanation is required. Patients may have unrealistic expectations and assessment by a clinical psychologist may be helpful.

In most cases, orthodontic treatment using fixed appliances will be required both pre- and postoperatively.

Aims of presurgical orthodontics
• General arch alignment • arch width correction • correction of anterior/posterior position of incisors • changes in overbite • correction of centrelines • create space for segmental surgery.

At this stage, the aim is to facilitate surgery and create tooth positions that are likely to be stable postoperatively, rather than to obtain 'ideal' cuspal relationships.

Fine adjustments and final tooth position are achieved postoperatively.

Treatment

Common problems requiring a combined orthodontic/ orthognathic surgical approach include: • severe skeletal pattern 2 • severe skeletal pattern 3 • severe anterior open bite • transverse skeletal asymmetry • congenital craniofacial deformity.

CHAPTER 14

ORAL AND MAXILLOFACIAL SURGERY

Tissue healing   382

Exodontia   384

Dentoalveolar surgery   388

Biopsy technique   398

Suturing   399

Laser surgery and cryosurgery   400

Infections   401

Swellings of mouth, face and neck   405

Bone pathology   407

Tumours – benign and malignant   408

Mouth cancer   410

Cysts of the jaws   412

Maxillary sinus   415

Preprosthetic surgery   419

Implants   421

Maxillofacial trauma   423

The temporomandibular joint (TMJ)   428

Facial and dental asymmetry   431

Orthognathic and cleft surgery   432

Reconstruction   436

Salivary gland surgery   437

TISSUE HEALING

Surgery by definition results in tissue damage; thus an understanding of factors influencing wound healing is important.

PHASES OF WOUND HEALING
Inflammatory phase (0–4 days after injury)
The *vascular* and *cellular* events in this phase produce a weak repair which derives most of its strength from fibrin.

Vascular events • Initial reflex vasoconstriction • subsequent vasodilation • fibrin and plasma leak into tissues.

Cellular events • Release of lysosomal enzymes from polymorphs • stimulation of macrophage phagocytosis • lymphocytic infiltration.

Proliferative phase (3–21 days after injury)
At the end of this stage the wound's strength has increased to 70% that of intact tissue. Fibroblasts produce ground substance and collagen precursors. Together with new capillary buds, fibroblasts form *granulation tissue*.

Remodelling phase (21 days after injury onwards)
Contraction of newly formed scar tissue eventually increases wound strength to 85%. Collagen is initially laid down in a disorganized fashion. Later, remodelling orientates this collagen into a less bulky form. Elastin is not replaced, and this results in a less supple scar.

HEALING BY PRIMARY AND SECONDARY INTENTION
Primary intention
Close approximation of wound edges produces a small haematoma. Subsequent granulation tissue and reorganization is therefore minimal. Healing results in a narrow scar with good tensile strength.

Secondary intention
Separation of wound edges produces a larger haematoma. This creates a larger volume within which a framework of fibroblasts and capillaries can grow and a greater surface area over which new

epithelium must spread. Healing leaves a weaker, more scarred wound, which contracts.

BONE HEALING

Healing by primary intention Occurs when there is less than 1 mm separation between bone ends, and rigid fracture fixation. This produces minimal callus.

Healing by secondary intention Results when there is a greater separation of bone ends. Osteoblasts (from periosteum, endosteum and blood) produce larger organizing callus extending between and beyond the ends of the fracture. This is emphasized more if fixation is not rigid.

Extraction socket healing

An example of secondary intention, combining mucosal and bone healing.

1st week • Inflammatory phase (*rubor, tumor, calor, dolor*) • followed by the start of proliferative phase, with ingrowth of fibroblasts and capillaries • epithelium migrates into the socket to begin covering granulation tissue • bone resorption from socket margins.

2nd week • Osteoid (immature bone, similar to callus) starts being laid down at socket margins • epithelialization usually complete.

4–6 weeks • Lamina dura (the socket wall) resorption usually complete.

FACTORS INFLUENCING HEALING

Tissue factors • Blood supply (reduced in smoking, diabetes) • drainage (e.g. venous, lymphatic – poor post-radiotherapy) • nutrition (e.g. low protein levels in debilitated patient).

Pre-existing infection

Acquired infection • General immune response reduced (elderly, concurrent disease, steroids, immunosuppressants) • local immune response reduced (radiotherapy, topical steroids) • adverse physical factors (barriers cut, tissue planes opened, reduced salivary flow) • microbes from patient (commensals or infective) • microbes from other patient (via instruments/working surfaces) • microbes from operator.

Operator Satisfactory healing is influenced by correct diagnosis and planning, e.g. an access flap to remove a maxillary root should

be designed to allow repair of an oral–antral fistula (see
Figure 14.9) should this be necessary.

EXODONTIA

Misguidedly often related to brawn. Strength is helpful, but
technique is everything! Knowledge of anatomy is the key.

LOCAL ANAESTHESIA (Chapter 6)

Adequate local anaesthesia is essential from the start, with
explanation and demonstration of the proposed technique.
Successful anaesthesia will be much easier to achieve if the dentist
establishes a good rapport with the patient. This should include an
indication of manoeuvres and pressure that the patient will
experience during extraction.

EXTRACTION TECHNIQUE

The initial movement is a *push* towards the tooth apex. This should
be combined with socket-expanding movements related to the
anatomy of the tooth and socket (Table 14.1). The beaks of the
forceps should be pushed carefully under the gingival margin onto
the tooth root, not just grasping the crown (Figure 14.1).

Feel and watch the tooth begin to move and increase expansion
movements. Remember that the non-extraction hand should be
working just as hard supporting the patient's head or mandible. In
the maxilla this can be achieved by grasping and fixing the
maxillary alveolus. In the mandible try to grasp the alveolus
between forefinger and thumb and wrap the remaining fingers
under the lower border. Having the patient bite on a rubber prop or
obtaining an assistant's help may be advantageous. Elevators
(p. 390) can be used to gain initial movements.

The movements required for specific teeth are listed in
Table 14.1.

PREVENTION AND MANAGEMENT OF
COMPLICATIONS

Potential complications of extraction include: • failed local
anaesthetic (LA) • soft-tissue injuries • nerve injuries • fractured

TABLE 14.1 Extraction technique

Tooth (Remember! All these suggested manoeuvres should be used with an apically directed push)	Movements
Mandibular teeth Third molars: two roots, variable First and second molar two roots – mesial and distal, may be divergent	Lingual and buccal expansion – 'figure of 8' movement when tooth mobile; may take time
First and second premolars: single ovoid root	Rotation in horizontal direction, small movements to begin with
Canines: long ovoid root	Slow labial and lingual expansion
Incisors: slim ovoid root	Little rotation towards the end
Maxillary teeth Third molars: three roots – frequently confluent and fused together	Consider elevator if access poor
First and second molars: three roots – mesiobuccal, distobuccal and palatal Divergent in first molar	Forceps grasp both buccal roots and the palatal, the main movement is buccal. Once the main buccal expansion has been achieved other movement can be employed
First premolar – two fine roots easily fractured Second premolar – single oval root	Again more buccal than palatal expansion – with less force; great care with first premolar. Consider elevator if access poor
Canine: very long oval root	Requires very slow buccal expansion to avoid fracturing buccal plate, some rotation
Incisors: single cone-shaped root	Mostly rotation

tooth • fractured buccal plate of bone • fractured maxillary tuberosity • displaced roots • lost tooth • maxillary–antral perforation • postextraction haemorrhage • dry socket • TMJ complications – trismus, acute subluxation, dislocation • pain – extraction of a painful tooth may not provide immediate relief • swelling – particularly following surgical extraction.

  Careful attention to detail can reduce potential complications.

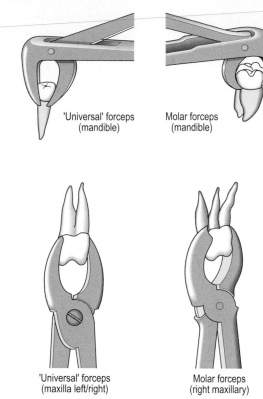

'Universal' forceps
(mandible)

Molar forceps
(mandible)

'Universal' forceps
(maxilla left/right)

Molar forceps
(right maxillary)

Figure 14.1 Application of extraction forceps.

Preoperative

Be fully aware of the patient's medical history, e.g. bleeding tendency, potential drug interactions. Select an appropriate mode of anaesthesia. Consider LA and sedation in anxious patients. Local pathology must be taken into account – consider a radiograph if there is a history of difficult extractions.

Perioperative

Check the treatment plan to ensure that the correct teeth are extracted – particularly important in extractions for orthodontic purposes. Rough or poor technique may cause excessive injury. Pay attention to the outer plate of the alveolus (particularly next to maxillary first molars and canines). If this is moving and attached to the tooth, dissect free from the overlying mucosa before the gingiva is torn.

The tooth may remain solid, or movement may be limited. If this happens, do not panic – rest and then expand slowly – consider radiograph. Thorough wound toilet is essential to remove residual debris such as small bony sequestra. Check the tooth after extraction to ensure that the entire root morphology is present.

Adequate haemostasis must be achieved. Socket compression between finger and thumb is essential. Biting on a small piece of damp gauze which fits into the edentulous gap helps stem haemorrhage. No patient should be discharged until haemostasis is achieved. If bleeding continues, try to identify specific bleeding point and suture it – consider haemostatic agents, e.g. Surgicel® or Sterispon®.

Postoperative

Non-steroidal anti-inflammatory agents are usually best for postoperative analgesia. They should be commenced immediately following the procedure and should be effective by the time the local anaesthesia is wearing off.

Postoperative haemorrhage may be *primary* (or immediate), *reactionary* (within 24 hours when reflex spasm of vessels relaxes) or *secondary* (7–14 days postoperatively – often infective); again, identify bleeding point and suture.

Infection may be *immediate* (i.e. surgery in infected area), *intermediate* (about 2 days – differential diagnosis dry socket) or *longer term* (consider retained root fragment, bony sequestrum or question original diagnosis).

DRY SOCKET (focal alveolar osteitis)

Incidence Incidence is about 2% of extractions. More common in mandibular than maxillary extraction sites. Also more common following surgical removal of teeth, e.g. lower third molars.

Aetiology The aetiology of dry socket is uncertain. Infection is probably not the primary cause (although some trials show reduced incidence of dry socket when antimicrobials are used). Some studies have shown excessive fibrinolytic activity; this may lead to premature loss of clot. Impaired vascular supply to the socket wall has been implicated. Both smoking and the use of oral contraceptives increase the incidence.

Diagnosis Pain occurs 24–48 hours postextraction, frequently with noticeable odour and bad taste. The alveolar socket wall is often exquisitely tender. Blood clot may be lost from the socket, but there is often little evidence of clinical infection.

Treatment Under local anaesthesia irrigate and look for debris and sequestra. Apply chlorhexidine (0.2%) by irrigation regularly to the socket. A pack impregnated with a eugenol or iodophor-based obtundant may be helpful if these more simple measures are unsuccessful. Such packing may retard long-term healing and so should be removed at the review appointment.

DENTOALVEOLAR SURGERY

SURGICAL REMOVAL OF TEETH

Extractions may become problematic when a portion of root or tooth cannot be removed from the alveolus. In this case, it may be necessary to cut the tooth and/or alveolar bone, to enable the remaining fragment to be removed.

Stages in the surgical extraction of the mandibular right first molar are illustrated in Figure 14.2.

Usually, a mucoperiosteal flap (1) must first be raised, as the roots (2) are usually beneath bone margins. Bone is thus exposed (3) and can be removed from the area around the root (4) with a bur. Bone should be removed initially from the coronal aspect of the root to try to create a point of application for an elevator (5). (Numbers refer to Figure 14.2.)

On occasion it is possible to elevate roots without raising a flap; e.g. a very broken down crown which can be removed piecemeal on a molar tooth. This allows sectioning of the remaining stump with a bur into individual roots, which can then be elevated separately.

Principles of flap design

When raising a mucoperiosteal flap, careful consideration must be given to the following to ensure viability postoperatively and promote satisfactory wound healing: • the base of the flap should be broader than its tip to provide an adequate blood supply • relieving incisions should not be made at acute angles • tissues should be handled with due care and attention • the design should enable sufficient access for surgery • postoperatively, the flap margins should rest on sound bone.

 Inexperienced operators frequently raise too small a flap. 'Keyhole' surgery should be avoided.

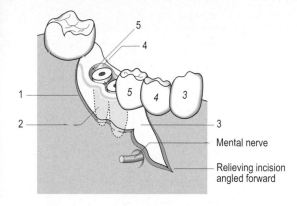

1 Buccal mucoperiosteal flap
2 Retained root mandibular first molar
3 Lateral plate of mandibular alveolus
4 Initial area of bone removal in a 'trench'
  around retained root
5 Example of a 'point of application' for
  elevator application

Figure 14.2 Stages in the surgical removal of the right first mandibular molar.

It is important to be aware of underlying anatomical structures as potential hazards when making an incision. In particular: • mandibular 4, 5 region buccally – *mental nerve* • mandibular 7, 8 region buccally – *branches of facial artery* • mandibular 8 region lingually – *lingual nerve* • maxillary 7, 8 region buccally – *pterygoid plexus* • palate – *palatal artery* – keep to the gingival margin to avoid this.

Elevators

These instruments are used to prise out teeth and pieces of root which cannot be grasped by forceps, or to facilitate forceps application (Figure 14.3).

The elevator point must engage the side of the root surface (usually within the periodontal ligament) and have a fulcrum point (usually alveolar bone). This combination is called the point of application and is the secret to successful elevation.

There are two types of elevator. The more common type is oval in cross-section, e.g. straight Warwick James'. It is this

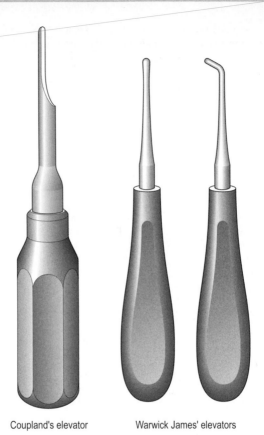

Coupland's elevator   Warwick James' elevators

Figure 14.3 Coupland's and Warwick James' elevators.

cross-sectional asymmetry that holds the key to its mode of action. The elevator point is maintained in contact with the root surface, and as the oval shaft is rotated against the inner rim of the alveolar margin, the root is rotated free.

The curved Warwick James' is an example of the hooked type of elevator. Again, the tip of the instrument is applied to the root surface and the root is literally 'hooked' out of the socket, using the alveolar margin as a fulcrum.

When elevating teeth remember: • support the jaw with your other hand • sufficient bone must be removed to allow the elevator a point of application and to allow the root a path of removal • the angle of approach of the elevator is crucial to enable the point to grip the tooth and the shank to have a fulcrum point on the bone • the elevator is a sharp-ended instrument. Use it with care. A finger rest is recommended. Carefully observe the tooth. Is the root moving as expected?

Bone removal

When surgically removing teeth, sufficient bone should be removed to create an application point on the tooth root. Bone may be removed using either a handpiece and bur or chisels. The latter are used only when operating under general anaesthesia in young patients (bone is less brittle). Care should be taken not to damage the roots of adjacent teeth or important anatomical structures. A sterile saline spray should be directed on the bur at all times to avoid overheating the bone. All bone fragments should be carefully removed to prevent postoperative infection. This is aided by efficient aspiration. Remove only sufficient bone to ensure adequate access to the tooth root.

IMPACTED THIRD MOLARS

The indications for removal of impacted third molars include:

Pericoronitis Recurrent inflammation of the overlying operculum, which is the most common indication for removal of third molars. Surgery should be delayed until the acute phase has been treated.

Caries Associated with a stagnation area; may result in caries in the third molar or distal aspect of the second molar.

Periodontal The operculum may predispose to acute necrotizing ulcerative gingivitis and more chronic problems.

Orthodontic Association with crowding is not proven; however, removal may be necessary for appliance therapy and orthognathic surgery.

Associated pathology e.g. a dentigerous cyst (i.e. cyst around unerupted tooth crown).

Impacted third molars have been shown to be an area of weakness more prone to mandibular fracture.

Symptoms arising from partly erupted third molars may be vague and every effort should be made to make a correct diagnosis. Signs and symptoms of impacted third molars may be similar to those of myofascial pain dysfunction syndrome, which should be actively excluded. Sometimes vague 'pressure' and 'discomfort' feelings may be cured by removing third molars, but beware of ascribing pain to buried teeth (particularly those which are covered completely with bone and discovered only on a radiograph).

There is controversy surrounding the removal of asymptomatic impacted third molars. Provided there is no communication between the tooth and the oral cavity, studies suggest the likelihood of problems is small.

Current thinking suggests the following approach to third molars: • Teeth presenting with symptoms other than those transiently associated with eruption – usually remove. • Teeth unlikely to contribute to the occlusion and jeopardizing the health of surrounding tissues (especially second molar) – usually remove. • Asymptomatic teeth, unerupted or partially erupted and surrounded by healthy attached gingivae – leave (needs review). Guidance on the removal of third molars has been issued in the UK by the National Institute for Health and Clinical Excellence (NICE) and the Scottish Intercollegiate Guidelines Network (SIGN).

Radiographs in third molar diagnosis

Careful radiographic examination should be undertaken in the assessment of third molars. A panoral view may be sufficient; intraoral views may be added to delineate further detail, e.g. inferior dental nerve proximity. Note the following:

Position
Angulation of the tooth relative to the occlusal plane, e.g. vertical, mesioangular, distoangular, horizontal, ectopic (grossly displaced).
Depth of impaction The relation of the maximum convexity of the most inferior part of the tooth crown to the margin of the alveolar bone.

Third molar
Tooth morphology e.g. proportion of crown to root, presence of caries, possibility of ankylosis.
Root morphology May be favourable (conical), or unfavourable (bulbous or hooked tip).

Surrounding structures
Inferior alveolar canal Position relative to tooth apices. In particular look for: • darkening of root (as it crosses the canal) • deflected roots (away from canal) • loss of continuity of canal roof (white line).
Trabeculation of bone Whether surrounding bone is sclerotic, normal or rarefied in type.

Pathology e.g. cysts, caries.

Other structures e.g. morphology of second molar (conical roots, so easily loosened), and presence of crown or distal amalgam that could be damaged.

Access Usually determined clinically (remember to assess aspects such as degree of opening possible); however, the radiograph may help by estimating the distance between the distal aspect of the second molar and the anterior border of the ramus of the mandible.

Removal of impacted third molar

Elevation of a buccal flap (Figure 14.4) The usual approach is via a buccal mucoperiosteal flap around the crown of the partially erupted 8. The gingival papilla between the 7 and 8 is included in the flap. From the gingival papilla, a relieving incision is continued down the side of the buccal alveolus (Figure 14.4i). For the distal part of the incision, it is important to have an understanding of the anatomy of the area immediately posterior to 8. If an incision were to be made directly posterior to 8, and in line with the alveolus, it would inevitably end up in the lingual sulcus, where the lingual nerve is vulnerable to damage. Thus the relieving incision should be angled laterally up the external oblique ridge (this is easily palpable and more lateral than you might think). The buccal flap may now be lifted to facilitate access to the impacted tooth. Difficulty is often encountered around the partially erupted crown where the mucoperiosteum is adherent.

Elevation of a lingual flap The incision described above also allows a lingual flap to be raised. Some think this is of importance in preventing lingual nerve injury. Others argue that less injury occurs without elevating this flap, and there is evidence that for non-specialist operators this may be the best for more simple surgical procedures. To raise a lingual flap it is most important to remain in the subperiosteal layer. This requires care as the alveolus overhangs the mandibular body on its lingual aspect, and there is a considerable concavity to deal with. If the periosteal elevator should pass through the periosteum by accident, and is then held as a retractor, the nerve may be trapped on the wrong side of the elevator, between the elevator and bone.

Surgical removal (Figure 14.4ii) Sufficient bone should be removed to allow visualization of the impacted tooth. The tooth itself is then sectioned so that it can be removed piecemeal. A tungsten carbide bur is used to cut as well as create a space to remove pieces separately. As with most practical procedures three-dimensional

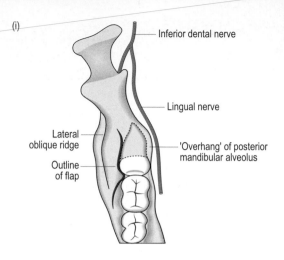

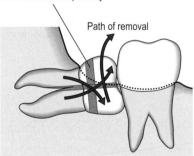

Figure 14.4 Removal of impacted third molar.

perception (particularly the location of the bur tip) is the key to preventing unwanted damage.

Nerve damage Nerve damage to inferior dental nerve and lingual nerve are potentially serious long-term complications of surgical third molar removal. This can be limited by adequate preoperative assessment and careful surgical technique.

All patients should, as part of the consent process, be warned about the possibility of nerve damage and of postoperative swelling and trismus. Document in case notes.

Closure Whilst sutures may contribute to postoperative discomfort, their placement is usually required to achieve satisfactory wound closure and an adequate gingival contour postoperatively.

Postoperative care Advice on a suitable analgesic (e.g. ibuprofen) should be provided to be commenced before the LA wears off (consider the use of a long-acting LA). Some advocate the use of chlorhexidine mouthwash, commencing 24 hours after extraction. The prescription of antibiotics following third molar extraction depends on individual circumstances, but is advised where extraction involves significant bone removal or chronic infection is evident.

Third molars should not be electively removed in the presence of acute soft tissue infection.

Patients should be provided with an information sheet and details of how to access care, should an emergency arise postoperatively.

MAXILLARY CANINE EXPOSURE/REMOVAL

Assessment This is usually done in conjunction with an orthodontist.

History Including planned orthodontics.

Examination Note displacement of other teeth, the state of the deciduous canine. Palpate to determine whether the crown is obvious palatally or labially.

Radiography Two intraoral views are usually required to permit parallax assessment (an anterior occlusal and one intraoral will also suffice). If the crown moves with the tube it lies palatal. Take care to notice if the canine lies across the arch of the alveolus (e.g. crown labial, root apex palatal). A panoral film can be useful. For estimation of the depth that the canine is in bone, a lateral cephalogram may help. Other views can distort how high the crown lies. Resorbed roots, particularly of lateral incisor, should be assessed and noted, as should the presence of cystic change around the crown.

Treatment Frequently requires day-case general anaesthetic.

Palatal flap around the necks of the standing teeth. This should start at the first maxillary molar and travel to the opposite canine (or molar if both canines involved).

Labial flap around the neck of the lateral incisor and the canine region with the relief incision over the alveolus in the first premolar region.

Canine exposure Bone is removed with great care to avoid damaging the crown or junction with the root. The whole of the greatest curvature of the crown is exposed and, for palatally placed teeth, an area of overlying mucoperiosteum is excised (a haemostatic coagulator is often needed). A suitable pack is placed – a dressing plate fabricated preoperatively is very useful to carry a periodontal dressing in the area of the exposed tooth. Labially placed teeth are probably best treated by bracket attachment with a gold chain leading out to the mouth and the flap sutured back in place (avoiding an apically repositioned flap).

Surgical removal Again necessitates bone removal and may require crown section with elevation in segments. Palatal impactions may be quite difficult, and correct patient positioning (head extended) may help.

APICECTOMY (see Figure 14.5)

> *Apicectomy* Surgical removal of the root apex, to allow the surgeon to visualize and gain access to the root canal. The main aim of the procedure is to establish an apical seal.

Indications for apicectomy • Failure of conventional endodontic therapy to eliminate apical infection • pathological change at the apex of a previously root-filled tooth, e.g. granuloma or cyst • failure during root canal treatment, e.g. overfilling, instrument fracture, lateral perforation • root unapproachable by conventional orthograde route, e.g. post-crowned tooth, calcified root canal • anatomical variations preclude normal endodontic therapy.

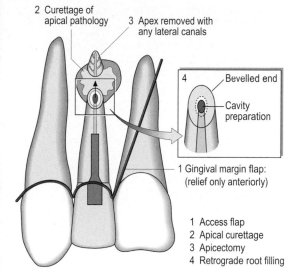

2 Curettage of apical pathology

3 Apex removed with any lateral canals

4 Bevelled end

Cavity preparation

1 Gingival margin flap: (relief only anteriorly)

1 Access flap
2 Apical curettage
3 Apicectomy
4 Retrograde root filling

Figure 14.5 Apicectomy of maxillary right lateral incisor.

Apicectomy alone cannot address the problems in complete root canal preparation and obliteration.

Technique

1. **Access flap** A mucoperiosteal flap is raised. A triangular flap is preferred, and careful repositioning and suturing minimize postoperative recession.
2. **Apical curettage** Any apical cystic tissue, granulation tissue or infection resulting from failed root canal therapy should be curetted and sent for histological assessment.
3. **Apicectomy** Section of the root apex with a slight anterior bevel to facilitate visualization of the root canal. In deciding how much apex to remove, several factors should be considered:
   - As much root as possible should remain to deal with occlusal loads.
   - Apical root (with the most potential for lateral canals) should be removed.

- Plan the root surgery to take account of the extent of apical pathology.
- Try not to remove so much apex as to expose any restorative post within the canal.

4. **Retrograde root filling** Where the apical seal is deficient, the root canal is cleaned out of old root filling and infected and necrotic dentine using an ultrasonic source and microtip. This enables the remaining apical root canal to be prepared without unnecessary loss of root or inadvertent perforation. The use of magnifying loupes is advantageous. A suitable cement, e.g. EBA (orthoethoxy benzoic acid), is used as a filling material. This should be a thick mix, well compressed by suitable instrumentation. Special microinstruments are available to facilitate this.

Even with the best retrograde root filling, the whole of the root canal is not prepared and sealed. Difficult cases are best approached from both ends, completely dismantling the restorative crown and post if this is technically possible. This allows an orthograde/retrograde approach. The canal is overfilled using gutta-percha and cement in an orthograde direction. This filling then protrudes at the root end and can be cut back under direct vision.

> ⚠ **Best treatment is always a well-placed orthograde root filling. Many of the 'indications' for apicectomy may be solved by a skilled endodontic practitioner with an orthograde approach alone.**

BIOPSY TECHNIQUE

Biopsy involves excision of tissue for histological examination.

Excisional biopsy The lesion is excised in its entirety. This should include a small margin of healthy tissue surrounding the lesion.

Incisional biopsy Removal of a representative portion of the lesion; should try to contain clinically healthy tissue at the margin. In potentially malignant lesions, the area most likely to show significant dysplasia should be included in the biopsy, e.g. the speckled part in a non-homogeneous leukoplakia.

Punch biopsy has gained favour with clinicians and patients alike.

Where the lesion is extensive, consideration should be given to sampling from more than one site.

Technique Try to infiltrate LA around the site, *not* directly into it. A suture placed through the tissue to be excised is preferable to grasping with forceps as this prevents crushing the sample. This also helps orient the specimen for the pathologist. An elliptical biopsy of the edge of a lesion should result in easy wound closure with two or three sutures.

> ⚠ **Full clinical details of the patient should be entered on the request form sent to the pathologist. Good communication with the pathologist is important in arriving at an accurate diagnosis.**

SUTURING

Sutures are used to hold flaps and tissue in apposition to facilitate wound healing. There are a variety of suture techniques possible, e.g. interrupted, vertical mattress, horizontal mattress, continuous.

Technique

To insert an interrupted suture The suture should always be passed from the free flap into the fixed tissue. The free edge of the flap is supported by toothed dissecting forceps; the needle is held in needle holders and inserted about 3 mm from the wound edge following the line of the needle curve. The needle is grasped as it emerges from the deep aspect of the flap and inserted in the underside of the opposing wound margin. It should be angled so that the needle emerges about 3 mm from the wound edge. The two ends of the suture are knotted so as to maintain the wound edges neatly in apposition. The standard knot tied with needle holders has two forward loops which are tightened and one loop turned back which is tightened. A further single loop may be necessary for added security. Don't cause over-tension – tissues should not be blanched.

Suture removal Non-resorbable intraoral sutures are normally removed 7 days postoperatively. To remove, the tied ends of the suture are grasped in non-toothed forceps. Fine point scissors or a stitch cutter is inserted under the knot and one side of the suture is cut. By gently pulling with the forceps the suture is removed. Any adherent debris may be removed with chlorhexidine solution before the suture is removed.

Suture materials

Resorbable Polyglycolic acid (e.g. Vicryl) is used for suturing within
   tissue layers (buried). Most surgeons use these routinely for
   surface oral mucosa as their use avoids the need for suture
   removal.
Non-resorbable Fine nylon or other monofilament suture is used for
   skin.

Needles

May be *cutting* (for skin and attached gingival) for ease in passing through tissue or *round bodied* (for mucosa) – avoids cutting out of tissue as the needle is passed through.

LASER SURGERY AND CRYOSURGERY

LASER SURGERY

> LASER stands for Light Amplification by the Stimulated
> Emission of Radiation.

As the energy emitted can be carefully controlled, lasers may be used to destroy soft tissue.

Laser types include: • carbon dioxide • neodymium:YAG (yttrium–aluminium–garnet) • argon laser • tunable dye laser • copper laser.

The last three types are well absorbed by pigmented substances and can be used selectively to destroy haemangiomas, sensitized tumours (tumour cells are identified by antibodies with pigment attached) and tattoos, at the same time sparing surrounding normal tissues.

Carbon dioxide laser

The light emitted from this laser is well absorbed by water, e.g. in soft tissue. The major intraoral application is the excision or ablation of potentially malignant lesions. Excision of soft tissue neoplasms is also possible with more powerful models. The depth of destruction can be controlled precisely, and small blood and lymphatic vessels are sealed (with possible prevention of tumour spread). The wound produced by a carbon dioxide laser is said to heal with less scarring than other wounds. Fewer myofibrils are generated in healing. This, together with retention of the connective tissue skeleton, reduces scar contraction. Carbon dioxide laser surgery may also be associated with less postoperative pain.

CRYOSURGERY

This involves the controlled destruction of tissues by freezing. *Liquid nitrogen*, *carbon dioxide* and *nitrous oxide* take in energy from their surroundings when they vaporize or expand. Formation of intra- and extracellular ice crystals leads to disturbances in osmotic and electrolyte balance and results in cell death at –20°C or below. Clinical cryosurgery may involve, for example, a 2-minute freeze and 5-minute thaw in two or three cycles.

Postoperatively, there is often a degree of swelling in soft tissue areas to which the cryosurgery has been applied. Cryosurgery does not give an opportunity for biopsy. There is a lack of scarring, probably related to the preservation of the connective tissue skeleton.

Applications include cryoanalgesia and cryoneurectomy for trigeminal neuralgia (e.g. of the mental nerve). It has also been used in the treatment of soft tissue lesions, e.g. haemangioma, and some intrabony lesions.

INFECTIONS

INFECTION OF DENTAL ORIGIN

Infections that are dental in origin frequently have a mixed bacterial aetiology, e.g. streptococci (aerobic and anaerobic) and *Bacteroides* (anaerobic).

Localized infections
The majority of dental infections remain localized.

Apical (dental) abscess The most common type of abscess arises from an infected pulp chamber (p. 232).

Periodontal abscess An infection within a periodontal pocket (p. 225).

Pericoronitis Pericoronitis is defined as infection under the operculum (i.e. the mucosa that covers a partially erupted tooth). Primary treatment is by irrigation under the operculum with chlorhexidine solution (0.2%). It may be necessary to remove the maxillary third molar to reduce occlusal trauma. Systemic antibiotics should be considered if there is evidence of trismus, lymphadenopathy, or spreading infection.

Spreading infection

Whilst most infections remain localized, an infection may spread. Pus from an infected tooth will spread along the path of least resistance. This may present as an extra- or intraoral sinus, but can on occasion spread along tissue and fascial planes to produce severe, life-threatening systemic infections. The pattern of spread associated with specific teeth often follows a distinct path, as indicated in Table 14.2 and Figure 14.6.

TABLE 14.2 Patterns of spread of odontogenic abscesses

Tooth	Potential spread
Maxillary teeth	
Molars and premolars	Swelling or sinus in buccal sulcus may spread to buccal space (lateral to buccinator)
Canine	Canine fossa – facial nasolabial fold area
Lateral incisor	May track to palate due to distal inclination of root, but usually labial
Central incisor	Labially – can give a swollen lip
Mandibular teeth	
Third molar (Beware! pericoronitis may track buccally along the inner aspect of buccinator to present in 5,6 region)	Has the potential to spread in many directions: submandibular space via lingual plate, pterygomandibular space, lateral pharyngeal space and on down the neck
Second molar	Spreading laterally, infection from the second/third molar may give severe trismus with an extension into the submasseteric space
First molar	Buccally, if lingual may be submental or submandibular depending on level of drainage and mylohyoid attachment
Premolars and canine	Buccally
Incisors	Labially

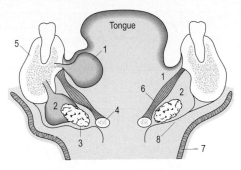

1 Sublingual space
2 Submandibular space
3 Submandibular salivary gland
4 Hyoid bone
5 Mandible
6 Mylohyoid muscle
7 Platysma muscle
8 Deep cervical fascia

Cross-section mandibular region premolar area

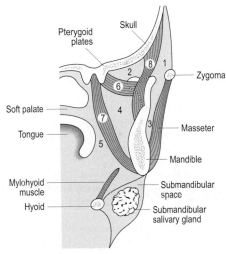

1 Superficial temporal space
2 Infratemporal space
3 Masseteric space
4 Pterygomandibular space
5 Lateral pharyngeal space
6 Lateral pterygoid muscle
7 Medial pterygoid muscle
8 Temporalis muscle

Cross-section mandibular ramus region

Figure 14.6 Potential spaces in spreading dental infections.

In all these spreading infections be alert to systemic conditions underlying the acute spread, e.g. diabetes, immune deficiency.

OTHER INFECTIONS OF THE HEAD AND NECK REGION

Facial cellulitis This presents with diffuse inflammation throughout subcutaneous tissues and deeper tissues. On examination, the skin feels firm with no fluctuance. Onset may be rapid, and there is no pus initially. Treatment is by surgical eradication of infected focus supplemented by systemic antibiotics. Careful observation is necessary, as abscess formation may occur, and this requires surgical drainage.

Osteomyelitis An acute or chronic infection of bone. Most commonly, both forms are associated with odontogenic infection and usually another factor promoting spread (e.g. immunosuppression).

Ludwig's angina This is a cellulitis involving floor of mouth spaces, which can quickly extend into the neck (deep cervical fascia, parapharyngeal space) and then the mediastinum. Tongue and floor of mouth are elevated. As it tracks down the pharynx 'hot potato speech' may develop. The real danger signs are difficulty swallowing and speech problems. Prompt referral and treatment is crucial as the airway can become compromised rapidly.

Necrotizing fasciitis This is rare in the head and neck. It is characterized by a rapidly progressive necrosis of fascia and subcutaneous fat that undermines and eventually causes necrosis of overlying subcutaneous tissues and skin.

Cavernous sinus thrombosis Veins in the facial region communicate with the cranial cavity, and, very rarely, infection may backtrack from the face up into the skull to the cavernous sinus.

Cancrum oris/noma This is associated with malnutrition (immunosuppression), and fusospirochaetal organisms similar to those associated with acute necrotizing ulcerative gingivitis are implicated in this condition.

INFECTION OF NON-DENTAL ORIGIN

Any of the spreading infections above may originate from non-odontogenic sources, including:

Salivary gland Suppurative parotitis.
Skin Infected sebaceous cyst, furuncle (suppurative folliculitis).
Bone Acute osteomyelitis, chronic osteomyelitis.
Other e.g. from nasal passages, paranasal sinuses.

PATIENT ASSESSMENT IN INFECTION

The factors identified in Chapter 2 relating to diagnosis apply
equally to a patient with an infection. However, the following
specific features should also be recorded:

History • speed of onset • malaise • rigors • effect on breathing and
swallowing • medical factors, e.g. drugs, diabetes.

Examination • temperature (axillary) • heart rate • trismus
• lymphadenopathy • spread, e.g. floor of mouth, tongue elevation,
neck involvement, airway/voice.
Delineate extent of swelling as a baseline.

Bacteriology • aspirate pus with a needle for an uncontaminated
sample – also helps preserve anaerobes • a pus specimen in a sterile
pot is better than a swab in transport medium • involve the
bacteriologist early if there is serious infection.

Other tests include radiography, vitality tests, urinalysis (diabetes).

Differential diagnosis

Differential diagnosis is particularly important. If temperature is
elevated postoperatively, consider: atelectasis and lung infection,
infection at the surgical site, urinary tract infection, deep vein
thrombosis (DVT), infection at site of indwelling line (see
Figure 14.12)

Management The basic principles in managing a patient with
infection involve: • accurate diagnosis • incision and drainage
• attention to the primary focus • appropriate antibiotic therapy
(p. 68).

SWELLINGS OF MOUTH, FACE AND NECK

A vast range of pathologies can present as a swelling. It is
essential to be able to identify efficiently the possible cause of
swellings.

History Record as described in Chapter 2. In particular note:
• duration • variation in size • pain – its nature and radiation • any
neurological involvement.

Examination Describe as follows:

Look • site • size • shape • surface (e.g. ulcerated) • colour.

Feel • consistency (e.g. fluid filled, soft, firm, hard) • relations
  (e.g. attachment to or displacement of other surrounding
  structures). Assess sensory changes (e.g. mental or infraorbital
  nerve).

Transillumination If cystic, or to determine if a hollow structure is
  filled, e.g. maxillary sinus.

Auscultation If a vascular anomaly is suspected, a bruit (flow
  murmur) may be heard.

Examine lymph nodes Lymphadenopathy is the most common
  cause of swellings in the neck. Examination of the lymph glands
  should be conducted in a systematic fashion using gentle
  palpation. Relax the patient, gently tilt the head forward and
  towards the side being examined. Start in the
  submental/submandibular area, standing behind the patient.
  Work around the angle of the jaw and up around the base of
  skull. Then work down around sternocleidomastoid (both sides)
  to the clavicle. Finally, palpate the anterior neck and then the
  posterior triangle of the neck.

Special tests

Vitality tests of surrounding teeth to elicit a possible dental
  cause.

Ultrasound examination may aid diagnosis by, for example,
  revealing whether the swelling is fluid filled.

Radiography Several views at different angles may be necessary.
  Advanced imaging techniques such as computed tomography
  (CT) scanning and magnetic resonance imaging (MRI) may
  provide valuable information (Chapter 4).

> ⚠ **Remember – common things occur commonly. Always
> list the possible diagnoses with the most likely first. To
> avoid missing possible diagnoses, think of what structures are
> contained in that anatomical area.**

INTRAORAL AND FACIAL SWELLINGS

A useful method of arriving at a differential diagnosis of a lump of
unknown origin is by use of a 'surgical sieve', based on possible
aetiological factors.

Infective The most common cause of lumps and swellings in the head and neck region.

Traumatic Common examples include oedema and haematoma following operation or accident, fibroepithelial polyp, denture hyperplasia, mucocele.

Inflammatory e.g. orofacial granulomatosis, angio-oedema.

Neoplastic (p. 461).

Endocrine e.g. hyperparathyroid disease and lesions of bone destruction (brown tumours), other giant cell lesions.

Developmental e.g. torus, haemangioma, lymphangioma, branchial cyst.

BONE PATHOLOGY

Fibrous dysplasia Discussed on page 510.

Paget's disease of bone Discussed on page 511.

Osteopetrosis Discussed on page 511.

Osteogenesis imperfecta Discussed on page 509.

Hyperparathyroidism Displays focal bone 'brown tumours' and is discussed further on page 506.

Ossifying fibroma The aetiology of this condition is uncertain. It may be a localized disorder of bone metabolism or a benign tumour. Often the only real difference between this swelling and fibrous dysplasia is the fibroma's discrete mass (clinically and on radiograph) and the relatively clear separation on surgical removal. Treatment is similar to that of fibrous dysplasia, but because of its discrete morphology, ossifying fibroma is more often removed in its entirety.

Giant cell lesions Describe a number of swellings whose only common feature is a preponderance of giant cells seen on histology of the lesion.

Reparative granuloma (peripheral giant cell lesion) Possibly related to trauma: usually responds to curettage.

Central giant cell tumour Can be aggressively destructive – but benign. May recur after curettage. Radiographs show multilocular radiolucency.

With both these lesions, hyperparathyroidism needs to be excluded from the diagnosis.

Other lesions with giant cells involved are cherubism (autosomal dominant inherited, resulting in bone remodelling in mandible and maxilla), aneurysmal bone cyst and occasionally fibrous dysplasia.

TUMOURS – BENIGN AND MALIGNANT

Due to the large variation in presentation of growths in the head and neck region, categorization is complex. The following is a basic classification of growths and tumours.

HAMARTOMAS

These arise before or soon after birth and grow with the patient; the swelling stops growing with the patient. They are not classified as tumours. Common examples include:

Pigmented naevi (moles) A collection of melanocytes.
Haemangiomas/lymphangiomas A collection of blood or lymph vessels.
Odontomes Differentiated as *compound odontomes* – normal relationship of enamel, dentine, cementum; and *complex odontomes* – diffuse masses of abnormal tooth tissue.

TUMOURS

Tumours may be differentiated into benign and malignant varieties (Table 14.3).

A tumour is an abnormal mass of tissue whose growth exceeds and is uncoordinated with that of surrounding tissues. Abnormal growth continues after the stimulation which initiated it has ceased.

Benign tumours

Benign tumours remain at their site of origin. Common examples include:

TABLE 14.3 Characteristic features of benign and malignant tumours

Benign tumours	Malignant tumours
Slow growing (usually)	Fast growing (often)
Well differentiated	Poorly differentiated
Infrequent mitoses	High mitotic rate
Little cytological variation	Nuclear and cellular pleomorphism
Remain localized	Abnormal mitoses Spread Metastasize

Lipoma (fat).
Neuroma (nerve).
Papilloma (epithelium).

Locally invasive tumours

As in benign tumours, growth is abnormal. There is, in addition, invasion into surrounding normal tissues. Examples include:

Ameloblastoma (enamel-producing organ).
Basal cell carcinoma (BCC) (skin), sometimes called 'rodent ulcer'.

Malignant tumours

In malignant tumours there is abnormal growth with the potential for local invasion and distant metastases. The latter may be via blood, lymphatics or body cavities. Carcinomas are malignant tumours of epithelial tissue. The most common malignant tumour in the oral cavity is the squamous cell carcinoma (p. 410). Sarcomas are malignant tumours of connective tissue, e.g. liposarcoma, osteosarcoma.

Odontogenic tumours

These are rare (some very rare). The majority are benign (some are more hamartomatous than tumours). Only a few are locally aggressive, and they do not usually metastasize. However, they should not be underestimated, as local spread to the skull base may kill.

Epithelial odontogenic tumours

Ameloblastoma The mean age of occurrence for this tumour is about 40 years, although they can arise at any age. They are most commonly found in the mandibular body/ramus region. They are locally invasive; this is particularly important in the posterior maxilla. Ameloblastoma normally presents as an expanded lesion of bone which is seen radiographically as a multilocular radiolucent area (see Table 4.15 for differential diagnosis of mutilocular radiolucencies). Treatment is by surgical resection of the tumour, taking a clear margin to ensure its eradication.

Calcifying epithelial odontogenic tumour This is clinically and radiographically similar to ameloblastoma, and is often associated with an unerupted tooth. It may also contain radio-opaque areas. Treatment is by surgical removal.

Mesenchymal odontogenic tumours

Odontogenic myxomas These are equally distributed between maxilla and mandible, and are most common at around 30 years of age. They present as a swelling which is usually radiolucent, often multilocular. Treatment is by surgical excision of the tumour and a small margin of surrounding tissue.

Cementifying fibromas Indistinguishable from ossifying fibroma.

Mixed odontogenic tumours
Odontomas (odontomes) Really hamartomas (p. 408).

Ameloblastic fibromas (including fibro-odontoma) Most common in young adults in the mandibular body/ramus region. Radiographs show a radiolucent lesion (with a calcified area if the odontome is present) which may be associated with an unerupted tooth crown. Treatment is by curettage.

MOUTH CANCER

The epidemiology and aetiology of squamous cell carcinoma are discussed on page 461.

ASSESSMENT

In addition to the usual features in examination and diagnosis (Chapter 2), particular note should be made of:

History • duration of symptoms • any sensory nerve deficit • pain • onset of difficulty opening mouth (trismus) • social habits and circumstances.

Examination This should include an exhaustive description of the primary lesion, which may be on an ulcer: • size • shape • colour • description of the ulcer edge • degree of induration (hardness) • whether bound down to other tissues • which tissues are involved clinically with the mass.

It may be useful to assess movement restriction, e.g. of the tongue, or the ability to open the mouth – remember this may be tumour invading muscle or motor nerve supply. Sensory function (e.g. mental, lingual and infraorbital nerves) needs to be checked, and, finally, the neck examined for lymph node involvement (p. 411).

Special tests The following special tests may be indicated in further assessment:

    Blood tests Full blood count (haemoglobin levels and nutritional status) and liver function tests (estimation of associated alcohol damage), calcium and phosphate analysis (to help determine obvious bone metastases).

Imaging Radiography of jaws and chest; in selected cases CT and MRI are considered (p. 48).

Biopsy (p. 398).

Examination under anaesthesia (EUA) Often enables the best assessment of more posterior or painful lesions and enables endoscopy for other (synchronous) lesions.

Squamous cell carcinoma can be graded using the TNM classification (p. 463).

TREATMENT

This requires a team approach. Surgeons work with oncologists as well as specialist nurses (e.g. Macmillan), speech and dietetic specialists. Considerable time needs to be spent with patients and their relatives to prepare them mentally and physically. They also need to feel part of the decision-making process.

A range of treatment options are available; they are influenced by the stage of the tumour as well as patient factors.

Potentially malignant lesions and carcinoma in situ Treatment is usually by surgery, which, for these lesions, often has minimal morbidity and allows histological examination of the specimen. Larger areas may be best treated with laser excision.

T1 and T2 lesions With these lesions, surgery or radiotherapy (either teletherapy [external beam] or brachytherapy [implants]) have similar cure rates.

Larger tumours involving deep tissues These lesions have a much reduced cure rate. The best hope for cure with improved chances for local/regional control is with radical surgery and reconstruction followed by postoperative radical radiotherapy. Despite advances in reconstruction, some areas remain major problems for postoperative rehabilitation, e.g. base of tongue tumours. In these circumstances, tumours may be treated by either brachytherapy, in which a radioactive source is loaded into tubes, located in the primary tumour, or external beam radiotherapy combined with concurrent chemotherapy. This may give as good a chance of cure with better functional outcome.

If bone is involved with tumour then surgery is usually preferred as radiotherapy is less successful in such cases.

Neck metastases If neck metastases are palpable, surgery is indicated. If there is no evidence of neck involvement on palpation

(N0), management is controversial. Options in management of such cases are: • watch and wait (advocated for sites with <10% change of occult metastasis) • selective neck dissection • external beam radiotherapy.

If there is a surgical need to gain access to the neck (e.g. access mandibulotomy or reconstruction demands), a sparing dissection may be necessary. About 56% of patients present with early clinical disease (T1 and T2) and an N0 neck. In patients with tongue cancer and an N0 neck, about 30% will have occult neck disease; advocates of prophylactic neck dissection hope to treat this group with surgery. Regional disease may present very quickly and be already advanced when it is discovered clinically. For this reason some are keen to treat at-risk patients (e.g. tongue and floor of mouth lesions) with N0 necks.

Results

There is very good evidence that early small lesions treated properly have the best prognosis. If nodal metastases are present, the overall chance of cure decreases by 50%. There is evidence of an increasing number of patients in whom, whilst the disease is controlled locally and regionally, distant metastatic disease results in death. Current research is investigating if the addition of chemotherapy into the treatment regimen may help some of these cases.

> ⚠️ **The need for early diagnosis cannot be overemphasized. Careful screening of the oral mucosa to detect potentially malignant and malignant lesions should be carried out routinely in any oral examination.**

CYSTS OF THE JAWS

> A cyst may be defined as a pathological cavity having fluid or semifluid contents, which has not been created by the accumulation of pus. It may or may not be lined by epithelium.

A basic classification of cysts is contained in Table 14.4.

TABLE 14.4 Classification of cysts		
EPITHELIAL CYSTS		
Odontogenic		
Developmental	Odontogenic keratocyst (primordial)	5–10%
	Dentigerous (follicular): eruption	10–15%
	lateral periodontal	
	gingival	
Inflammatory	Radicular: apical	}>60–70%
	lateral	
	residual	
	Paradental	
Non-odontogenic		
	Nasopalatine	5–10 %
	Nasolabial (soft tissue)	
NON-EPITHELIAL BONE CYSTS		
	Solitary bone cyst (haemorrhagic, idiopathic or traumatic)	
	Aneurysmal bone cyst	
	Stafne's bone cyst	

PATHOGENESIS

One theory suggests that central cell degeneration in a proliferating mass of epithelial cells sets up an osmotic pressure gradient and causes prostaglandin release. This promotes fluid accumulation. The other theory suggests death and degeneration of granulation tissue and then a similar progression.

Odontogenic keratocysts tend to grow quickly and recur (25–60% of cases). This recurrence may be associated with rapid epithelial cell turnover in the cyst wall, common satellite cysts and a fragile cyst wall.

Clinically cysts may present with a blue tinge in the overlying mucosa.

TREATMENT

A number of treatment options exist for cysts.

Orthograde root canal therapy (p. 287)
There is good evidence that smaller apical radicular cysts will regress completely with adequate orthograde root canal therapy.

Enucleation and primary closure

If technically possible, this is the operation of choice as, if healing progresses uneventfully, no further intervention is needed. In smaller lesions the only problem usually encountered in raising the access flap is dissecting the soft tissue of the flap from the cyst wall tissues. Larger lesions may have to be dissected from antral lining, nasal floor or other structures, e.g. inferior dental nerve. Postoperative infection may be a problem if a large blood-filled cavity is left.

Marsupialization

In this procedure, the cyst is opened to allow continuity with the oral mucosa. Although it is technically easy, marsupialization may involve the patient in considerable postoperative care as the cavity must be cleaned regularly. It is advantageous in large mandibular lesions where surgical removal would put the inferior dental nerve at risk and may allow preservation of adjacent teeth (Figure 14.7).

Unfortunately, marsupialization does not allow the whole lesion to be submitted for pathological examination. A high degree of

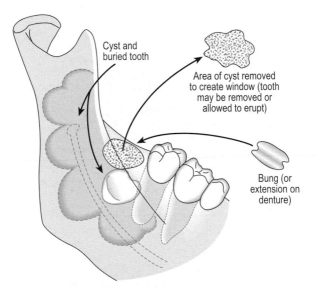

Figure 14.7 Marsupialization of large mandibular cyst.

suspicion should always remain when dealing with marsupialized cysts, and close follow-up with radiographic review is essential if other very rare pathologies, e.g. neoplasia, are not to be missed.

MAXILLARY SINUS

The maxillary sinus (Figure 14.8) can be visualized as pyramidal in shape with the apex of the pyramid projecting laterally into the zygomatic process of the maxilla. The base is formed by the lower part of the lateral wall of the nose (in detail, by the uncinate process of the ethmoid, descending part of the lacrimal bone, the inferior concha and the perpendicular plate of the ethmoid). The ostium draining the sinus enters the middle meatus. Cilia of the epithelium lining the sinus waft continuously to this exit. The mucoid film is replaced every hour. The healthy sinus does not contain microorganisms.

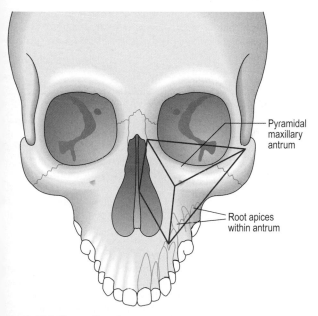

Pyramidal maxillary antrum

Root apices within antrum

Figure 14.8 The maxillary sinus.

History

Think of the surrounding structures forming the pyramid. Look for pain, tenderness or swelling (which will be facial, intraoral, buccal or palatal). There may be nasal discharge, nose bleed or escape of oral liquid into the nose via the maxillary antrum. This last symptom suggests an *oral–antral fistula*. Eye symptoms include pain, epiphora and visual disturbance. Sensation of the skin or mucosa may be abnormal.

Examination

Pathology originating in the maxillary sinus may result in:
• swelling and tenderness leading to obliteration of the normal anatomy, e.g. nasolabial fold, buccal sulcus • loosening of maxillary teeth; in the edentulous patient denture fit is altered • maxillary teeth next to the sinus may be tender.

The patency of the nasal airway should be checked, and the passage examined for the presence of a mass. Eye signs include proptosis, injection (reddening) and movement problems.

Special tests

• Vitality tests • fine needle aspiration of cells and fluid
• radiography including occipitomental views at 15° and 30° as well as suitable intraoral views • CT and MRI may be indicated • sinus endoscopy.

ORAL–ANTRAL FISTULA (OAF) CLOSURE

A maxillary premolar or molar root may extend from the alveolus into the maxillary antrum. When the tooth is removed, an oral–antral communication may be created. Many of these communications close spontaneously by normal healing of the socket. Sometimes, however, it is necessary to close the fistula surgically. A number of options for closing oral–antral communications exists. It is important to address any antral infection prior to any attempt at closure. Preoperative washouts can be very helpful.

Buccal flap with periosteal release (Figure 14.9)

This is the most common flap used to cover an OAF from a tooth socket. The two relieving incisions buccally (1) are placed to diverge only slightly so that the flap will fit the usual space of one tooth diameter. A flap of mucosa and periosteum is then everted to expose the periosteum at the base, which is then detached (2) by an incision parallel to the base. The incision should cut only through the periosteum, leaving the flap pedicled on the relatively elastic mucous membrane and submucous tissue, which contain the blood supply. The flap is then pulled over the tooth socket to meet the palatal mucosa and trimmed to size before suturing in position (3) (numbers relate to Figure 14.9).

Palatal rotation flap

This flap is based on the greater palatine artery, and when swung into position leaves an area of denuded palatal bone.

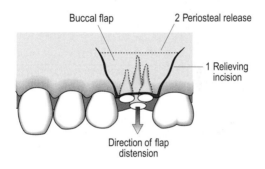

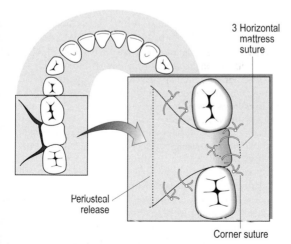

Figure 14.9 Periosteal release buccal flap repair of oral–antral fistula.

Buccal fat pad transfer

This is an excellent reserve reconstruction for OAFs that have been subject to difficult or repeated attempts at closure. The fat pad is easy to find but mobilization should be done with care to preserve bulk and avoid the pterygoid plexus of veins. It can then be sutured into position. The fat pad becomes covered by oral mucosa by seeding of oral squames and growth from the margins.

Postoperative care

Patients should be instructed not to blow their nose, to prevent any back pressure on the repair. Antibiotics are usually prescribed – broad-spectrum variety preferred – with scrupulous oral hygiene. Nasal inhalations using steam and a decongestant may help. Advise analgesics in the immediate postoperative period.

DISPLACEMENT OF A FRACTURED ROOT INTO THE MAXILLARY ANTRUM

A potential complication of the extraction of maxillary posterior teeth is displacement of a fractured root into the maxillary antrum. Should fracture occur: • remember which root you were working with, particularly in multirooted teeth • is the fractured root still visible? • if you can see it, can it be retrieved by careful suction? • decide whether you will persevere in removing the root • if not, and referral is some time in the future, then repair the OAF; sometimes a simple mattress suture is sufficient as an emergency measure in a small OAF. Alternatively, suture a small pack over the socket to give a watertight seal at the site where the tooth has disappeared into the antrum • suitable radiographs of the socket area (at different angles) should be taken.

To retrieve the root

Raise an adequate flap designed to close the OAF following exposure and removal of the root. Remove appropriate bone to expose the root. Often the lateral socket/alveolus wall is a good place to look first. Roots can slip through this lateral wall and lie between periosteum and bone in the buccal sulcus. Radiographs will not define this problem easily. Careful examination of the lateral wall whilst raising the flap will help. If the root is well in the sinus, consider prompt referral to a specialist.

FRACTURED MAXILLARY TUBEROSITY

Fracture of the maxillary tuberosity may occur during extraction of a posterior molar. If the bone cannot be dissected from the roots, it should be carefully dissected from the overlying mucosa and the tooth and tuberosity removed together. An extensive communication with the antrum results but careful preservation of the mucosa leaves ample tissue to achieve a watertight closure. Postoperative treatment is as for OAF closure.

PREPROSTHETIC SURGERY

The purpose of preprosthetic surgery is (in close communication with the prosthodontist) to correct any architectural problems in the oral cavity which may lead to denture instability or retention problems. Conditions in which preprosthetic surgery may be required are shown in Figure 14.10.

BONE IRREGULARITIES
Maxillary and mandibular tori

Tori are localized developmental bony exostoses. Mandibular tori are located lingually in the premolar regions whilst palatal tori are found in the midline. Their presence may prevent insertion of a denture and they can be recontoured surgically.

Local alveolar ridge architecture problems

Often result from previous poor extraction technique (e.g. buccal plate removed along with tooth), resulting in overhanging areas and concavities. Bone irregularities can be recontoured by surgery or grafting.

Resorption problems

In the maxilla Resorption reduces the lateral and anteroposterior dimensions of the alveolus. Gross discrepancies can be corrected surgically.

In the mandible Both alveolar ridge shape and relationship with maxilla change. The alveolar ridge may have: • an overall lack of height and width • knife edge or flabby ridges • concavities,

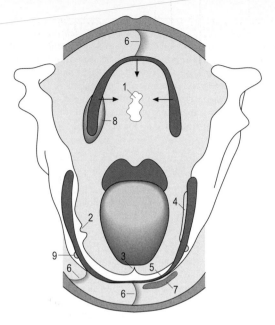

Hard tissue

1 Palatal torus
2 Mandibular torus
3 Genial tubercles
4 Prominent mylohyoid ridge
5 Thin knife edge ridge

Soft tissue

6 Fraenula (various sites)
7 Denture-induced hyperplasia
8 Enlarged fibrous tuberosity
9 Superficial mental nerve

Figure 14.10 Potential problems amenable to preprosthetic surgery.

particularly in the body region • more prominent genial tubercles • prominent mylohyoid ridges • an exposed mental nerve.

SOFT TISSUE PROBLEMS

Problems that may require surgical correction include denture-induced hyperplasia, loss of sulcus depth or prominent fraenula. Denture hyperplasia may regress following gross trimming of the denture and abstention from denture wear (if this is possible). However, there is often a residual fibrous mass which requires surgical trimming. Take care not to remove too much mucosa in this situation. This is a delicate balance between removal, scar formation and loss of sulcus depth.

Vestibuloplasty is used to deepen the sulcus; it can be problematic and may involve grafting.

The management of local architecture problems and some soft tissue abnormalities too gross for prosthodontic management may be aided by placement of implants.

IMPLANTS

Implants are alloplastic materials that can be incorporated into the jaw bone. Materials include titanium, titanium coated with hydroxyapatite, or plasma-sprayed titanium.

Dental implants are mainly used for support of prostheses. Commonly, two fixtures are inserted anteriorly into the mandible to support a full denture. Implants to replace single teeth are now commonly used. Facial or cranial implants can also be placed around the orbits or in the mastoid area to support other prostheses. Implants are locked solidly into bone by virtue of a direct interface between bone and implant – *osseointegration*. Achieving and maintaining this interface is essential for implant survival. For intraoral implants this means scrupulous oral hygiene.

FACTORS INFLUENCING IMPLANT SUCCESS

Implant factors They must be inert and biocompatible with oral tissue.

Surgical factors The precise fit of implant to bone is important, as is atraumatic surgery – in particular avoiding thermal injury to bone. The implant should be correctly sited to ensure optimal loading by the prosthesis. This requires careful cooperation with the prosthodontist.

Soft tissue The mucosa around the implant should be thin, relatively immobile and healthy – attached mucoperiosteum is best.

Bone The bone needs to be of sufficient depth to accept an implant. This may be a problem where there is gross resorption. There is usually sufficient bone in the edentulous maxilla in front of the maxillary sinus and in the mandible anterior to the mental nerve (Figure 14.11).

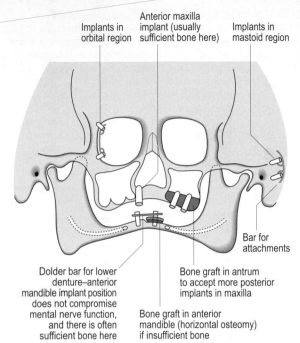

Implants in orbital region

Anterior maxilla implant (usually sufficient bone here)

Implants in mastoid region

Bar for attachments

Dolder bar for lower denture–anterior mandible implant position does not compromise mental nerve function, and there is often sufficient bone here

Bone graft in antrum to accept more posterior implants in maxilla

Bone graft in anterior mandible (horizontal osteomy) if insufficient bone

Figure 14.11 Implants in the oral cavity and other sites.

There are various manoeuvres to deal with lack of suitable amounts of bone: • anterior mandibular osteotomies and bone grafting with the implant as a stabilizer • surgical repositioning of the inferior dental nerve, prior to implant placement • sinus lift bone grafting to increase the bone available in the posterior maxilla. Bone density is reduced in the maxilla; because of this, a longer 'sleep' period may be required before loading of the implant. There is a slightly greater overall failure rate in the maxilla.

Implant design is advancing. Implants which can be immediately loaded have been developed, as have shorter implants for use in areas with reduced amounts of bone available.

Postoperative A 'sleep' period may be required to allow osseointegration. The site must be protected from trauma by overlying dentures.

Prosthetic factors Prosthetic aspects of implants are discussed on page 330.

MAXILLOFACIAL TRAUMA

EMERGENCY RECEIVING

Dealing with patients suffering facial trauma can be difficult. There are three main points which need to be considered together:
• cervical spine • airway • bleeding.

The importance of these is closely followed by consideration of any other injury of significance to life, e.g. *hidden haemorrhage* from intra-abdominal injury, fractured pelvis, femur, etc. Head injury must be considered, particularly if there is deterioration in the level of consciousness determined by history (from friend) or observation (Glasgow Coma Scale).

If the patient arrives in obvious respiratory distress or with torrential haemorrhage these will obviously take precedence.

> ⚠ **For more major injuries you will be part of a team.**
> **However, many more minor referrals may come straight**
> **to you. Never forget to look for associated injuries. A patient with**
> **a 'simple' fractured zygoma may have fallen as a consequence of**
> **the blow and have sustained a significant head injury.**

MAXILLOFACIAL EMERGENCY ACTION

Airway/cervical spine

Emergency action will be as part of a team. It is essential to have good light and suction. Oral or nasopharyngeal airways may help. Endotracheal intubation (if possible) definitively secures the passage. Beware base of skull fractures when cannulating the nose. Tracheostomy or cricothyrotomy may be needed, if other measures fail.

Any suspicion of neck injury (beware – a lowered consciousness level may make history and examination difficult) makes temporary immobilization with collar or sandbags essential. The following objects may be causing upper airway obstruction: foreign bodies such as teeth or denture fragments, vomit or blood. Anterior mandibular fracture and loss of tongue control may be helped (as a temporary measure, under LA) by wire ligatures applied to the teeth on the displaced fragment to permit repositioning. A tongue suture and anterior traction can be applied. A maxillary fracture may cause displacement of the maxilla downwards and backwards, and this can cause airway obstruction. Simple digital repositioning can allow the patient to breathe.

Bleeding

Torrential nasal haemorrhage following mid-face fractures is rare but frightening. A mobile maxilla is best dealt with by disimpaction and resiting using finger pressure, directed up and anteriorly on the palate. Posterior nasal packs can then be placed (pass Foley catheters and inflate) and, finally, the nose should be packed under pressure in layers.

Circulation

Fluid replacement is essential (colloid or crystalloid) and often needed rapidly. Fluid replaced should be guided by the anaesthetist in charge. Signs of circulatory collapse are rarely due to maxillofacial injuries alone – check elsewhere.

CONSOLIDATION

Once any emergency stabilization has been accomplished, a more complete assessment may be undertaken.

History Remember to use witness accounts if necessary, e.g. was the patient ever conscious following the traumatic event?

Examination If injuries are severe, keep reassessing the cervical spine (stabilization), airway (patency), vital signs (haemorrhage) and coma status. Usually one team member is assigned to this ongoing assessment.

Specific oral and facial examination

Extraoral Assess any facial lacerations. Observe facial contours from above. Check/palpate: • forehead • orbital rims • arch of zygoma • nasal contour and patency • medial canthal attachment and any telecanthus (separation of inner eyelid attachment) • mandibular borders • mandibular movement.

Check skin sensation changes: • *supraorbital and supratrochlear* – forehead sensation • *zygomaticofacial and temporal* – lateral face and temporal region • *infraorbital* – cheek, lateral nose, upper lip and teeth/gingivae of the maxilla • *mental* – lower lip.

If there is an eye or orbital injury consider ophthalmological referral. The most important test is acuity (each eye is tested for ability to read a series of standardized size texts).

Note specific signs such as: • bilateral 'racoon eyes', indicating base of skull fracture • cerebrospinal fluid (CSF) leak • bruise behind ear (Battle's sign), indicating base of skull fracture.

Intraoral Note: • areas of swelling and bruising • palpable steps in the bone contour • obvious occlusion derangements • gently 'springing' suspected areas of mandible and maxilla • injuries to the teeth (p. 185).

All fractures of consequence are usually diagnosed *clinically*.

Radiographs (Chapter 4) Radiographic examination aids clinical assessment of fractures. The most common views are: • *maxilla –* occipitomental (15° and 30°), lateral facial • *zygomatico-orbital –* occipitomental (15° and 30°) • *mandible –* orthopantomogram, PA mandible. The availability of CT scanning in the emergency situation has improved overall, particularly in trunk and head injury. CT scans are particularly helpful in assessment of maxillary orbital and naso-orbital and ethmoidal injuries. Figure 14.12 shows a patient after major trauma or surgery.

Glasgow Coma Scale (GCS)

Levels of consciousness are measured using the Glasgow Coma Scale (Table 14.5).

The scores for best motor response, best verbal response and eye opening should be added together. The total for a normal patient is 15. This gives a method of repeatable assessment so improvement or deterioration can be noted. Care must be used in assessing patients who may also be hypotensive, intoxicated with drugs (including alcohol) or hypoxic.

Lacerations

Good documentation is essential, not least for medico-legal purposes. A diagram with measurements is best.

Facial skin has a very good blood supply from a rich interconnecting subdermal plexus of vessels. This means that pieces

TABLE 14.5 The Glasgow Coma Scale					
Best motor response		Best verbal response		Eyes open	
Obeys commands	6				
Localizes pain	5	Orientated	5		
Normal flexion to pain	4	Confused conversation	4	Spontaneously	4
Abnormal flexion to pain	3	Inappropriate words	3	To speech	3
Extension to pain	2	Incomprehensible	2	To pain	2
None	1	None	1	Do not open	1

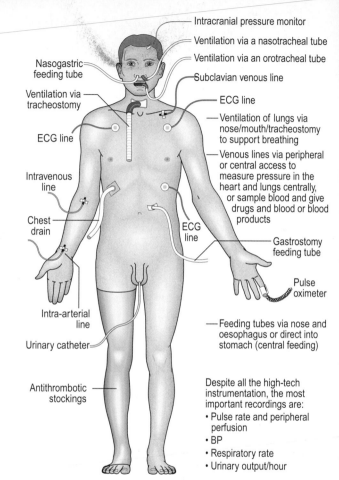

Figure 14.12 Patient following major trauma/surgery.

of skin survive on the face which may not in other areas. Never discard skin unless you are very sure of the final reconstruction.

Cleaning is very important. Any cleaning solutions should be used only on the intact skin (beware entry into the eyes). In the wound itself use normal saline. Take care to recognize tattooing, particularly with road dirt. A large scalpel blade to scrape skin margins, or used tangentially on abrasions can be very helpful.

Underlying structures need consideration, particularly: • facial nerve (VII) • parotid duct • tarsal plates and eyelid muscles • cartilage skeleton of the pinna.

Treatment may be possible under LA (e.g. block anaesthesia at supraorbital, infraorbital or mental nerves) but can be very time consuming. Large involved areas or younger patients may need a GA for optimal management.

Remember to check tetanus prophylaxis.

FACIAL SKELETON FRACTURES
Classification

Fractures may be classified generally as: • simple • compound • comminuted • greenstick • pathological.

Mandibular fractures Classified according to site: • condyle • angle • body • symphysis • dentoalveolar • coronoid • ramus.

Maxillary (middle third of face) fractures described as: • Le Fort I • Le Fort II • Le Fort III (Figure 14.13).

Zygomatic complex fractures Classified as: • arch • zygomatico-orbital • orbital.

Nasal fractures Classified from anterior progressing posteriorly: • cartilaginous • cartilage + nasal bones • complex naso-orbital–ethmoidal.

Treatment

As with any bone fracture, treatment involves: • reduction • fixation and immobilization • prevention of infection • return to function (see Figure 14.14).

Treatment may be *closed* or *open*, depending on the need to expose the fracture site for accurate reduction and fixation. The amount of fracture distraction usually determines whether a closed manipulation with external fixation will suffice. External fixation may be maxillo-mandibular wire fixation using the dentition to help locate the bite and stabilize a relatively undisplaced jaw fracture, or external pin fixation connected across a fracture site.

Other factors influencing choice of fixation for fracture treatment include recovery facilities, expertise in dealing with patients whose jaws are wired closed and patient preference. In most situations the main consideration is anatomical reconstruction. If indicated, open approaches and internal fixation (using plates and screws to hold the reduced fracture in place) usually achieve this best.

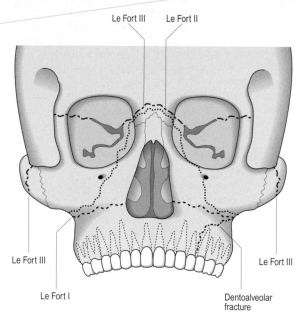

Figure 14.13 Fractures of the maxilla.

Access to the facial skeleton is often gained via intraoral incisions to avoid facial scars. The buccal sulcus in the maxilla and mandible is often used with a facial degloving technique to reach the fracture site.

More severe zygomatico-orbital fractures, orbital, naso-orbital–ethmoidal and craniofacial fractures may need facial incisions such as: lateral eyebrow, lower eyelid, crowsfoot, or a more extensive bicoronal 'scalping' approach.

THE TEMPOROMANDIBULAR JOINT (TMJ) (FIGURE 14.15)

ACQUIRED CONDITIONS OF THE TMJ
Myofascial pain dysfunction syndrome (p. 472)
Osteoarthrosis (p. 473)
Arthritis (p. 473)
Meniscal incoordination (p. 472)

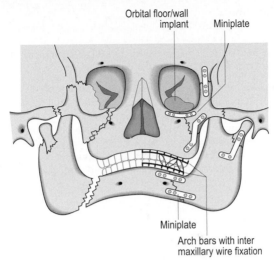

Figure 14.14 Stabilization of facial fractures.

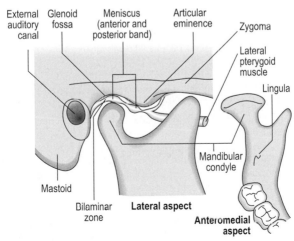

Figure 14.15 Anatomy of the temporomandibular joint.

Dislocation

This is movement of the mandibular condyle over the articular eminence of the glenoid fossa. The condyle is prevented from returning to the fossa by 'protective' vertical muscle spasm (masseter and medial pterygoid).

Treatment Acute dislocation can be reduced by placing the thumbs on the lower molar teeth and rotating downwards and backwards. Sedation may relax muscle spasm and aid relocation.

Patient education to avoid opening too wide may be of benefit in cases of recurrent dislocation. A variety of surgical procedures, which include eminectomy and eminence augmentation, have been described when persistent dislocation is a problem.

Fracture

Subcondylar (condylar neck) May be high (possibly intracapsular) or low. These are amongst the most common mandibular fractures.

Intracapsular In children under 5 years old this is the only possible fracture because of the anatomy of the developing mandible (there is no real condylar neck, and a soft, large condylar head). There may be a risk of ankylosis.

Treatment This depends on the occlusion. If the occlusal alignment is disrupted in a minor fashion, arch bars and elastic traction may be successful. Fracture dislocations and fractures of the condyle with loss of ramal height and occlusal problems probably should be considered for open reduction.

Ankylosis

True Caused by joint pathology (usually trauma or infection). True ankylosis may be bony or fibrous. Usually, there is some movement (1–3 mm) even in gross bony fusion.

False Caused by pathology outside the joint such as: • myogenic, e.g. postoperative damage to muscles • neurogenic, e.g. cardiovascular accident (stroke) • psychogenic, e.g. hysteria • bone impingement, e.g. coronoid exostosis • fibrous adhesions, e.g. post trauma and infection • tumours, e.g. oral squamous cell carcinoma invading medial pterygoid muscle.

Treatment This is by surgery, where indicated, to release the anatomical obstruction. Reconstruction may be necessary, e.g. costochondral graft. In childhood, surgery should be performed as soon as practicable to reduce secondary developmental deformity.

CONGENITAL CONDITIONS OF THE TMJ

These are rare, e.g. hemifacial microsomia, which has a varying lack of development of the condyle and ascending ramus associated with other bony underdevelopment (e.g. ossicles of middle ear, zygoma and temporal bone) and surrounding muscles of mastication and facial nerve.

FACIAL AND DENTAL ASYMMETRY (FIGURE 14.16)

DIFFERENTIAL DIAGNOSIS

Congenital (intrauterine growth) e.g. hemifacial microsomia, cleft lip and palate (p. 377).

Developmental (growth post birth) e.g. hemifacial hypertrophy, condylar trauma ± ankylosis.

Occlusal cant – an intact occlusion that facial growth (or lack of growth) has adapted to circumstances, resulting in a slope between one side of the occlusion and the other.

Open bite – lack of occlusion which may result from recent trauma, excessive growth or continuing habit, e.g. thumb sucking. May be compensated in a growing child. Compensation often leads to a facial asymmetry as growth is held back in one area (e.g. unilateral condylar trauma).

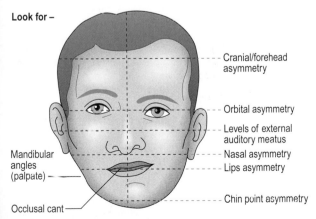

Look for –

- Cranial/forehead asymmetry
- Orbital asymmetry
- Levels of external auditory meatus
- Nasal asymmetry
- Lips asymmetry
- Chin point asymmetry

Mandibular angles (palpate)

Occlusal cant

Figure 14.16 Facial and dental asymmetry.

Careful analysis will determine the correct diagnosis. For example, unilateral condylar trauma with ankylosis in the growing child will not show a deformed pinna. Orbital and cranial asymmetry is found in hemifacial microsomia.

ORTHOGNATHIC AND CLEFT SURGERY

ORTHOGNATHIC SURGERY

Surgery to the facial skeleton can radically alter function and appearance; often undertaken in collaboration with specialists in orthodontics, restorative dentistry and prosthodontics.

Indications

Function This may be interceptive surgery during growth to encourage further, more normal, growth as in costochondral grafting in hemifacial microsomia and muscle reconstruction in cleft surgery. Functional correction may also be indicated once growth has ceased, e.g. to correct an anterior open bite, an overjet/overbite problem, or a crossbite which may improve mastication and speech.

Aesthetics Of increasing importance. In some cases, psychiatric or psychological assessment and guidance will be needed.

Facial disproportion May arise from soft or hard tissue discrepancies. These may be in any dimension: anterior–posterior, vertical or lateral.

Planning Careful planning and assessment is required before undertaking orthognathic surgery. The function of a planning clinic is to facilitate communication between the various specialties. Orthodontic aspects of orthognathic surgery are discussed on page 379.

History Include as detailed an account of the patient's problems from their perception as possible.

Examination

Head and neck assessment An idea of overall proportions is obtained, with the face in repose, especially the lips. The head should be in the natural head position (sit upright, relax and look straight ahead into a mirror).

Intraoral assessment • orthodontic • restorative and prosthodontic.

Other assessments • speech • nasal function • hearing • psychological • maxillofacial technical assessment.

Special tests • radiographs, e.g. lateral and anterior–posterior cephalograms, orthopantomograms • photographs • 3-D imaging • dental models • facebow transfer.

Planning takes into account all the information gleaned. Model surgery (Figure 14.17) allows visualization of proposed procedures.

Treatment

Hard tissue discrepancy Myriad osteotomies and ostectomies are possible; some more common procedures are listed in Table 14.6 Grafting or bone sculpture is performed to augment or reduce areas.

Soft tissue discrepancy This may be corrected either at the time of hard tissue correction or later. *Augmentation* is possible with flaps, fat transfer, collagen and similar injection/implants. *Reduction* involves excision, lipectomy, liposuction.

CLEFT LIP AND PALATE

The management of cleft lip and palate is discussed on page 377.

Cleft surgery

A complete cleft of lip and palate crosses many structures with developmental, functional, aesthetic and psychological consequences. Various surgical procedures are involved in reconstruction to improve alignment, function and appearance with

---

TABLE 14.6 Classification of surgery to correct facial deformity (Numbers refer to Figure 14.17)

Mandibular surgery	
Sagittal split osteotomy	1
Vertical subsigmoid osteotomy	2
Body ostectomy	
Genioplasty	3

Maxillary surgery	
Le Fort I osteotomy	4
Le Fort II osteotomy	5
Le Fort III osteotomy	6

Segmental surgery
- Premaxillary osteotomy: premaxilla moved
- Posterior maxillary osteotomy: allows posterior alveolar segments to be repositioned
- Lower labial segment surgery: allows for repositioning of lower six anterior teeth

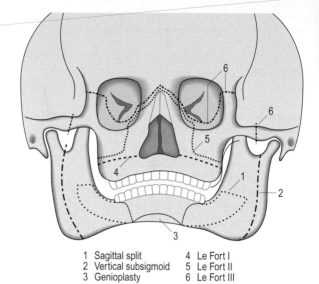

1 Sagittal split   4 Le Fort I
2 Vertical subsigmoid 5 Le Fort II
3 Genioplasty   6 Le Fort III

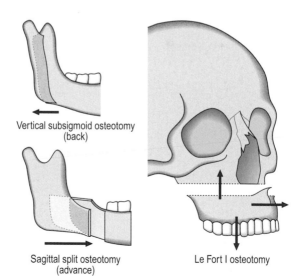

Vertical subsigmoid osteotomy
(back)

Sagittal split osteotomy
(advance)

Le Fort I osteotomy

Figure 14.17 Orthognathic surgery procedures.

particular attention to muscle reconstruction in soft palate and lip. Surgery will result in scarring which impedes growth and development. Developments in technique have focused on improving function by reconstructing the anatomy while reducing scarring. This is thought to maximize growth potential and function.

The anatomy of cleft lip and palate are shown in Figure 14.18.

Surgical interventions include • first 6 months of life – lip/nose and soft palate reconstruction • within 12 months – palate totally closed • evidence of middle ear problems – drainage operations • speech problems – may need palatal revision/pharyngoplasty • alveolar cleft – bone graft • alveolar collapse/jaw deformity – orthognathic surgery • residual nasal/lip problems – revision surgery.

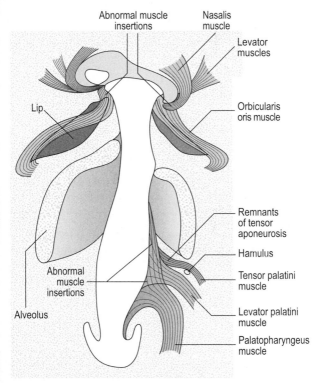

Figure 14.18 Anatomy of cleft lip and palate.

As discussed on page 378, this outlines the need for a comprehensive team approach to the management of cleft lip and palate patients. This management should take place in a regional centre.

RECONSTRUCTION

A variety of techniques and materials are available to aid in reconstruction and repair of tissue defects in the head and neck region.

Techniques for reconstruction include: • no intervention – leave to granulate, e.g. soft tissue defect on the hard palate • obturation – e.g. prosthesis in maxillary defect • skin grafting (full or partial thickness) • local flaps • regional flaps • free flaps.

FLAPS

Random pattern This type of flap relies on random pattern blood vessels in the subcutaneous tissue for survival, e.g. the standard apicectomy flap with one or two buccal relieving incisions (see Figure 14.5).

Axial pattern These flaps can be of much greater length as the pedicle is designed to incorporate specific vessels (artery and vein). Axial pattern flaps may be rotated into the desired position based on this peninsula of skin with the specific vessels enclosed. Island flaps just have the axial vessels in the pedicle (which makes them quite delicate, but more mobile); e.g. the palatal island flap based on the greater palatine artery (and tiny associated veins), which can be rotated round to reconstruct defects in the palate.

A variant on this concept uses an axial blood supply to an underlying muscle, which then supplies overlying skin right to the end of the muscle length; e.g. in a pectoralis major myocutaneous flap, skin is taken from the lower chest wall based on the underlying pectoralis muscle and rotated up to be passed under skin flaps in the neck and used to reconstruct a defect in the mouth.

Free flap This sort of reconstruction has an isolated vascular pedicle (as in an island flap); however, this pedicle is divided and the vessels reanastomosed to arteries and veins in the neck, e.g. the radial forearm fasciocutaneous flap. These techniques allow a greater choice of reconstructive flaps based on delicate pedicles which do not have to travel long distances.

The selection of which flap to use in a reconstruction depends to some extent on what tissues have been removed. There are free flaps that can replace skin, bone or muscle, or any combination of these; e.g. free fibula reconstruction of the mandible, with or without skin, depending on the need for any soft tissue replacement.

GRAFTS

Autogenous grafts Use the patient's own tissue: • skin grafts – split-skin graft, full-thickness skin graft • bone grafts – cancellous, corticocancellous • grafts grown in tissue culture 'to order', e.g. skin for patients with extensive burns.

Allografts Tissue from a human donor specially prepared to reduce abnormal antigens: • bone grafts • cartilage grafts.

Heterografts Tissue from another species, again treated to reduce any recipient immune reaction. Specially bred animals, with genetically manipulated compatibility genes to overcome rejection problems, may make these grafts more popular.

Alloplastic materials These should be biocompatible. Materials uses include:

Internal fixation plates and screws Titanium, stainless steel, cobalt–chromium.

Resorbable materials Sutures, internal fixation screws and plates: polyglycolic acid (Dexon), polyglycolic/polylactic acid (Vicryl), poly-*p*-dioxanone (PDS).

Orbital wall/floor reconstruction material Vicryl sheet, PDS sheet, titanium mesh.

Bone substitutes Ceramics, hydroxyapatite.

Contour materials Gore-tex, Proplast.

Soft tissue crease/wrinkle obliterative materials Collagen.

SALIVARY GLAND SURGERY

Salivary gland disorders are discussed on page 465.

SURGICAL MANAGEMENT

Surgical management of salivary glands includes:

Enucleation

Of, for example, benign minor salivary gland pathology (e.g. mucocele).

Operations on the duct

Meatoplasty To open up a constricted orifice.

Removal of stone Most commonly performed in the submandibular duct. The more proximal (near the gland), the more difficult to remove the stone. Place a suture behind the stone and put on tension to prevent posterior displacement. Incise through floor of mouth mucosa. Blunt dissection reveals the duct (beware vessels and lingual nerve). Identify stone in duct and incise wall. Remove stone. No sutures.

Excision of gland

Parotidectomy Usually performed superficial to the facial nerve. In tumour surgery an attempt is made to leave a cuff of normal parotid tissue round the tumour. There is usually at least one branch of facial nerve adjacent to the tumour, and this means a very careful dissection and no formal cuff of gland in this area of the excision. Transient damage to at least this branch of the facial nerve is usually expected. Sensory nerve damage to greater auricular (cervical plexus) and auriculotemporal (trigeminal) nerves may also occur. *Frey's syndrome* – sweating of the overlying cheek skin as a result of salivary stimulation (gustatory sweating) – results from secretomotor nerves which previously supplied the salivary gland, healing to innervate the sweat glands. May arise as a complication of surgery.

Submandibular gland excision This is performed much more often for infection (sialadenitis) associated with stone obstruction (sialolithiasis).The nerves at risk from this dissection are the marginal mandibular (branch of the facial – VII – nerve), the lingual (branch of the trigeminal – V – nerve) and very rarely the hypoglossal – XII – nerve.

CHAPTER 15

ORAL MEDICINE

Oral infections   440

Recurrent oral
ulceration   447

Vesiculobullous
lesions   451

White patches   455

Potentially malignant
lesions and conditions   457

Pigmented lesions of the
oral mucosa   459

Mouth cancer   461

Miscellaneous lesions   464

Salivary gland
disorders   465

Effects of drugs on the
teeth, oral mucosa and
salivary glands   471

Disorders of the
temporomandibular
joint   471

Facial pain   473

Oral manifestations of
systemic disease   478

HIV infection and
AIDS   484

Halitosis (oral
malodour)   487

ORAL INFECTIONS

BACTERIAL INFECTIONS

A wide variety of bacterial infections may have oral lesions, although with the exception of dental caries (p. 152) and periodontal disease (p. 199), they are all relatively uncommon.

Tuberculosis

Oral involvement with *Mycobacterium tuberculosis* is infrequent and is usually secondary to open pulmonary tuberculosis. Primary infections of the oral mucosa are rare, although recently incidence has increased, mainly amongst human immunodeficiency virus (HIV)-seropositive patients.

Clinical features Most commonly a persistent ulcer with indurated margins on the dorsal surface of the tongue, although other sites may be affected. Pain is a variable feature.

Investigations and diagnosis Biopsy, submitting half the specimen for routine histopathology and the other half for culture on an appropriate medium (e.g. Lowenstein–Jensen medium). Histopathological examination demonstrates the presence of caseating granulomata. Ziehl–Neelsen stain may reveal small numbers of acid- and alcohol-fast mycobacteria.

Treatment Oral lesions respond to treatment of underlying pulmonary tuberculosis.

Occasionally, infection with atypical mycobacteria is reported – most likely as a lymphadenitis in childhood. Increasing incidence of atypical mycobacterial infection (e.g. *Mycobacterium avium-intracellulare*) seen among immunocompromised patient groups.

Gonorrhoea

Sexually transmitted disease caused by *Neisseria gonorrhoeae*. Oral lesions occur as a result of orogenital contact with an infected partner. Particularly common amongst male homosexuals. Affected patients may complain of a dry, burning sensation with associated altered taste sensation and halitosis.

Clinical features Presentation is variable. May include pyrexia, diffuse mucosal erythema involving the mouth and oropharynx, oral ulceration and grey/yellow pseudomembranes – readily removed to reveal a bleeding surface. Cervical lymphadenopathy may also be a prominent feature.

Investigation and diagnosis Swabs from suspected oral lesions submitted for culture.

Treatment High-dose penicillin or tetracycline.

Syphilis

Systemic infection caused by the spirochaete *Treponema pallidum*. Incubation period 10–90 days. Infection may be acquired or congenital. Acquired syphilis divided into three stages: primary, secondary and tertiary. Incidence of syphilis is rising. Oral lesions are relatively uncommon.

Clinical features

Primary syphilis Characterized by a painless round or ovoid ulcerated lesion (chancre), which develops at the site of entry. Lips are the most common site for extragenital lesions. Painless, rubbery cervical lymphadenopathy may be a feature. *Treponema pallidum* is readily recovered from the chancre and therefore the lesion is highly contagious. The chancre resolves within 2–3 months.

Secondary syphilis Develops 1–4 months after healing of the primary chancre. Characterized by a generalized macular skin rash. Oral lesions, classically superficial ulcers or mucous patches, are highly contagious. May coalesce to form serpiginous lesions, '*snail track ulcers*'. Resolves within 2–6 weeks. Disease may then enter a latent phase which can become active as the tertiary stage of the disease. Alternatively the latent phase may last a lifetime.

Tertiary syphilis Uncommon in the Western world. Most distinctive lesion is the gumma – a chronic granulomatous reaction with central necrosis. In the mouth it presents in the midline of the hard palate, and perforation into the nasal cavity may ensue. Of low infectivity. Atrophic glossitis may also occur in this stage.

Congenital syphilis Lesions include tooth malformations (*Hutchinson's incisors* and *mulberry molars*) caused by infection of the developing tooth germs; saddle deformity of the nose; frontal bossing.

Investigation and diagnosis Dark ground microscopy of exudate from primary chancre or secondary mucous patches. This is of limited value for oral lesions as other spirochaetes are commensals in the mouth. Definitive diagnosis is by serological tests: *Treponema pallidum* haemagglutination assay (TPHA) and fluorescent treponemal antibody (FTA) test.

Treatment High-dose penicillin or tetracycline.

FUNGAL INFECTIONS

The oral mucosa may be affected by a variety of fungal diseases, including: • candidosis • histoplasmosis • cryptococcosis • paracoccidioidomycosis. With the exception of candidosis, all are uncommon in the UK. This section will concentrate on candidal infections.

Candidosis (candidiasis)

Candida species can be isolated from the mouths of up to 70% of the normal population, where it exists as a commensal organism. Of 150 different species, only seven are of pathogenic significance. Most common is *Candida albicans*; other common isolates include *C. tropicalis, C. glabrata, C. parapsilosis, C. guilliermondii, C. krusei* and *C. pseudotropicalis*.

A variety of local and systemic factors predispose to the development of candidal overgrowth and overt clinical infection (Table 15.1).

Classification of oral candidosis – see Table 15.2.

Clinical features

Pseudomembranous White/yellow plaques on the oral mucosa. These can be removed to reveal an erythematous base which may bleed.

Erythematous Erythematous areas on the oral mucosa. Most commonly affects dorsal surface of the tongue, palate, buccal mucosa.

TABLE 15.1 Local and systemic factors predisposing to candidal infection

Local factors
- Trauma
- Denture wearing
- Poor denture hygiene
- Xerostomia

Systemic factors
- Radiotherapy
- Antibiotic therapy
- Corticosteroid therapy
- Extremes of life – infancy and old age
- Diabetes mellitus
- Nutritional deficiency (iron, folate and vitamin B_{12})
- Immunosuppression
- Cigarette smoking
- High carbohydrate diet

TABLE 15.2 Classification of oral candidosis	
Primary oral candidoses	
Acute	Pseudomembranous
	Erythematous
Chronic	Pseudomembranous
	Erythematous
	Hyperplastic
Candida-associated lesions	Denture-induced stomatitis
	Angular cheilitis*
	Median rhomboid glossitis

Secondary oral candidoses
This term encompasses a complex and rare group of conditions in which superficial chronic mucocutaneous candidosis occurs in conjunction with endocrine abnormalities (hypoparathyroidism, hypothyroidism, hypoadrenocorticism (Addison's disease) and diabetes mellitus) or immunodeficiency

*Staphylococci and streptococci may also be involved in the aetiology of some cases of angular cheilitis.

Chronic hyperplastic Chronic, discrete adherent white plaque-like lesions. Most commonly occur at the commissures. May also affect other parts of the oral mucosa.

Denture-induced stomatitis Chronic erythema and oedema of the mucosa in contact with the fitting surface of the upper denture. Often coexists with angular cheilitis. Three subtypes have been described (Newton's classification): • I – pinpoint hyperaemia (some have suggested that this is simply a response to chronic trauma) • II – diffuse erythema • III – granular (papillary hyperplasia).

Angular cheilitis Soreness, erythema and fissuring at the angles of the lips.

Median rhomboid glossitis Elliptical or rhomboid area of papillary atrophy centrally placed, anterior to the circumvallate papillae. Less commonly, it may have a hyperplastic or lobulated appearance.

Investigation and diagnosis Essentially clinical although confirmation can be obtained with the investigations shown in Table 15.3. Screen for nutritional deficiencies and diabetes – FBC, ferritin, folate, vitamin B_{12} and glucose.

Treatment Eliminate predisposing factors if possible, e.g. reduce refined carbohydrate intake. Appropriate denture hygiene, store dentures in hypochlorite solution overnight.

TABLE 15.3 Investigations in candidal infections

	Swab	Smear	Biopsy
Pseudomembranous	+	+	–
Acute erythematous	+	+	–
Chronic erythematous	+	+	–
Chronic hyperplastic	–	–	+
Denture-induced stomatitis*	+	+	–
Angular cheilitis	+	+	–
Median rhomboid glossitis	+	+	+

*Swab and smear from palate and fitting surface of denture.

Antifungal agents • *topical* – nystatin, amphotericin, miconazole • *systemic* – fluconazole, itraconazole. Azole antifungal agents should be avoided in patients taking warfarin or lipid-regulating drugs due to significant drug interactions.

VIRAL INFECTIONS

A wide range of viruses are responsible for causing oral lesions. These include: • herpes simplex virus (HSV) types 1 and 2 • herpes zoster • Epstein–Barr virus (EBV, see hairy leukoplakia) • Coxsackie viruses • paramyxoviruses • human papillomaviruses.

Primary herpetic gingivostomatitis

Caused commonly by herpes simplex type 1. Type 2, which is more commonly associated with genital herpes, accounts for a proportion of cases. Transmission is via direct contact with recurrent skin lesions or infected saliva. In infancy and childhood, the disease may be subclinical and is self-limiting. May be attributed to teething. In adulthood the infection is usually more severe.

Clinical features Initial pyrexia, malaise, painful mouth and throat, associated cervical lymphadenopathy. Subsequent development of widespread intraoral vesicular lesions which rapidly rupture to form small irregular superficial ulcers with erythematous haloes. If the gingivae are affected they appear inflamed and bleed readily. Lesions are entirely self-limiting and resolve within 10–14 days.

Investigation and diagnosis Primarily based on history and clinical features. Can be confirmed by: • polymerase chain reaction (detection of HSV DNA) • detecting virus in a smear • viral culture • demonstration of a fourfold rise in antibody titre is a largely historical investigation.

Treatment
Mild cases Treat conservatively with symptomatic measures such as oral fluids, prevention of secondary infection and analgesics.

Moderate and severe cases or infections occurring in immunosuppressed patients Systemic antiviral drugs (aciclovir or famciclovir) are useful particularly if started early in the course of the disease.

Recurrent herpetic infection
Approximately 30% of patients subsequently develop recurrent infections, most commonly in the form of *herpes labialis* (cold sores). The virus lies dormant in the trigeminal ganglion and is reactivated by a variety of precipitating factors including: • fever, • trauma • exposure to sunlight • stress • menstruation • immunosuppression.

Lesions affect the mucocutaneous junction of the lip or involve the nostril. Recurrence is heralded by a prodromal burning or prickling sensation in the area followed by the formation of small vesicles which enlarge, coalesce and then rupture. Lesions then crust over and heal spontaneously. Less commonly recurrence can manifest intraorally as clusters of small superficial ulcers usually affecting the hard palate.

Treatment Lesions of herpes labialis can be treated with topical penciclovir 1% or aciclovir 5% cream applied every 2 hours during the prodromal stage.

Chickenpox
Primary infection with varicella zoster virus (VSV). Highly contagious; spread by droplets. Incubation period 14–21 days.

Clinical features Often a subclinical infection occurring primarily in children. Fever, malaise, anorexia, skin eruption affecting the face and trunk, cervical lymphadenitis. Skin lesions initially present as papules which evolve into vesicles, pustules and scabs. Commonly occur as crops – lesions are seen at varying stages of evolution. Oral lesions are characterized by small ulcers – may predate the appearance of the skin rash.

Investigation and diagnosis Diagnosis is largely clinical. Rising antibody titre may confirm clinical suspicion.

Treatment Symptomatic as disease is self-limiting. In immunosuppressed patients systemic antiviral agents (aciclovir, famciclovir or valaciclovir) may be given.

Shingles

Localized reactivation of herpes zoster in sensory ganglion leading to vesicular eruption affecting the skin dermatome supplied by that nerve. Most cases affect the elderly or immunosuppressed.

Clinical features Usually involves thoracic dermatomes, with only about 30% involving divisions of the trigeminal nerve – usually mandibular division. Localized pain, often described as a burning sensation and/or altered sensation in the distribution of the nerve, commonly precedes the appearance of the skin eruption. Skin lesions are initially erythematous – subsequently develop vesicles which form scabs after a few days. Unilateral oral ulceration when mandibular or maxillary divisions of the trigeminal nerve involved.

If ophthalmic division affected an urgent ophthalmological opinion should be arranged due to the risk of corneal ulceration and subsequent blindness.

Investigation and diagnosis Primarily a clinical diagnosis. Confirmed by isolation of VSV in vesicular lesions or testing for specific immunoglobulin M (IgM) to VZV.

Treatment Systemic high-dose aciclovir (800 mg five times daily for 7 days); less effective once the vesicular rash appears. Aciclovir and systemic corticosteroids may be helpful in reducing incidence of postherpetic neuralgia.

Herpangina

Relatively common infection caused by various Coxsackie viruses (A7, 9, 16; B1–5). Occurs most commonly in children – may be mistaken for teething. Characterized by pyrexia, dysphagia, sore throat and multiple small vesicles on the soft palate and uvula which rupture to leave superficial ulcers.

Treatment No specific treatment. Management aimed at controlling symptoms (soft diet, fluids, prevention of secondary infection and analgesics).

Hand, foot and mouth disease

Common viral infection predominantly affecting young children. Occurs in small epidemics. Caused by various Coxsackie viruses, particularly A16 (less commonly A5 or 10). May be subclinical infection. Characterized by low-grade pyrexia, malaise, anorexia, multiple shallow ulcers of the labial and buccal mucosa often indistinguishable from primary herpetic gingivostomatitis although no gingival involvement; papular or vesicular rash on the palms and soles. Management as for herpangina.

Human papillomavirus (HPV)

The human papillomaviruses are a group of more than 70 different types of virus. Several types are associated with specific oral lesions.

Squamous cell papilloma Common benign tumour found most frequently in patients in third to fifth decades. Most commonly presents on the soft palate although may also affect dorsum and lateral surfaces of tongue or the lower lip. Clinically presents as a pedunculated or sessile cauliflower-like swelling. HPV 6 or 11 found in up to 80% cases.

Verruca vulgaris Common skin lesion, particularly in children. Occasionally may affect oral mucosa. Usually appears as a firm, sessile, white, exophytic lesion on the lip and may be associated with autoinoculation from pre-existing skin lesion. Predominantly associated with HPV types 2 or 4.

Condyloma acuminatum Usually presents on anogenital mucosa, although may also present on oral mucosa. Present as multiple white or pink nodules which may coalesce to form soft sessile swellings. Associated with HPV types 6, 11 or 16. More common in HIV-seropositive patients.

Focal epithelial hyperplasia (Heck's disease) Rare benign lesion of oral mucosa characterized by multiple painless papules most commonly on the lower lip and may extend onto the vermillion border. More common in certain ethnic groups (e.g. Inuit and Indians from North and South America). Possible genetic predisposition. Associated with HPV type 13 or 32.

RECURRENT ORAL ULCERATION

Oral ulceration

Ulceration is defined as a break in the continuity of an epithelial lining. Causes are summarized in Table 15.4.

Recurrent aphthous stomatitis

Recurrent aphthous stomatitis (RAS) is a common oral condition of unknown aetiology affecting approximately 20% of the population. Three types are recognized, although it is unclear if

TABLE 15.4 Causes of oral ulceration	
Traumatic	Mechanical Chemical Thermal Radiation Artefactual
Idiopathic	Recurrent aphthous stomatitis including Behçet's syndrome
Infection	Viral Bacterial Fungal
Associated with systemic disease	Haematological disorders Crohn's disease Ulcerative colitis
Associated with dermatological diseases	Lichen planus Vesiculobullous disorders
Neoplastic	Squamous cell carcinoma and other tumours
Drug-induced	Cytotoxic agents Nicorandil

they represent variants of the same disease or are distinct entities:
• minor, 80–85% • major, 10–15% • herpetiform, 5%.

Clinical features are shown in Table 15.5.

Aetiological factors Can be considered as *host* or *environmental* factors. Evidence for aetiological factors can be summarized as:

Genetic Family history in up to 45% cases. High concordance rate among identical twins. Several HLA associations reported.

Nutritional deficiencies Haematological deficiencies (most commonly iron, although may also be associated with vitamin B_{12} and folic acid). Found in approximately 20–30% of patients with RAS. Some reports also suggest increased incidence of vitamin B_1 and B_6 deficiencies.

Systemic diseases RAS may occur in association with a variety of systemic disorders, e.g. coeliac disease, Crohn's disease, ulcerative colitis and cyclic neutropenia.

Endocrine In a small proportion of female patients RAS may be more severe during the luteal phase of the menstrual cycle, related to the increased levels of progestogens and decreased oestrogens. Remissions often occur during pregnancy.

Stress/anxiety Conflicting reports in the literature; this issue remains unresolved.

TABLE 15.5 Clinical features of minor, major and herpetiform oral ulceration

	Minor	Major	Herpetiform
Sex ratio	M = F	M = F	F > M
Age of onset (years)	10–19	10–19	20–29
No. of ulcers	<10	<5	10–100
Size of ulcers	<10 mm	>10 mm	1–2 mm Larger if ulcers coalesce
Duration	4–14 days	>30 days	>30 days
Recurrence rate	1–4 months	< monthly	< monthly
Sites affected	Labial and buccal mucosa, tongue	Labial and buccal mucosa, tongue, palate, pharynx	Labial and buccal mucosa, soft palate, floor of mouth
Scarring	Uncommon	Common	Possible if ulcers coalesce

Trauma Minor trauma may initiate ulceration in susceptible patients. Influences the site of ulceration.

Allergy Some reports suggest associations between RAS and exposure to dietary allergens, although further study is required in this area.

Infection Conflicting data on the role of oral streptococci as direct pathogens or antigenic stimuli for production of antibodies that cross-react with keratinocyte determinants. Similarly, some investigators have suggested a role for VSV and HSV although the results require confirmation.

Smoking Negative association between RAS and cigarette smoking. Onset of RAS in some patients may coincide with cessation of smoking.

Investigation and diagnosis Full blood count, assays of ferritin, vitamin B_{12} and folate to exclude nutritional deficiency. In areas where there is a high prevalence of coeliac disease, or if the patient has features suggestive of malabsorption, coeliac serology (antiendomysial antibody or tissue transglutaminase antibodies) is appropriate as a screen to exclude coeliac disease. No specific diagnostic tests. In patients who are rarely free of ulcers, allergy may be a contributing factor and patch testing can identify dietary and/or environmental allergens.

Treatment No specific management available for the majority of patients. Correct haematinic deficiencies. In general, symptoms can be reduced although no treatment consistently prevents recurrences (Table 15.6).

Behçet's syndrome

Comprises a triad of: • recurrent aphthous stomatitis • genital ulceration • posterior uveitis.

Only about 42% of cases show the classic triad although >90% have oral ulceration. Diagnosis is usually made if two of these features are present. Any of the three variants of aphthous stomatitis may occur although there is an increased prevalence of herpetiform and major aphthae. Other manifestations, occurring with varying frequency, now recognized as components of the syndrome include: • cutaneous lesions • neurological problems • joint lesions • intestinal lesions • haematological abnormalities • vascular lesions.

Age of onset mainly third decade. Male preponderance (M : F, 2.3 : 1). There is a significant geographic variation, with the syndrome being more common in the Eastern Mediterranean and Japan.

Clinical features are shown in Table 15.7.

Investigations and diagnosis No universally agreed diagnostic criteria. Diagnosis is essentially clinical. Exclude nutritional deficiency as a contributing factor. Strong association with HLA B51 may support the diagnosis.

Treatment Overall treatment with immunosuppressive agents, e.g. steroids, azathioprine, colchicine, tacrolimus, thalidomide. Oral

TABLE 15.6 Treatment options in recurrent oral ulceration	
Antiseptic mouthwashes	Chlorhexidine 0.2% Benzydamine hydrochloride
Antibiotics	Tetracycline mouthwash
Topical steroids	Hydrocortisone pellets Triamcinolone paste Betamethasone mouthwash Beclometasone spray
Systemic steroids	Prednisolone
Other	Azathioprine Dapsone Colchicine Thalidomide

TABLE 15.7 Features of Behçet's syndrome

Oral	Minor, major or herpetiform aphthae
Ocular	Uveitis, optic atrophy, retinal vasculitis
Genital	Ulceration
Dermatological	Pustules, erythema nodosum
Neurological	Symptoms resembling multiple sclerosis, pseudobulbar palsy
Joint disease	Recurrent arthralgia involving large joints
Miscellaneous	Thromboses, depression, renal disease, anorexia, colitis

ulceration can be managed as for RAS. Ophthalmological opinion to exclude ocular involvement should be sought as this may lead to visual impairment or blindness.

VESICULOBULLOUS LESIONS

Classified as intraepithelial or subepithelial (Table 15.8). Table 15.9 shows the immunopathological features of vesiculobullous disorders.

Angina bullosa haemorrhagica (localized oral purpura)

Clinical features Predominantly affects elderly people. Characterized by the rapid formation of blood-filled blister, usually on soft palate although may occur on any other part of the oral mucosa. Blister ruptures to leave a superficial ulcer, which is

TABLE 15.8 Classification of vesiculobullous lesions

Intraepithelial	Subepithelial
Pemphigus	Angina bullosa haemorrhagica
Viral infections	Mucous membrane pemphigoid
• Herpes simplex	Bullous pemphigoid
• Herpes zoster	Dermatitis herpetiformis
• Coxsackie	Lichen planus
Epidermolysis bullosa	Erythema multiforme
(simplex types)	Epidermolysis bullosa (gravis and dystrophic types)
	Linear IgA disease

TABLE 15.9 Immunopathological features of vesiculobullous disorders

Disease	Direct immunofluorescence	Indirect immunofluorescence
Pemphigus	Intercellular IgG and C3	Titre correlates with disease severity
Mucous membrane pemphigoid	Linear IgG and C3 at basement membrane zone	Essentially negative
Bullous pemphigoid	Linear IgG and C3 at basement membrane zone	Positive in ~75% of cases
Linear IgA disease	Linear IgA and C3 at basement membrane zone	Negative
Dermatitis herpetiformis	Granular deposits of IgA and C3 at tips of dermal papillae	Negative

entirely self-limiting. Unknown aetiology, no coagulation defect identified. Association with use of steroid inhalers has been suggested.

Investigation and diagnosis Check clotting screen and full blood count to ensure normal haemostatic components. Rarely may require biopsy to differentiate from pemphigoid.

Treatment Reassurance and use of an antiseptic mouthwash for symptomatic relief.

Pemphigus

Serious, rare autoimmune skin disease with several different variants: • pemphigus vulgaris • pemphigus vegetans • pemphigus foliaceous • pemphigus erythematosus. The latter two variants rarely, if ever, have oral manifestations.

Pemphigus vulgaris The most common and most severe variant. Predominantly affects females. Presents in middle age. More common among those of Ashkenazi Jewish and Mediterranean descent.

Clinical features Characterized by widespread bullous lesions affecting mucous membranes and/or skin. Oral lesions occur in almost all patients and may be the presenting feature in up to 50%. In some cases oral lesions may be the only manifestation of the disease predating the development of skin lesions for a considerable time. Positive Nikolsky sign, although this is not pathognomonic of pemphigus. Intact intraoral bullae are rare. Tend to rupture shortly after they form to leave irregular areas of non-specific ulceration. Pain is often a prominent feature. Despite widespread involvement scarring is uncommon. Untreated, the disease may be fatal due to extensive skin involvement leading to fluid and electrolyte imbalance.

Investigation and diagnosis Routine histopathology of perilesional tissue together with direct and indirect immunofluorescence. IgG and C3 bind to component of desmosomes (predominantly desmoglein 3). Circulating antibody titre reflects severity of disease and can be used as a marker of disease activity.

Treatment Immunosuppressive therapy with systemic steroids ± azathioprine or other immunomodulating drugs.

Pemphigus vegetans Considered to be a milder variant of pemphigus vulgaris. Characterized by the formation of hyperplastic vegetations of granulation tissue when bullae rupture. Oral lesions occur in approximately 50% of cases.

Mucous membrane pemphigoid Chronic subepithelial bullous disorder principally affecting the elderly. More common among females (F : M, 2 : 1). Lesions can occur on oral and genital mucosa, conjunctiva and skin. Characteristically heals by scarring, particularly on the conjunctiva.

Clinical features Oral mucosa almost invariably involved while skin lesions are uncommon. Bullae are thick walled and therefore may remain intact for several days before rupturing to leave superficial areas of ulceration. May also present as desquamative gingivitis. Ocular involvement is potentially serious and may lead to blindness.

Investigation and diagnosis Histopathology demonstrates subepithelial bulla formation. Immunofluorescence – IgG and C3 at basement membrane.

Treatment Topical steroids are generally effective for oral lesions. Systemic steroids and/or dapsone in severe cases.

Bullous pemphigoid Primarily a bullous disorder of skin with oral lesions occurring in only one-third of patients. A disease of the elderly – most patients >60 years. Males and females equally affected. Skin lesions on limbs and trunk may begin as a non-specific urticarial rash several weeks before the appearance of vesiculobullous lesions. Clinically the oral lesions are indistinguishable from those of mucous membrane pemphigoid although they heal rapidly without scarring.

Erythema multiforme

Self-limiting acute vesiculobullous disease affecting skin and/or mucous membrane. Usually affects young adult males. Aetiology unknown in most cases, although recognized precipitating factors include:

● infections – HSV, *Mycoplasma pneumoniae*
● drugs – sulphonamides, barbiturates, thiazide diuretics, tetracyclines, carbamazepine
● other – radiotherapy, malignancy, pregnancy.

Clinical features Wide spectrum of disease severity and presentation. May affect mouth, skin and other mucosal surfaces, alone or in any combination. Prodromal symptoms of upper respiratory tract infection followed by appearance of skin and/or mucosal lesions. Variety of skin lesions may occur, most commonly affecting hands and feet, including an erythematous maculopapular rash. Vesiculobullous lesions and classical 'target' or 'iris' lesions. Oral lesions are characterized by haemorrhagic crusting of the lips together with extensive bullous lesions which rapidly rupture to form widespread painful erosions. Ocular involvement may lead to conjunctival scarring and blindness. Symptoms usually subside within 2 weeks although recurrences may occur.

Investigation and diagnosis Diagnosis usually based on clinical picture but can be confirmed with biopsy.

Treatment Identify and eliminate precipitating factor if possible (e.g. aciclovir if episodes known to be triggered by herpes simplex infection). Prevent dehydration. Systemic steroids (± azathioprine) in severe cases.

Epidermolysis bullosa

Complex group of syndromes with over 30 different types of varying severity. Inherited as autosomal dominant or recessive conditions. Most severe forms become evident shortly after birth and are generally incompatible with life while milder forms may not become apparent until adolescence or adulthood. Characterized by fragility of skin, leading to formation of bullae in response to minor trauma. In severe forms bullae may arise spontaneously. Healing occurs with scarring. Systemic steroids, phenytoin and vitamin E may be of benefit in some patients.

Dermatitis herpetiformis

Uncommon autoimmune-mediated blistering disease of skin that usually affects middle-aged males. Related to coeliac disease and gluten hypersensitivity. Most patients have no evidence of malabsorption although most have at least histological evidence of jejunal involvement. Skin lesions characterized by an intensely itchy papulovesicular rash on the trunk and limbs. Oral lesions range from asymptomatic erythematous areas to extensive erosive patches. Incidence of oral lesions may be up to 70%.

Linear IgA disease

Rare blistering disease of skin which may be a variant of dermatitis herpetiformis. Gluten hypersensitivity may be a feature although this is less common than in patients with dermatitis herpetiformis. Oral lesions include persistent non-specific ulceration.

WHITE PATCHES

Classification (Table 15.10)

White sponge naevus

Benign keratin defect; autosomal dominant mode of inheritance with incomplete penetrance and variable expression.

TABLE 15.10 Classification of white patches	
Genetic	White sponge naevus
	Darier's disease
	Dyskeratosis congenita
	Pachyonychia congenita
	Hereditary intraepithelial dyskeratosis
Traumatic	Chemical burn
	Mechanical (frictional)
	Thermal burn: smokers' keratosis, nicotinic stomatitis
Infection	Candidosis (pseudomembranous and hyperplastic types)
	Hairy leukoplakia
	Syphilitic leukoplakia
Idiopathic	Leukoplakia
Dermatological	Lichen planus
	Lupus erythematosus
Metabolic	Associated with renal failure
Neoplastic	Squamous cell carcinoma

Clinical features Diffuse, ill-defined, thickened white lesions most commonly affecting buccal mucosa. Less commonly labial mucosa, tongue and floor of mouth. A proportion of patients have similar lesions involving nasal, rectal or genital mucosa.

Investigation and diagnosis Biopsy will confirm diagnosis although often clinical features are sufficient.

Treatment Reassurance. No specific treatment required.

Darier's disease (follicular keratosis)
Rare condition transmitted by an autosomal dominant pattern of inheritance although many cases may arise as new mutations. Skin lesions initially appear as multiple small papules, particularly on the forehead, scalp and neck, which subsequently become grey/brown as they ulcerate and crust over. Lesions become foul smelling when secondarily infected. Oral lesions occur in about 50% and appear as minute white papules which coalesce. Common sites include palate and gingivae.

Pachyonychia congenita
Uncommon disease inherited as an autosomal dominant condition. Characterized by dystrophic changes affecting the nails which are present at birth or develop shortly after; hyperhidrosis and palmoplantar keratosis in 40–60%. Oral lesions are usually present and consist of white, opaque thickening of the dorsum and lateral margins of the tongue. Involvement of the buccal and labial mucosa is less commonly seen.

Dyskeratosis congenita
Rare inherited condition (X-linked) characterized by hyperpigmentation of skin, dystrophy of the nails and oral leukoplakia. Oral lesions most commonly appear in early childhood and initially present as multiple vesicles/ulcers followed by the development of white plaques, which may later undergo malignant transformation.

Chemical burns
Various chemicals or drugs used in self-medication may produce burns if held in contact with the oral mucosa (e.g. aspirin and choline salicylate). Presents as an irregular white patch with oedema, necrosis of the epithelium, sloughing and ulceration. The lesion resolves within several days following removal of the irritant.

Frictional keratosis

Localized white patch lesion that forms in response to chronic low-grade trauma from irritants such as cheek biting, sharp cusps or ill-fitting dentures. Lesion will resolve if source of irritation is removed.

Smokers' keratosis

Regular use of tobacco often results in appearance of discrete white plaques on the oral mucosa, typically affecting buccal mucosa at the commissures, tongue or palate. Chemical irritation may also be involved in the aetiology of these lesions.

Nicotinic stomatitis

Seen frequently in heavy pipe smokers. Presents as diffuse grey/white thickened appearance affecting the posterior palate with numerous red papules, in the centre of which are the dilated orifices of swollen mucous glands. Regresses rapidly on cessation of smoking habit. Not considered to have any malignant potential.

Renal failure

Rarely, oral keratosis, predominantly affecting the floor of mouth and tongue, may be a feature of chronic renal failure. The white plaques regress on treatment of the renal disease.

The following white patch lesions are discussed elsewhere: *leukoplakia* (p. 457), *candidosis* – pseudomembranous and hyperplastic types (p. 442), *hairy leukoplakia* (p. 484), *lichen planus* (p. 478), *lupus erythematosus* (p. 480), *neoplasia* (p. 461).

POTENTIALLY MALIGNANT LESIONS AND CONDITIONS

A lesion can be regarded as potentially malignant if it is associated with a significantly increased risk of cancer. However, it must be stressed that most mouth cancers arise de novo with no recognizable preceding premalignant state.

Potentially malignant lesions of the oral mucosa include:
• leukoplakia • erythroplakia • chronic hyperplastic candidosis
• lichen planus (p. 478) • oral submucous fibrosis • sideropenic dysphagia.

Leukoplakia and erythroplakia

Leukoplakia is defined as a white patch or plaque on the oral mucosa that cannot be removed by scraping and cannot be characterized clinically or pathologically as any other disease. The definition has no histological connotation. Thus the diagnosis is essentially one of exclusion.

Erythroplakia is defined as a bright red velvet plaque on the oral mucosa which cannot be characterized clinically or pathologically as being due to any other condition.

While the term leukoplakia does not imply a particular type of behaviour, a small percentage of such lesions can be considered premalignant and a few may even be invasive tumours at initial presentation. Thus the lesion is highly significant. Unfortunately it is not possible to predict the behaviour of an individual lesion although some clinical and histological features are associated with an increased risk of malignant transformation.

The histological features of oral leukoplakia vary considerably, with some lesions having essentially benign appearances while others may show varying degrees of epithelial dysplasia (mild, moderate or severe) or carcinoma in situ.

Features of epithelial dysplasia include • nuclear hyperchromatism • loss of polarity • increased nuclear–cytoplasmic ratio • pleomorphism • disordered maturation • basal cell hyperplasia • drop-shaped rete pegs • premature keratinization • reduced intercellular adhesion • increased or abnormal mitoses.

The clinical appearance of such lesions does not allow prediction of the presence or severity of epithelial dysplasia with any degree of certainty, although erythroplakias and nodular leukoplakias are more likely to be dysplastic than homogeneous leukoplakias.

Reported rates of malignant transformation vary from 0.3% to 17.5% over periods of about 10 years. In western Europe an overall figure of 2–6% is considered a realistic estimate of the risk.

Factors associated with increased rate of malignant transformation
Site of lesion Floor of mouth, ventral surface of tongue and lingual alveolar mucosa are higher-risk areas and often termed 'sublingual keratoses'. Some studies have suggested that up to 25% may be invasive carcinoma at time of initial diagnosis and a further 25% will undergo malignant transformation.
Presence of epithelial dysplasia The degree of dysplasia is widely believed to be an important factor although there is no definitive proof to support this assertion.
Clinical nature of lesion Nodular or speckled leukoplakias have a higher tendency for malignant transformation than homogeneous leukoplakias.

Chronic hyperplastic candidosis (candidal leukoplakia)

Homogeneous or nodular white patch lesion most commonly affecting the commissures, although may also involve cheeks, palate or tongue. Male:female, 2:1. Homogeneous lesions are often asymptomatic whereas nodular lesions may give rise to intermittent discomfort. Frequently associated with other oral candidal lesions (angular cheilitis and *Candida*-associated denture stomatitis).

Predisposing factors • tobacco usage • nutritional deficiency • poor denture hygiene • steroid inhaler use.

Approximately 50% show features of epithelial dysplasia and malignant transformation rates vary from 10 to 40% – significantly higher than that for leukoplakia in general.

Management Biopsy is considered mandatory for all white/red lesions, as clinical features are unreliable for diagnostic purposes. Elimination of predisposing factors and systemic antifungal therapy may be prescribed where indicated on histology. Small lesions or those with features of severe dysplasia may be removed surgically. Long-term follow-up is essential for all such lesions, with periodic biopsy, particularly if there is a change in the appearance of the lesion.

Oral submucous fibrosis

Insidious chronic disease affecting the oral mucosa; occasionally may extend to involve the pharynx and oesophagus. Characterized by progressive fibrosis. Occurs almost exclusively in peoples from the Indian subcontinent and Myanmar although sporadic cases have been reported in other countries. Aetiology unclear – strong association with betel chewing. Tobacco and vitamin deficiencies are other factors. Clinically the mucosa has a blanched opaque appearance with fibrous bands most commonly affecting the lips, buccal mucosa and tongue. Epithelial dysplasia is a common finding; histological evidence of carcinoma observed in 5–6%.

PIGMENTED LESIONS OF THE ORAL MUCOSA

Causes are listed in Table 15.11.

Exogenous causes of pigmentation

Superficial mucosal staining May be caused by various foods and tobacco products.

TABLE 15.11 Causes of oral mucosal pigmentation

Exogenous	Endogenous

Superficial mucosal staining	Developmental
	  Racial
	  Pigmented naevi
	  Peutz–Jeghers syndrome

Black hairy tongue	Acquired
	  Endocrine associated:
	  • Addison's disease
	  • Ectopic ACTH production
	  Associated with chronic irritation
	  Drug-induced
	  Associated with HIV infection
	  Melanotic macules

Foreign bodies Amalgam tattoo Graphite Road grit	Neoplastic Malignant melanoma
Heavy metal salts Lead Mercury Bismuth	

ACTH, adrenocorticotrophic hormone.

Black hairy tongue Benign condition characterized by overgrowth of the filiform papillae together with lack of normal desquamation and associated discoloration, which may vary from brown to black. Discoloration may be related to overgrowth of bacteria and fungi which produce pigment. May be exacerbated by use of tobacco. Generally asymptomatic although some patients become alarmed by the appearance. Occasionally may cause nausea due to stimulation of the soft palate.

Foreign bodies (e.g. amalgam, graphite from pencils, road grit following road traffic accident.) Amalgam tattoo characterized by blue/black area of pigmentation on the mucosa. May occur following fracture of amalgam restoration during extraction of a tooth and inclusion in the healing socket. Alternatively fragments of amalgam may become implanted in the soft tissues during removal of restoration or insertion of retrograde root filling at time of apicectomy.

Heavy metal salts (e.g. mercury, lead, bismuth and silver.) Deposition of heavy metal salts along gingival margin in occupationally exposed individuals – now uncommon.

Endogenous causes of pigmentation

Melanin is the most common endogenous pigment associated with mucosal pigmentation. Oral lesions associated with the other endogenous pigments (haemosiderin and lipofuscin) are relatively uncommon.

Developmental causes of melanin pigmentation

Racial pigmentation
Peutz–Jeghers syndrome (p. 482)

Acquired causes of melanin pigmentation

Associated with endocrine disease Addison's disease, Nelson's syndrome and tumours secreting ACTH (most commonly bronchogenic carcinoma).

Drug-induced Antimalarials, anticonvulsants, phenothiazines and oral contraceptives.

Reaction to chronic irritation Most commonly associated with smoking although it may also be seen in lesions that are a response to chronic mechanical trauma, e.g. hyperkeratotic lesions.

Melanotic macule Flat localized area of brown pigmentation often on the lower lip or buccal mucosa. Analogous to a freckle on skin.

Associated with HIV infection

Neoplastic

Malignant melanoma Highly malignant melanin-containing tumour that may affect skin, mucosa and the eye. Rare tumour in the oral cavity with most cases involving the posterior hard palate and maxillary alveolar ridge. Most cases occur after the age of 30 years. Usually presents as a deeply pigmented lesion which may be ulcerated and bleeding. Progressively increases in size although growth may be very rapid. Bone involvement is often a prominent feature. Lymph node and distant metastases are common. Treatment is by radical excision but the overall prognosis is poor.

MOUTH CANCER

Marked geographic variations in incidence worldwide. In the UK mouth cancer accounts for only 1–2% of all malignant tumours whereas in some parts of India and Sri Lanka it may account for 30–40%. Ninety to 95% of all mouth cancers are squamous cell carcinomas. Mainly seen in middle aged and elderly but as yet unexplained increasing incidence among younger adults.

Aetiological factors

Tobacco All forms of smoking tobacco (cigarettes, cigars and pipe smoking) are associated with an increased risk of mouth cancer, particularly if reverse smoking is practised. Chewing betel quid, with added tobacco, accounts for the high incidence of mouth cancer in south Asia. Similarly use of snuff and chewing tobacco increases the risk.

Alcohol Increased risk in association with alcohol consumption. Alcohol also acts synergistically with tobacco and multiplies the risk of mouth cancer.

Diet and nutrition Poor diet increases risk. Increased risk of oesophageal and oropharyngeal tumours in patients with Brown Kelly–Paterson syndrome (primary sideropenic anaemia).

Ultraviolet light Important risk factor for carcinoma of the lip.

Chronic Candida *infection* Chronic hyperplastic candidosis is considered to be a premalignant condition although other chronic *Candida* infections are not associated with an increased risk of mouth cancer.

Immunosuppression Increased risk of lip cancer among renal transplant recipients.

Syphilis Previously reported association may be related to carcinogenic nature of treatment (e.g. arsenicals). In addition, epithelial atrophy, which is a feature of the later stages of the disease, may render the mucosa more susceptible to carcinogens.

Chronic trauma Mechanical trauma from ill-fitting dentures and a poorly maintained dentition as well as poor oral hygiene have all been suggested as possible aetiological factors, although convincing evidence is lacking. Experimentally, in animals, it has been shown that mechanical trauma can act as a promoter although not an initiator. Thus it is possible that these factors play a similar role in the development of mouth cancer in humans.

Clinical features Clinical presentation varies considerably. Early mouth cancers are very often asymptomatic. Common patterns of presentation include the following:

Early lesion: • painless solitary ulcer • exophytic growth • white patch • erythroplakia • erythroleukoplakia • chronic crusted lesions on the vermillion border of the lip.

Advanced lesion: • pain • exophytic mass • necrotic, bleeding or warty surface • deep, cratered ulcers with indurated edges • bone invasion leading to possible altered sensation and pathological fracture.

Prognosis Factors that are considered to influence the prognosis of mouth cancer are:

Early versus late diagnosis Early diagnosis is by far the most important factor affecting outcome.

Extent of disease Several clinical staging systems exist; the most widely used is the TNM classification (Table 15.12).

Site In general terms lesions at the back of the mouth have a poorer prognosis than those situated more anteriorly – probably related to later diagnosis of tumours at the back of the mouth. Additionally, early metastasis is a feature of tumours affecting the base of the tongue. In contrast, cancers of the lip have the best prognosis as they are frequently detected at an early stage and are less aggressive tumours.

Pathology The value of histological grading of mouth cancers is controversial due to potential errors in sampling tumours, which are often microscopically heterogeneous.

Age With increasing age, patients are less able to cope with extensive surgery and/or radiotherapy. Diminished cell-mediated response associated with age may also play a role.

Treatment Surgery and/or radiotherapy (p. 411).

TABLE 15.12 TNM classification					
T *Primary tumour*		**N** *Lymph node status*		**M** *Distant metastases*	
T0	No evidence of primary tumour	N0	No nodes involved clinically	M0	Absent
T1	Greatest diameter <2 cm	N1	Single ipsilateral node <3 cm diameter	M1	Present
T2	Greatest diameter 2–4 cm	N2	Single ipsilateral node >3 cm and <6 cm Multiple ipsilateral nodes <6 cm		
T3	Greatest diameter >4 cm	N3	Bilateral nodes or ipsilateral nodes >6 cm		
T4	Tumour >4 cm with gross local invasion				

Verrucous carcinoma

Regarded as a variety of low-grade squamous cell carcinoma with distinctive clinical appearance and behaviour. Most commonly affects the buccal sulcus and buccal mucosa in the elderly. Established aetiological link with tobacco and betel chewing.

Clinical features Markedly exophytic white plaque-like lesion. Slow growing and erodes rather than invades underlying tissues, including bone.

Treatment Surgical excision is the preferred method of treatment as radiotherapy may induce anaplastic transformation.

MISCELLANEOUS LESIONS

Geographic tongue (benign migratory glossitis)

Common condition of unknown aetiology, characterized clinically by irregular partially depapillated areas on the anterior two-thirds of the tongue, often with distinct white margins. These lesions regress and reappear on other parts of the tongue. Frequently asymptomatic although may be some discomfort, particularly on eating hot or spiced foods. Occasionally may affect other parts of the oral mucosa (migratory stomatitis or erythema migrans). If symptomatic, other causes of glossitis should be considered.

Fissured tongue (scrotal tongue)

Common abnormality which is often associated with geographic tongue. Often asymptomatic and seen frequently in Down syndrome. Clinical features consist of multiple prominent fissures of variable depth. Exclude nutritional deficiency if tongue painful. Also a component of Melkersson–Rosenthal syndrome (triad of fissured tongue, facial nerve palsy and lip/face swelling).

Sarcoidosis

Granulomatous disorder of unknown aetiology with multisystem involvement. Occurs most commonly in young adults, more common in females. Serum angiotensin-converting enzyme level usually elevated. Clinical presentation depends on which organ systems are involved:

Lungs Hilar lymphadenopathy
Skin Erythema nodosum
Eyes Uveitis
Heart Conduction defects

Oral Salivary gland swelling, lip/cheek swelling (orofacial granulomatosis-like picture), hyperplasia of gingivae, painless red nodules.

SALIVARY GLAND DISORDERS

XEROSTOMIA

Possible causes: • aplasia of the major salivary glands (very rare) • psychogenic (anxiety, depression, hypochondriasis) • drug-induced (atropine and atropine analogues, antihypertensive agents, tricyclic antidepressants, phenothiazines, antihistamines, lithium) • postirradiation • Sjögren's syndrome • sarcoidosis • dehydration (e.g. diabetes mellitus, renal failure, fluid loss) • HIV salivary gland disease.

Sjögren's syndrome

Chronic inflammatory disease with autoimmune basis. Characterized by lymphocytic infiltrate involving exocrine glands. Classified into two types – primary (previously known as sicca syndrome) and secondary. Oral complications of Sjögren's syndrome include: • increased incidence of dental caries • predisposition to oral candidosis • ascending bacterial sialadenitis • an increased incidence of lymphoma. The incidence of lymphoma is greatest among patients with primary Sjögren's syndrome.

Clinical features see Table 15.13.
Primary Xerostomia (dry mouth), xerophthalmia (dry eyes).
Secondary Xerostomia, xerophthalmia, connective tissue disorder – most commonly rheumatoid arthritis. Other possible connective

TABLE 15.13 Features of primary and secondary Sjögren's syndrome

	Primary	*Secondary*
Connective tissue component	Absent	Present
Xerostomia	More severe	Less severe
Recurrent sialadenitis	More common	Less common
Xerophthalmia	Severe	Less severe
Rheumatoid factor positive	50%	90%
Anti-Ro positive	5–10%	50–80%
Anti-La positive	50–70%	2–5%

tissue disorders include systemic lupus erythematosus, primary biliary cirrhosis, mixed connective tissue disorder.

Investigation and diagnosis No single test will consistently and reliably establish the diagnosis although the following investigations may provide supportive evidence of a positive diagnosis of Sjögren's syndrome: • salivary flow rate (stimulated parotid flow rate normally >1.5 ml/min) • Schirmer test – assesses lacrimal flow (positive if ≤5 mm wetting in 5 min) • immunological investigations – rheumatoid factor, antinuclear factor, anti-Ro (SS-A) and anti-La (SS-B) • sialography – variable degrees of sialectasis are found in patients with Sjögren's, although this abnormality is not specific • scintigraphy – both uptake and excretion of the radioactive isotope sodium pertechnetate is diminished • labial gland biopsy - histological features which support the diagnosis include focal lymphocytic sialadenitis, duct dilation, acinar loss and periductal fibrosis. American–European diagnostic criteria are summarized in Table 15.14.

Treatment Treatment is largely non-specific and simply aimed at controlling symptoms. Maintain adequate hydration. Salivary substitutes (e.g. Oralbalance gel, Saliva Orthana and Glandosane). Salivary stimulants: chewing gum, glycerine and lemon (but avoid in dentate patients due to low pH). Pilocarpine acts as a systemic salivary stimulant and may prove useful, although clearly patients must have some residual functional salivary gland tissue. Preventive dental care – fluoride rinses and avoidance of sugary foodstuffs. Denture hygiene measures because of increased risk of candidosis. Treat acute episodes of bacterial sialadenitis with appropriate antibiotics. Long-term follow-up indicated in view of increased incidence of lymphoma, which may present as persistent salivary gland swelling.

SALIVARY GLAND NEOPLASMS

Relatively uncommon – constitute only 3% of all tumours. Approximately 80% occur in the major glands, 20% in minor glands. Overall, while only a minority of tumours occur in minor glands there is a greater proportion of malignant tumours in minor glands than in major glands. While tumours of the submandibular, sublingual and minor glands are less common than parotid tumours, there is an increased risk of malignancy at these sites. Table 15.15 gives the classification of salivary gland tumours.

TABLE 15.14 American–European classification criteria for Sjögren's syndrome

I Ocular symptoms – a positive response to at least one of the following questions:
- Have you had daily, persistent, troublesome dry eyes for at least 3 months?
- Do you have a recurrent sensation of sand or gravel in the eyes?
- Do you use tear substitutes more than three times a day?

II Oral symptoms – a positive response to at least one of the following questions:
- Have you had a daily feeling of a dry mouth for more than 3 months?
- Have you had recurrently or persistently swollen salivary glands as an adult?
- Do you frequently drink liquids to aid swallowing dry food?

III Ocular signs – objective evidence of ocular involvement defined as positive result in at least one of the following two tests:
- Schirmer test (≤5 mm in 5 min)
- Rose Bengal score ≥4 (van Bijsterveld's scoring system)

IV Histopathology – a focus score of >1 on labial gland biopsy
A focus is defined as an agglomerate of at least 50 mononuclear cells; the focus score is defined by the number of foci in 4 mm^2 of glandular tissue

V Salivary gland involvement – objective evidence of salivary gland involvement, defined as a positive result in at least one of the following investigations:
- Unstimulated salivary flow (<1.5 ml in 15 min)
- Salivary gland scintigraphy demonstrating reduced uptake and/or excretion
- Sialography demonstrating sialectasis

VI Autoantibodies – the following autoantibodies present in serum: Antibodies to Ro (SS-A) and/or La (SS-B) antigens

In patients without any potential associated connective tissue disorder the presence of any four of the above six items is indicative of primary Sjögren's syndrome.
In patients with a connective tissue disorder, item I or item II together with two other items from III, IV and V is indicative of secondary Sjögren's syndrome.

Pleomorphic adenoma

Most common salivary gland tumour (60% of all parotid tumours and 45% of all minor gland tumours); 90% occur in the parotid, with the tail of the parotid being the favoured site. Most patients in fifth and sixth decades. Slightly more common among females. Painless, slow-growing rubbery mass. As the name implies there is considerable variation in histological features, with intermingled

TABLE 15.15 Classification of salivary gland tumours	
Benign	*Malignant*
Pleomorphic adenoma	Mucoepidermoid carcinoma
Monomorphic adenomas:	Acinic cell carcinoma
• adenolymphoma	Adenoid cystic carcinoma
• oxyphilic	Polymorphous low-grade adenocarcinoma
• basal cell	Carcinoma arising in pleomorphic
• tubular	adenoma
• clear cell	
• trabecular, etc.	

epithelial elements and mesenchymal tissue. Connective tissue capsule is poorly developed in some areas with outgrowths of the main tumour mass extending beyond the capsule.

Monomorphic adenomas
Various subtypes according to histological pattern. Less common than pleomorphic adenomas (20% of all parotid tumours, 10% of minor gland tumours).

Adenolymphoma
Most common of the monomorphic adenomas. Most patients >50 years; male : female, 1.5 : 1. Vast majority occur in the parotid. Bilateral in up to 10% of cases. Painless, firm to palpate. Clinically indistinguishable from other benign parotid tumours. Well-encapsulated, papillary cystic structure with two histological components, namely epithelial and lymphoid tissue.

Mucoepidermoid carcinoma
Accounts for 5% of all salivary neoplasms. Occurs mainly in parotid. Peak incidence fourth and fifth decades. More common in females. Variable grades of malignancy, which influences rate of growth. *Low-grade tumours* usually present as painless, slowly enlarging lesions not unlike a pleomorphic adenoma. *Tumours of high-grade malignancy* grow rapidly and local pain may be an early feature. Facial nerve paralysis may also occur. Lymph node and distant metastases common. Prognosis influenced by grade of tumour.

Acinic cell carcinoma
Uncommon tumour arising mainly in parotid. Clinical presentation is similar to that of a pleomorphic adenoma. Behaviour unpredictable.

Adenoid cystic carcinoma

Usually affects middle-aged and elderly; accounts for 15% of minor gland tumours, 2–3% of parotid tumours. Slow-growing tumour which may initially be clinically indistinguishable from a pleomorphic adenoma. Local pain, ulceration of overlying mucosa, fixation to deeper structures and facial nerve palsy (in case of parotid tumour) may be features. Widely infiltrative with perineural spread. Cribriform or 'Swiss cheese' pattern.

Carcinoma arising in pleomorphic adenoma

Most arise in parotid tumours that have been present for 10–15 years. Characteristic sudden increase in rate of growth.

SALIVARY MUCOCELES

Two types:

Mucous extravasation cysts Account for 90% of cases and occur as a result of extravasation of mucus from a damaged minor gland duct.

Mucous retention cysts Less common and due to retention of mucus within a salivary gland or duct.

Clinical features Most cases arise in the lower lip, although less commonly may affect buccal mucosa, floor of mouth and tongue. Extremely uncommon in upper lip. Painless, bluish translucent, fluctuant submucosal swelling. Readily ruptured to release viscous mucus. Recurrence common.

Treatment If symptomatic – excision with underlying minor gland.

BACTERIAL SIALADENITIS

Usually occurs in association with local (e.g. calculus, mucus plug or duct stricture) or systemic causes of reduced salivary flow (e.g. diabetes mellitus, Sjögren's syndrome or following radiotherapy). Previously a relatively common postoperative complication due to dehydration, although this is now rare. Ascending infection from oral flora. The main organisms involved are *Staphylococcus aureus*, α-haemolytic streptococci, *Streptococcus viridans* and anaerobes.

Clinical features Pain and swelling of the affected gland. Associated pyrexia, malaise, cervical lymphadenopathy and occasional erythema of the overlying skin. Pus may be expressed from the involved gland duct orifice.

Investigation and diagnosis Pus for culture and sensitivity.

Treatment Antibiotics (flucloxacillin is the drug of choice, or erythromycin if the patient has an allergy to penicillin). Encourage drainage by use of sialogogues. General supportive measures such as ensuring adequate fluid intake and analgesia. After acute infection has resolved, sialography should be performed to exclude predisposing factors such as calculi, mucus plugs or duct strictures.

MUMPS

Common viral infection caused by a paramyxovirus which predominantly affects children. Transmitted by droplet spread. Incubation period of 14–21 days.

Clinical features Prodromal fever, malaise, trismus and sore throat followed by acute, tender, usually bilateral, swelling of the parotid glands. In a minority of cases the submandibular glands may be involved. Usually self-limiting and resolves within a week although, rarely, complications such as pancreatitis, encephalitis, orchitis or oophoritis may develop.

Investigation and diagnosis Usually based on characteristic history and clinical features. Diagnosis can be confirmed by serology (elevated IgM to 'S' and 'V' antigens).

Treatment Bed rest, analgesia, antipyretic and adequate fluid intake.

SIALOSIS (SIALADENOSIS)

Uncommon benign, non-inflammatory, non-neoplastic swelling of major salivary glands, most commonly affecting parotid glands although may also affect submandibular glands. Generally idiopathic although recognized associations include the following: • drug-induced (e.g. isoprenaline, phenylbutazone and antithyroid agents) • diabetes mellitus • thyroid disease • pregnancy • malnutrition • anorexia and bulimia nervosa • cirrhosis and liver disease.

Clinical features Usually soft, non-tender bilateral swelling of the parotid glands.

Histological features Include serous acinar hypertrophy, oedema of the interstitial stroma and striated duct atrophy.

Management Identify and correct predisposing factors if possible.

EFFECTS OF DRUGS ON THE TEETH, ORAL MUCOSA AND SALIVARY GLANDS

Discoloration of teeth • chlorhexidine • tetracycline • iron.

Oral candidosis • broad-spectrum antibiotics • corticosteroids (systemic and topical) • cytotoxic drugs.

Oral ulceration • aspirin applied topically • penicillamine • nicorandil.

Gingival hyperplasia • phenytoin • calcium channel blockers (e.g. nifedipine, diltiazem) • ciclosporin.

Erythema multiforme • sulphonamides • barbiturates • penicillin • carbamazepine.

Lichenoid reactions • oral hypoglycaemic agents • non-steroidal anti-inflammatory agents • beta-blockers • diuretics • allopurinol • methyldopa.

Mucosal pigmentation • antimalarials (e.g. mepacrine, chloroquine) • phenothiazines • oral contraceptives.

Xerostomia • antihistamines • tricyclic antidepressants • monoamine oxidase inhibitors • diuretics • anticholinergic agents (e.g. atropine-like drugs) • anti-Parkinsonian agents (e.g. benzhexol, benzatropine).

Salivary gland pain and swelling • phenothiazines • antithyroid drugs • insulin.

DISORDERS OF THE TEMPOROMANDIBULAR JOINT

See also craniomandibular disorders (p. 327).

Common disorders of the TMJ

• Myofascial pain dysfunction syndrome • internal joint derangement • degenerative disorders, e.g. osteoarthrosis • trauma.

Rare disorders of the TMJ

• Inflammatory – infection, rheumatoid arthritis, psoriatic arthropathy • ankylosis • congenital problems • neoplasms.

> ⚠ Craniomandibular disorders are complex from a diagnostic and management viewpoint. For this reason, patients are probably best treated in a combined clinic where experts in oral medicine and surgery, restorative dentistry and pain management formulate a common approach to patient management.

MYOFASCIAL PAIN DYSFUNCTION SYNDROME

Very common problem. Multiplicity of synonymous terms: • TMJ pain dysfunction syndrome • craniomandibular dysfunction • facial arthromyalgia • mandibular stress syndrome • mandibular dysfunction.

Widely considered to be more common in females, although this is a misconception and is a simple reflection of more females seeking treatment. Epidemiological studies suggest that there is equal prevalence in males and females.

Symptoms Dull intermittent or continuous ache, localized to muscle area. Pain may increase in severity with function. Headache is often an associated feature.

Signs Tenderness on palpation over muscles, which may elicit patient's symptoms. May be limitation of mandibular movement. Possible evidence of clenching or grinding habit (wear facets).

Treatment options • explanation and reassurance • physiotherapy (e.g. short-wave diathermy, ultrasound) • occlusal splint therapy (wide variety of splints suggested) • pharmacotherapy (NSAIDs and/or tricyclic antidepressant).

ANTERIOR DISC DISPLACEMENT WITH REDUCTION

Symptoms Joint noises. The presence of pain around the joint is a variable feature.

Signs Click on opening and closing (reciprocal click). Full range of movement.

Treatment Normally no treatment other than reassurance required.

ACUTE ANTERIOR DISC DISPLACEMENT WITHOUT REDUCTION

Symptoms Acute onset of limitation of opening. Previous history of opening click that suddenly resolved. Pain on opening is a variable feature.

Signs Opening less than 35 mm. Contralateral excursion of the mandible less than 7 mm. Unassisted opening within 4 mm of assisted opening. Deviation to affected side on opening.

CHRONIC ANTERIOR DISC DISPLACEMENT WITHOUT REDUCTION

Symptoms Significant limitation of opening for a variable period. Previous history of joint click.

Signs Opening >35 mm. Assisted opening >5 mm more than unassisted opening.

Treatment Occlusal splint therapy, muscle relaxant (e.g. dosulepin), arthroscopy, surgery.

OSTEOARTHROSIS

TMJ may be affected in up to one-third of cases. Characterized by crepitus and pain localized to the preauricular area with no radiation. Limitation of movement which becomes more apparent with function. Changes in the condylar head are apparent radiographically. Treatment is not usually surgical but aimed at symptomatic relief (e.g. NSAIDs and intra-articular steroid injections).

RHEUMATOID ARTHRITIS

Approximately 70% of patients with rheumatoid arthritis have clinical and/or radiographic evidence of TMJ involvement, although this is rarely symptomatic. Other causes of arthrosis are psoriasis, gout and ankylosing spondylitis. Treatment is as for osteoarthrosis and physiotherapy may be of benefit.

FACIAL PAIN

ORAL DYSAESTHESIA ('BURNING MOUTH SYNDROME')

> Burning sensation or other abnormal sensation affecting the oral soft tissues in the absence of clinically evident mucosal disease.

More commonly affects females (F : M, 7 : 1). Classified into three broad types according to temporal pattern of symptoms:

Type 1 Asymptomatic on waking; symptoms increase in severity during the day. Associated with a good prognosis.

Type 2 Symptoms present on waking and continue throughout the day. Often associated with significant anxiety or depressive element. Prognosis poorer than Type 1.

Type 3 Intermittent symptoms and often involves unusual sites, e.g. floor of mouth. May be associated with aetiological factors such as allergy.

Aetiological factors in oral dysaesthesia are described in Table 15.16.

Investigation Haematological investigations (FBC, assays of ferritin, folate and vitamin B_{12}) to exclude nutritional deficiency. Random blood glucose to exclude diabetes. (In known diabetics glycosylated haemoglobin can be used as an assessment of glycaemic control.) Microbiology for *Candida*. Prosthodontic assessment. Evaluation of psychological status (anxiety and depression). If an allergic component is suspected, arrange patch testing although this is an uncommon cause.

TABLE 15.16 Aetiological factors in oral dysaesthesia ('burning mouth syndrome')	
Nutritional deficiencies	Iron, folate and vitamin B_{12} Vitamins B_1 and B_6
Undiagnosed or poorly controlled diabetes mellitus	
Denture factors	Inadequate tongue space Unstable dentures Inadequate freeway space Hypersensitivity to acrylic monomer
Mucosal infections	Candidosis and candidal carriage
Xerostomia	
Parafunctional activity	Tongue thrusting Clenching Bruxism
Psychological factors	Anxiety Depression Cancer phobia
Drugs	Captopril
Allergy	Denture base materials Food additives

Treatment Reassure patient regarding the benign nature of the problem. Correct underlying organic predisposing factors. If symptoms persist following correction of above and a psychogenic element is suspected, antidepressant drug therapy is often helpful in controlling symptoms. In such cases a tricyclic antidepressant (e.g. amitriptyline or dosulepin) is the drug of choice although selective serotonin reuptake inhibitors (e.g. fluoxetine or venlafaxine) may be of value.

ATYPICAL FACIAL PAIN (PERSISTENT IDIOPATHIC FACIAL PAIN)

Essentially a diagnosis of exclusion.

International Headache Society Diagnostic criteria:

- pain in the face, present daily and persisting for all or most of the day
- pain confined at the outset to one side of the face; deep and poorly localized
- pain not associated with sensory loss or other physical signs
- pain investigations including radiography do not identify any relevant abnormality.

While the pain is generally not sufficiently severe to disturb sleep, patients may report early morning wakening as part of a depressive element. Atypical odontalgia is considered to be a variant of atypical facial pain. Predominantly affects females in the fourth or fifth decade of life.

Clinical features No organic cause to explain pain. High incidence of depression and anxiety.

Treatment Tricyclic antidepressant (e.g. dosulepin or amitriptyline) or selective serotonin reuptake inhibitor (e.g. fluoxetine or venlafaxine).

TRIGEMINAL NEURALGIA

A true neuralgia is characterized by severe paroxysmal pain lasting seconds in the distribution of one or more branches of the trigeminal nerve. Most commonly affects the maxillary or mandibular divisions with less than 5% cases affecting the ophthalmic division. Most patients are >50 years although it rarely occurs in younger age groups. Pain is often described as like an electric shock, lancinating, stabbing or piercing in nature. Some patients describe a trigger zone which may be either extraoral or intraoral. Thus patients may avoid washing or shaving a particular area on the face for fear of precipitating an attack of pain.

Clinical features Normal examination apart from possible presence of trigger area.

Investigation and diagnosis Exclude odontogenic source for pain. Response to carbamazepine is generally diagnostic. Presence of abnormal neurological signs should raise the suspicion that the pain is due to underlying CNS pathology. In young individuals it may be indicative of underlying systemic disease, e.g. multiple sclerosis or posterior cranial fossa tumour. Thus an MRI scan may be indicated in younger patients and in those who do not respond to medical therapy.

Treatment Treatment options are listed in Table 15.17.

GLOSSOPHARYNGEAL NEURALGIA

Uncommon condition characterized by severe lancinating pain in the distribution of glossopharyngeal nerve. Thus pain experienced in the base of the tongue and pillars of fauces. May be triggered by swallowing, coughing and chewing. Treatment based on principles similar to those for trigeminal neuralgia.

TABLE 15.17 Treatment options in trigeminal neuralgia	
Medical	*Surgical*
Carbamazepine	*Peripheral nerve procedures*
Phenytoin	Bupivacaine, alcohol or glycerol injections
Baclofen	Cryosurgery of peripheral nerve
Gabapentin	Neurectomy
Oxcarbazepine	
	Procedures involving trigeminal nerve ganglion
	Alcohol or glycerol injection
	Fogarty balloon compression
	Radiofrequency thermocoagulation
	Central procedures
	Microvascular decompression of main sensory root
	Rhizotomy

GIANT CELL ARTERITIS (TEMPORAL ARTERITIS)

Vascular pain syndrome which predominantly affects elderly patients and manifests as unilateral temporal and/or jaw pain, often reported as a burning sensation. May affect any artery in the head and neck, often the temporal and occipital branches of the external carotid. Involvement of retinal or ciliary vessels may cause blindness.

Clinical features Affected arteries may be thickened or tender and may show diminished pulsation. Claudication involving the muscles of mastication may also be a feature. May be associated fever, malaise, anorexia and weight loss. May be part of polymyalgia rheumatica.

Investigation and diagnosis Elevated ESR and C-reactive protein levels during acute phase. Normochromic, normocytic anaemia in 50% of cases. Temporal artery biopsy demonstrates infiltration of arterial wall with giant cells. The typical histological features do not affect the artery uniformly and therefore a negative result does not exclude the diagnosis. Early diagnosis and treatment is important in view of the potentially serious ophthalmic complications.

Treatment Systemic steroids without delay – high-dose prednisolone (60–80 mg daily).

PERIODIC MIGRAINOUS NEURALGIA (CLUSTER HEADACHE)

Characterized by severe unilateral pain predominantly affecting the orbital, supraorbital or temporal regions. Males more commonly affected. Pain occurs in discrete bouts, each typically lasting 30–90 minutes, and is often sufficiently severe to waken patient. Episodes often accompanied by rhinorrhoea, nasal congestion, lacrimation, facial sweating or conjunctival injection. Most patients appear agitated or restless during attacks. Some patients report that alcohol may be a precipitant. Episodes occur in bouts which can last for several days or weeks and then are followed by a variable period of remission.

Treatment Treatment can be considered under two headings: treatment of acute episode and prophylaxis.

Acute episode Sumatriptan, oxygen.
Prophylaxis Indometacin, beta-blockers, methysergide, calcium channel blockers, lithium.

ORAL MANIFESTATIONS OF SYSTEMIC DISEASE

ORAL MANIFESTATIONS OF SKIN DISEASE
Lichen planus and lichenoid reactions

Lichen planus is a common mucocutaneous disorder involving skin and/or oral mucosa, mainly affecting middle-aged and elderly females. Oral lesions are seen in about 50% of patients presenting with skin lesions while skin lesions are seen in only 10–30% of those presenting with oral manifestations. Skin lesions generally resolve within 18 months whereas oral mucosal lesions have a more chronic course, often persisting for several years. While most cases of oral lichen planus follow an entirely benign course, malignant transformation has been reported in a small proportion of cases and this appears to be more common in the atrophic and erosive types. Most studies quantify the risk of malignant transformation as approximately 1% over a 5–10 year period. (For aetiology, see Table 15.18.)

Clinical features Cutaneous lesions are characterized by itchy, violaceous, polygonal papular lesions with fine white streaks on the surface (*Wickham's striae*). The most common sites are the flexor aspect of the wrists, forearms and legs. Skin lesions may be induced by trauma (*Koebner phenomenon*). Nail involvement occurs in around 10% of cases and hair loss may also be a feature.

Lichenoid reactions have similar clinical features as lichen planus and in many cases it may be impossible to differentiate between the two lesions. Asymmetrical lesions, palatal involvement and recent drug therapy may be suggestive of a lichenoid reaction rather than lichen planus.

TABLE 15.18 Factors suggested as important in the aetiology of lichen planus

Exogenous factors	Systemic factors
Dental materials, e.g. amalgam, mercury, gold	Graft versus host disease
Food allergens	Nutritional deficiencies
Drugs e.g. diuretics, β-blockers, NSAIDs, oral hypoglycaemics	Diabetes mellitus
Infection	Liver disease
• Bacterial plaque	
• *Candida*	
Stress	
Tobacco	
Trauma	

Several patterns of oral lesions are recognized although different variants may coexist in the same patient:

Reticular Most common variant characterized by fine lace-like network of white striae; usually present bilaterally on the buccal mucosa and less commonly on the lateral margins of the tongue. Frequently asymptomatic.

Plaque Lesions resemble leukoplakia although a reticular pattern may often be observed at the periphery of the lesion.

Papular Relatively uncommon. Small white papules usually on the buccal mucosa.

Atrophic Diffuse erythematous areas, often with reticular lesions at edges.

Erosive or ulcerative Painful, irregular, persistent superficial erosions of variable size. Often coexists with non-erosive lesions.

Bullous Very rare variant.

Desquamative gingivitis A common variant affecting the gingivae.

Histological features • acanthotic or atrophic epithelium • liquefaction degeneration of the basal cell layer • inflammatory cell infiltrate in the deeper layers of the epithelium • dense subepithelial band of chronic inflammatory cells (predominantly T lymphocytes) with well-defined lower border.

Treatment Asymptomatic lesions require no active treatment. A wide variety of treatments have been advocated for management of symptomatic lesions although none is universally successful. Treatment options are listed in Table 15.19.

TABLE 15.19 Treatment options for symptomatic lichen planus

Antiseptic mouthwashes:
   chlorhexidine gluconate
   benzydamine hydrochloride (Difflam)
Corticosteroids:
   Topical:
      triamcinolone (Adcortyl in Orabase)
      betamethasone (Betnesol)
      beclometasone (Becotide)
   Intralesional:
      triamcinolone (Kenalog)
   Systemic:
      prednisolone
Azathioprine

Lupus erythematosus

Several different forms exist; on this basis it is classified into two main types: • systemic lupus erythematosus (SLE) • chronic discoid lupus erythematosus (CDLE).

Systemic lupus erythematosus (SLE)

An autoimmune disorder largely of unknown aetiology although a few cases may be drug induced (hydralazine, phenytoin). Females more commonly affected (F : M, 9 : 1). Characterized by the presence of non-organ-specific autoantibodies and widespread clinical manifestations which may involve virtually all tissues. Features typically include a photosensitive erythematous skin rash over the nose and malar eminences (butterfly pattern), arthritis and anaemia, although cardiac, respiratory, renal, hepatic, pancreatic and neurological manifestations may also occur. Thus the actual clinical presentation varies according to which organs are involved.

Oral lesions may be seen in up to one-third of patients and are similar to those of lichen planus with erythematous lesions and superficial erosions. Erosive oral lesions are often difficult to treat and may only respond to high-dose systemic steroids. Sjögren's syndrome may also be a complication of the disease.

Chronic discoid lupus erythematosus (CDLE)

Predominantly a mucocutaneous disorder with no systemic abnormalities. Similar butterfly rash to that seen in SLE. In addition ears, scalp and hands may be affected. Typical skin lesions consist of well-defined scaly erythematous macules which may heal by scarring and leave areas of hypopigmentation. Oral lesions occur in up to 50%. Buccal mucosa and vermillion border of the lip are common sites. Classically oral lesions consist of a central erythematous or erosive area with peripheral radiating white striae. Oral lesions generally respond to treatment with topical steroids.

Vesiculobullous disorders (p. 451)

ORAL MANIFESTATIONS OF GASTROINTESTINAL DISEASE

Crohn's disease

A chronic granulomatous disorder of unknown aetiology originally described as affecting the terminal ileum although it is now recognized that the disease can affect any part of the gastrointestinal tract from mouth to anus. General symptoms include abdominal pain, pyrexia, malaise, weight loss and disturbance of bowel habit with rectal bleeding. Extraintestinal manifestations (e.g. erythema nodosum, arthritis and uveitis) are also recognized. Oral lesions may predate the development of bowel symptoms or may be the only feature of the disorder.

Clinical features • recurrent aphthae • diffuse lip or cheek swelling • cobblestone appearance of buccal mucosa • mucosal tags • full-width gingivitis • granulomatous angular cheilitis • vertical fissures of the lips.

Orofacial granulomatosis (OFG)
Clinical and histological features identical to those of oral Crohn's disease and considered to be a diagnosis of exclusion (Crohn's disease, sarcoidosis). Increasing evidence to suggest that OFG is a hypersensitivity response to dietary and/or environmental allergens, particularly benzoic acid and cinnamon.

Ulcerative colitis
Chronic inflammatory disorder of unknown aetiology affecting the colon.

Clinical features Characterized by diarrhoea, passage of blood and mucus per rectum, weight loss and abdominal pain. Arthritis, uveitis and erythema nodosum may also be features of the disease.

Oral lesions may occur and include: • recurrent oral ulceration (secondary to nutritional deficiency or specific effect of underlying disease process) • pyostomatitis gangrenosum • pyostomatitis vegetans.

Treatment Specific treatment of the underlying intestinal disease often results in improvement in oral lesions.

Brown Kelly–Paterson syndrome (Plummer–Vinson syndrome)
Uncommon syndrome occurring principally in postmenopausal women. Components of the syndrome: • dysphagia due to postcricoid web, which is premalignant • iron deficiency anaemia with glossitis, koilonychia and angular cheilitis.

Gardner's syndrome
Autosomal dominant condition.

Hard tissue 'tumours' Bony exostoses, compound odontomes and/or supernumerary teeth.

Soft tissue 'tumours' Sebaceous cysts, subcutaneous fibromas, polyposis of the large intestine which almost invariably undergoes malignant change.

Peutz–Jeghers syndrome

Autosomal dominant condition. Mucocutaneous pigmentation; skin pigmentation may fade in adult life although mucosal pigmentation persists. Intestinal polyposis with very low malignant potential, which principally affects the small bowel.

ORAL MANIFESTATIONS OF NEUROLOGICAL DISEASE

Facial nerve palsy

The upper part of the face receives bilateral upper motor neurone innervation from both cerebral hemispheres whereas the lower part of the face receives upper motor neurone innervation only from the contralateral hemisphere. Thus an upper motor neurone lesion affects only the lower part of the face on the opposite side while a lower motor neurone lesion affects the whole of the face on the same side (see Table 15.20 for causes of sensory loss).

Upper motor neurone lesions • cerebrovascular accident • multiple sclerosis.

Lower motor neurone lesions • Bell's palsy • trauma • cerebellopontine angle tumours • malignant parotid gland tumour • otitis media • sarcoidosis.

Bell's palsy

Acute onset over several hours. Some patients report pain 1 or 2 days before onset of facial paralysis. Most patients recover spontaneously over a period of several weeks. Protect cornea while

---

TABLE 15.20 Causes of trigeminal nerve sensory loss

Intracranial	Extracranial
Multiple sclerosis	Trauma to peripheral branches of
Connective tissue diseases	trigeminal nerve
Cerebral tumours	Osteomyelitis
Cerebrovascular diseases	Neoplasia
Benign trigeminal neuropathy	Carcinoma of nasopharanx
Paget's disease	Carcinoma of the maxillary antrum
Sarcoidosis	Leukaemic deposits

palsy is present. If patient seen within 5 days of onset, systemic steroids may reduce the likelihood of incomplete recovery – prednisolone 80 mg daily for 5 days and tail-off dose over the next 5 days. Recent evidence implicates herpes simplex in many cases and therefore treatment with high-dose aciclovir orally may also be indicated.

ORAL MANIFESTATIONS OF HAEMATOLOGICAL DISEASE
Anaemia

> Reduction in the concentration of haemoglobin below the normal level considering age and gender of the patient.

Oral features include: • recurrent oral ulceration • atrophic glossitis • angular cheilitis • candidosis • oral dysaesthesia • Brown Kelly–Paterson syndrome.

Leukaemias

> Neoplastic proliferation of white cell precursors which may occur in either acute or chronic forms.

Cells affected include lymphocytes, monocytes or granulocytes. In general oral lesions in acute leukaemia are more common and more severe than those seen in association with chronic leukaemias.
Oral problems include: • bleeding and petechial haemorrhage • mucosal pallor • increased predisposition to infections (e.g. candidosis, herpes) • ulceration • gingival swelling.

Myeloma
Disseminated malignant neoplasm of plasma cells. Principally affects middle aged and elderly with slight male predominance. Multiple discrete osteolytic lesions in the skull and, less commonly, jaws. Macroglossia due to infiltration with amyloid.

Leucopenia
Reduced numbers of total circulating white blood cells ($<4 \times 10^9$/l). Possible causes include leukaemia, aplastic anaemia, drug-induced, autoimmune disease, HIV infection. Oral lesions include increased

susceptibility to infection, mucosal ulceration and exacerbation of periodontal disease.

Cyclic neutropenia

Rare form of leucopenia characterized by reduction in neutrophil count in 3–4-week cycles. Oral problems are as above.

HIV INFECTION AND ACQUIRED IMMUNE DEFICIENCY SYNDROME (AIDS)

Oral lesions occur commonly in HIV-seropositive patients. In general they are not specific to HIV infection and simply reflect the immunocompromised state. Thus many of the oral lesions occur in patients who are immunosuppressed for other reasons. The prevalence of oral lesions among HIV-seropositive patients is dramatically reduced by highly active anti-retroviral therapy (HAART).

The current classification of these lesions is based on the strength of association with HIV infection (Table 15.21). Three groups are recognized:

Group I Lesions strongly associated with HIV infection
Group II Lesions less commonly associated with HIV
Group III Lesions seen in HIV infection.

Erythematous and pseudomembranous candidosis

Most common oral fungal infections seen in association with HIV infection. Various studies report the frequency of oral candidosis as ranging from 7 to 93%. Erythematous candidosis generally occurs early in the disease process whereas pseudomembranous candidosis is a later manifestation, occurring when the patient is severely immunosuppressed. Both forms are highly predictive of the development of AIDS. Clinical features of fungal infections (p. 442).

Hairy leukoplakia

Usually asymptomatic. Characterized by bilateral vertically corrugated white patches on the lateral margins of the tongue. May affect the ventral surface, where it assumes a more homogenous appearance. Rarely may involve other parts of the oral mucosa (buccal mucosa and palate) although when it affects these unusual sites it is also always present on the lateral margin of the tongue. Originally considered to be pathognomonic of HIV infection, although as the lesion has been described in other

TABLE 15.21   Lesions associated with HIV infection
Group I: lesions strongly associated with HIV infection
Candidosis:
erythematous
pseudomembranous
angular cheilitis
median rhomboid glossitis
Hairy leukoplakia
Kaposi's sarcoma
Non-Hodgkin's lymphoma
Periodontal diseases:
linear gingival erythema
acute necrotizing ulcerative gingivitis
acute necrotizing ulcerative periodontitis
Group II: lesions less commonly associated with HIV infection
Atypical ulceration
HIV-associated salivary gland disease (HIV-SGD):
Xerostomia and/or swelling of the major salivary glands
Necrotizing ulcerative stomatitis
Thrombocytopenic purpura
Viral infections:
Cytomegalovirus
Herpes simplex virus
Human papillomavirus
Varicella zoster
Group III: lesions seen in HIV infection
Bacterial infections
Drug reactions
Fungal infections
Neurological disturbances:
Facial nerve palsy
Trigeminal neuropathy

immunosuppressed patient groups (e.g. organ transplant recipients, patients receiving chemotherapy for acute leukaemia) it is now simply regarded as a marker of underlying immunodeficiency. Characteristic histological features; believed to represent an opportunistic infection of the oral mucosa by EBV. Definitive diagnosis is by detecting presence of EBV within the lesional tissue by in-situ hybridization. May respond to treatment with aciclovir although when treatment is discontinued the lesion inevitably recurs. Marker of poor prognosis in HIV-infected patients.

Kaposi's sarcoma

Before the advent of AIDS and HIV infection Kaposi's sarcoma (KS) was seen mainly among elderly Jewish males of eastern European or Mediterranean descent, and an endemic form was recognized in southern Africa. AIDS-associated KS is seen almost exclusively in male homosexuals and is rare among other risk categories for HIV infection. Presents as red or purple maculopapular lesions. Approximately 50% occur intra- or periorally with the most common site in the mouth being the junction of hard and soft palate. Caused by infection with human herpes virus 8 (HHV8). KS is usually very responsive to radiotherapy. Alternative treatments include chemotherapy (systemic and intralesional), surgical excision, laser excision and cryosurgery.

Non-Hodgkin's lymphoma
Uncommon but well-recognized complication of HIV infection. Typically presents as a rapidly enlarging, firm, rubbery swelling. Common intraoral sites include fauces, palate and gingivae. Lesions can ulcerate and may be associated with destruction of tooth support. Treatment is generally with radiotherapy and/or chemotherapy.

Linear gingival erythema
Characterized by an intense linear band of erythema along the gingival margin, which may also extend onto the attached gingivae. Severity of inflammation is out of proportion to the state of oral hygiene. Spontaneous gingival bleeding may also be a feature.

Acute necrotizing ulcerative gingivitis
Characterized by gingival pain, bleeding on probing or spontaneous bleeding and interdental ulceration with craterlike defects.

Acute necrotizing periodontitis
Rapid localized or generalized periodontal destruction with severe pain, bone loss, tooth mobility and periodontal pocketing.

HIV salivary gland disease
More common in HIV-infected children than adults. Characterized by xerostomia and/or swelling of the major salivary glands. Clinical

parallels with Sjögren's syndrome although characteristic autoantibody profile is lacking. Histological features similar to Sjögren's syndrome.

HALITOSIS (ORAL MALODOUR)

Relatively common complaint with a wide variety of possible causes summarized in Table 15.22. Where sepsis is responsible the organisms are usually anaerobic. In some patients there is no objective evidence of malodour and the patient's perception of halitosis may be a manifestation of an underlying psychogenic problem.

Diagnosis Largely clinical based on history and examination. Overall assessment of the halitosis can be undertaken by simply smelling the exhaled breath or objective measurement of volatile sulphur compounds (e.g. hydrogen sulphide and methyl mercaptan) using a halimeter.

Treatment • Treat underlying cause where possible. • Avoid smoking and pungent foodstuffs. • Antiseptic mouthwashes.

Table 15.22 Causes of halitosis (oral malodour)

Xerostomia
Periodontal disease
Oropharyngeal sepsis
Nasal sepsis (e.g. sinusitis or foreign body)
Smoking
Various foodstuffs (e.g. garlic, onions)
Drugs
Systemic disease (diabetes, respiratory tract infection, renal failure, hepatic failure)
Psychogenic

CHAPTER 16

GENERAL MEDICINE OF RELEVANCE TO DENTISTRY

Introduction 490

History taking 490

Cardiovascular system 491

Respiratory system 493

Gastrointestinal (GI) system 494

Haematological system 498

Renal disease 503

Endocrine disorders 505

Locomotor system disease 509

Neurological disorders 513

Psychiatric disorders 516

Dermatology 517

Immune system disorders 518

References 519

Further reading 519

INTRODUCTION

This is an exciting time for dentistry with the medical–dental interface assuming increasing importance. There are more people taking more prescribed drugs, people with chronic diseases are living longer, and understanding of the oral manifestations of systemic diseases is increasing. Indeed, it has been suggested that oral diseases may impact on systemic conditions (e.g. periodontitis and cardiovascular disease). All of these factors make the dental team's input to the wider healthcare team a vital one. Thus it is imperative that dentists and DCPs should keep up to date with their understanding of medicine and related issues.

HISTORY TAKING

The art of history taking is central to good medical and dental practice (see Chapter 2). The goal is to obtain appropriate information from the patient to facilitate any physical examination and to arrive at a diagnosis. Within this, past medical and drug history and systemic inquiry are essential elements. Past medical history should cover the following: • hospital admissions and operative procedures (including anaesthetic reactions) • allergies • medications taken currently and in the past • illnesses (including arthritis, heart failure, hypertension, asthma, bleeding disorders, myocardial infarction, angina, pacemakers, rheumatic fever, stroke, epilepsy, diabetes mellitus, renal disease, hepatic disease [esp. hepatitis]) • human immunodeficiency virus (HIV) exposure.

When patients use technical terms to describe their illnesses or diagnoses, it is incumbent upon the dentist to clarify the meaning of such terms with the patient. Make no assumptions! Systematic review is essential if important aspects of medical care are not to be overlooked. Patients often have weird and wonderful ideas about what facts are important, and so specific questioning is essential. Shorter inquiries may be appropriate depending on the patient and circumstances, but a full review should include the following:

General Weight loss or gain, anorexia, energy level, fevers and night sweats.
Dermatological Hair or nail changes, scaling, dryness, pigmentation, jaundice, pruritus (itching), lesions ± biopsy.
Haematological Bruising, bleeding, nodes, lumps, anaemia.
Endocrine Goitre, hot/cold intolerance, voice changes, hair pattern, polydipsia (increased thirst), polyuria (increased production of urine), development of breasts and sexual characteristics.

Neurological Headache, fainting, nausea, vomiting, vertigo, dizziness, pains at any body site, loss of smell, taste, or vision, muscle weakness or wasting, paraesthesia (change in sensation) or anaesthesia (loss of sensation), loss of coordination, tremors, seizures, spectacles, diplopia ('double vision'), blind spots, tunnel vision, pain, swelling, redness or dryness of the eyes, decreased hearing, tinnitus (ringing in the ears).

Respiratory Epistaxis (bleeding from the nose), rhinorrhoea (mucoid discharge from the nose), cough, sputum production, dyspnoea (breathlessness), wheezing, cyanosis, pleuritic pain.

Cardiovascular Palpitations, chest pain ± radiations, number of pillows used, hypertension, cyanosis (blue coloration), haemoptysis (coughing up blood), oedema, varicose veins and phlebitis, congenital or acquired cardiac anomalies, murmurs, exercise tolerance, claudication.

Gastrointestinal Appetite, food intolerance, flatus and flatulence, indigestion, abdominal pain ± radiations, nausea, vomiting, haematemesis (vomiting blood), constipation or diarrhoea, stool colour, consistency and quality, steatorrhoea, mucus, haemorrhoids, hepatitis and jaundice, alcohol abuse, ascites, oral mucosal and dental problems.

Genitourinary Urinary frequency, hesitancy, changes in stream, difficulties starting or stopping stream, dysuria, haematuria, urinary tract infections, impotence, sexually transmitted diseases.

Obstetrics/gynaecology Parity and complications of pregnancy, abortions or miscarriages, menstrual history, premenstrual syndrome (PMS), dysmenorrhoea, menorrhagia, date of last menstrual period, menopause, postmenopausal bleeding.

Musculoskeletal Fractures, arthritis, joint pain and swelling, muscle pain and weakness, limitation of movement and deformity.

Psychiatric Mood and appearance, anxiety, depression and personality disorders, insomnia, early morning wakening, hallucinations, delusions.

CARDIOVASCULAR SYSTEM

Ischaemic heart disease

Particularly common in the UK (affects 1 in 6 men aged 40–44 years; 1 in 3 men aged 55–59 years). Due to gradual reduction in the lumen diameter of the coronary arteries by atheroma. This results in a decrease in oxygenation of parts of the heart muscle, especially when the heart is undergoing increased demands of exercise, and leads to the classical pain of angina pectoris. Risk factors include raised serum cholesterol, raised blood pressure and cigarette smoking. Patients with unstable angina should be managed as inpatients. Patients with stable angina may have an attack precipitated by the fear of dental treatment. Their anti-angina medication (e.g. glyceryl trinitrate spray/tablet) should be readily available. Epinephrine-containing local anaesthetic agents are *not* contraindicated when proper injection technique is adhered to.

Cardiac failure
The end-point of many cardiovascular diseases is characterized by peripheral oedema, venous congestion and breathlessness.

Hypertension
In excess of 20% of the adult population is estimated to have hypertension (i.e. BP >140/90 mmHg). Prevalence increases with increasing age. Risk factors include: age, ethnic origin, obesity, inactivity, family history. More than 80% of cases are idiopathic or 'essential'; the remainder secondary to other diseases, e.g. renal. Several drugs used in the treatment of hypertension (e.g. thiazide diuretics, calcium channel blockers and angiotensin-converting enzyme [ACE] inhibitors). Diuretics can cause lichenoid reactions of the oral mucosa (see p. 478), calcium channel blockers can cause gingival hyperplasia and ACE inhibitors may cause a stomatitis.

Cardiac murmurs
Prophylaxis of infective endocarditis in congenital and acquired heart valve disease and previous cases of rheumatic fever is clearly of significance in dental practice. The current recommendations for antibiotic prophylaxis are described on page 72. However, many cardiologists are now taking a more liberal approach to the necessity for prophylaxis and it is important that all patients with such a history are assessed by a cardiologist, using modern cardiac imaging techniques, to determine current treatment need.

> Patients with a history of cardiac murmur or endocarditis requiring antibiotic prophylaxis for dental treatment should be referred to a cardiologist for assessment using modern imaging techniques.

RESPIRATORY SYSTEM

Asthma

Bronchial hyper-reactivity may be worsened by anxiety or nervousness and so dental patients should always bring their inhalers when they attend for treatment. This will normally be salbutamol which acts acutely to relieve wheezing. Patients may additionally use steroid inhalers which only cause adrenal suppression (albeit mild) in high doses over long periods. Drug reactions are more common in asthmatics, and non-steroidal anti-inflammatory drugs (NSAIDs) should be avoided.

Inhaled and systemic steroid use may predispose to oral candidosis (see p. 442). Patients should be encouraged to rinse out with tap water after using their steroid inhaler to minimize the amount of residual steroid in the oral cavity.

Infection and chronic obstructive pulmonary disease (COPD)

Respiratory infections may complicate the care of patients with any pre-existing respiratory disease, but particularly COPD. Most are now treated acutely with antibiotics rather than by long-term prophylactic antibiotics. Antibiotic therapy may be complicated by co-prescribing in dental practice, causing emergence of resistant organisms or reduced clinical response. Accordingly, patients should always be questioned closely about concomitant or recent antibiotic use.

The incidence of pulmonary tuberculosis is increasing again worldwide and multiple drug resistance is emerging.

Bronchial carcinoma

A common tumour in smokers. Bronchial carcinoma may rarely secrete adrenocorticotrophic hormone (ACTH) and be a cause of oral mucosal melanosis.

> ⚠ **Fifty per cent of regular long-term smokers will die early from a disease or diseases related to smoking. Dental team members will be involved increasingly in smoking cessation advice to patients. Patients should be asked their smoking status at the initial consultation and offered advice to stop, with the assistance of appropriate treatments. Such support and advice should be offered at regular opportunities thereafter (p. 163).**

Cystic fibrosis

An inherited condition seen in children with increased mucus viscosity and recurrent chest infections. Increasingly, children are surviving into adulthood.

Sarcoidosis

An idiopathic (possibly infective) cause of granulomatous inflammation, which may cause gingival enlargement, lip swelling, salivary gland enlargement and facial palsy.

GASTROINTESTINAL (GI) SYSTEM

Oral manifestations may be:

Primary A direct extension of the disease process into the mouth, e.g. lip swelling in Crohn's disease.

Secondary An indirect effect of the disease process, e.g. sialosis in anorexia nervosa.

Any GI disorder that may cause malabsorption (e.g. vitamin B_{12}, folic acid or iron) or chronic blood loss (with resultant loss of iron) may present with oral manifestations as a result of *haematinic deficiency*. The most common features are mucosal atrophy, oral ulceration and angular cheilitis. Most haematinic deficiencies are *latent*, i.e. not yet apparent as a reduction in the haemoglobin level. Assays of vitamin B_{12}, folic acid and ferritin (in addition to a full blood count) are therefore mandatory in investigating many oral mucosal diseases.

Dysphagia

Difficulty in swallowing is a relatively common complaint and should be treated seriously with appropriate referral. Causes include benign stricture, oesophageal carcinoma, achalasia, oesophageal spasm (with pain, which may mimic angina pectoris and be precipitated by anxiety), tonsillitis, pharyngeal pouch, bulbar or pseudobulbar palsy, and the psychiatric state of globus. The dental professional's responsibility lies in excluding oral causes such as stomatitis and oral cancer. Brown Kelly–Paterson (Plummer–Vinson) syndrome (iron deficiency anaemia, postcricoid webs and a premalignant condition for oesophageal carcinoma) may present with dysphagia and may also have oral manifestations due to the haematinic deficiency.

Dysphagia is an ominous symptom and patients reporting this should be referred for urgent assessment to exclude oesophageal cancer.

Gastro-oesophageal reflux disease (GORD)

May cause oesophagitis and heartburn (a dull retrosternal ache). Predisposing factors include hiatus hernia, pregnancy, obesity and smoking. Reflux may also be habitual, e.g. bulimia nervosa. Chronic acid reflux may cause oral problems including mucosal irritation (ranging from tongue coating to mucosal erythema and ulceration) and non-carious tooth surface loss (p. 280).

Gastric carcinoma

More common in certain population groups (e.g. Japanese) and patients with blood group A, atrophic gastritis, pernicious anaemia and previous gastric surgery. 10% have a family history. It should be excluded in patients with left supraclavicular lymphadenopathy (Virchow's node).

Gastritis and peptic ulceration (PU)

Gastritis is inflammation of the mucosa lining of the stomach. Three major causes are: infection with *Helicobacter pylori*, NSAID use and autoimmune conditions. Peptic ulceration is divided into two main groups – gastric (GU) and duodenal (DU). May be asymptomatic, mildly discomforting or cause severe abdominal pain. The advent of treatment to eradicate *H. pylori has* transformed the management of peptic ulcer disease. *H. pylori* may be screened for by serology (blood test), urea breath test and biopsy urease test (following endoscopic biopsy of the gastric mucosa).

NSAIDs should not be prescribed for dental pain in patients with peptic ulceration. Paracetamol (± codeine) may be prescribed safely. Also, two commonly prescribed antibiotics in dentistry (amoxicillin and metronidazole) may be used for the eradication of *H. pylori* and this may influence the choice of antibiotics for dental use in patients undergoing eradication therapy. Omeprazole (a proton pump inhibitor drug used to stop acid production) is a rare cause of stomatitis.

Coeliac disease

Characterized by diarrhoea, steatorrhoea, weight loss and failure to thrive – normally in children. It is caused by mucosal villous atrophy in the jejunum (with resultant failure to absorb folic acid) as a result of immunologically mediated injury (IgA formed to the alpha-gliaden component of gluten cross-reacts with the intestinal mucosa). Screening for coeliac disease is best carried out by serological assessment for tissue transglutaminase and/or anti-endomysium antibodies. Diagnosis is confirmed by a jejunal biopsy showing sub-total villous atrophy (STVA). An increased incidence of intestinal lymphoma is recognized. Symptoms and signs improve after gluten withdrawal from the diet.

Oral manifestations include oral ulceration (as a primary manifestation and also due to folic acid deficiency) and dermatitis herpetiformis (a vesiculobullous disorder caused by IgA deposition at the basement membrane zone of the oral mucosa; also occurs on the skin).

Irritable bowel syndrome

A common and complex GI disorder. Symptoms of altered bowel habit, abdominal pain and bloating are explained by disturbance of gastrointestinal motility. A diet deficient in fibre is important in the causation, and psychological factors are frequently evident. Patients with psychogenic orofacial pain disorders often include irritable bowel syndrome in their profile.

Crohn's disease

A chronic non-caseating granulomatous inflammation affecting any part of the GI tract. The terminal ileum and proximal colon are the most commonly affected sites. Oral manifestations are described on page 480. Folic acid and iron deficiency states may occur alone or in combination in Crohn's disease with resultant secondary manifestations. Systemic steroids are frequently employed in the management of Crohn's disease and so 'steroid cover' should be considered in these patients in the dental operative context (p. 507).

Ulcerative colitis

A chronic inflammatory disease of the colon. Chronic blood loss, causing iron deficiency, may lead to secondary oral manifestations such as recurrent aphthous stomatitis. Other oral manifestations include stomatitis gangrenosum and pyostomatitis vegetans. Occasionally, the TMJs may be involved in a seronegative arthritis; the eyes may manifest inflammatory changes as uveitis. Systemic steroids are frequently employed in the management of ulcerative colitis; therefore 'steroid cover' should be considered in the dental operative context (p. 507).

Colorectal cancer

A very common malignancy in the UK. It may manifest, prior to overt abdominal signs, as an iron deficiency state with resultant oral mucosal problems such as recurrent aphthous stomatitis.

When oral mucosal problems such as aphthae appear in middle-aged or elderly patients, *haematinic deficiencies* must be excluded. Where such a deficiency is identified, the underlying causative disease state *must* be diagnosed. The alert dental professional can play a significant role in identifying important systemic diseases at an early stage.

 Dental professionals are uniquely placed to identify the oral manifestations of systemic diseases – often by way of 'early warning'.

Antibiotic-associated pseudomembranous colitis

A recognized risk (albeit very small) every time an antibiotic is prescribed. The role of clindamycin has probably been overstated in the past and now cephalosporins are frequently implicated. Diarrhoea often complicates antibiotic prescribing but persistent symptoms with abdominal pain should be viewed with great suspicion and appropriate hospital referral instituted. The overgrowth of *Clostridium difficile* is treated with oral vancomycin for 7–10 days, accompanied by aggressive intravenous rehydration.

Hepatic disease

Clearly blood-borne viral infections are of great concern to the dental profession. Jaundice is the main sign of liver disease and is best seen as yellow discoloration of the sclerae. The skin and oral mucous membranes may also be involved.

Acute viral hepatitis may be caused by a large number of viruses including hepatitis A, B, C and D viruses and Epstein–Barr virus.

Chronic hepatitis is defined as inflammatory disease of the liver lasting longer than 6 months; causes include: • hepatitis B virus (HBV) infection • autoimmune chronic active hepatitis • chronic non-A, non-B hepatitis • alcohol abuse • drugs, e.g. isoniazid • metabolic, e.g. Wilson's disease.

Chronic liver disease is of dental relevance for the following reasons: • bleeding problems due to impaired synthesis of clotting factors • bleeding problems due to increased platelet consumption (hypersplenism) • possible transmission of blood-borne viruses • impaired metabolism/excretion of drugs (e.g. local anaesthetic agents) • dangers of surgery under general anaesthesia as some GA agents are contraindicated • dangers of surgery with resultant dehydration and hepatorenal syndrome • dangers of surgery with biochemical imbalance and induction of hepatic encephalopathy.

Preoperative assessment of patients with chronic liver disease is complex; even basic dentistry is probably best carried out in a specialist regional centre. Assessment includes: • knowledge of underlying diagnosis and ensuring strict cross-infection control • coagulation screen and full blood count (platelet numbers) • correction of coagulopathy as indicated with vitamin K injections or fresh frozen plasma infusion; platelet transfusion • early involvement of experienced anaesthetist since the proper choice of induction and anaesthetic agents is essential; forward planning of regimen for i.v. fluids and acid–base balance • knowledge of appropriate drug prescribing – e.g. paracetamol may be contraindicated; LA agents are liver metabolized; dose reduction of most drugs should be considered.

Consider additional local precautions for postoperative bleeding by way of sutures, packs, etc.

Pancreatic disease

Inflammation of the pancreas may be either acute or chronic.

Acute pancreatitis caused by gallstones, alcohol or other drugs. Carries an overall mortality of around 15% and complications include shock, adult respiratory distress syndrome (ARDS), disseminated intravascular coagulopathy (DIC), diabetes mellitus, renal failure and hepatic failure.

Chronic pancreatitis is of greater relevance to dentistry. The most common cause is alcohol abuse. Management involves adequate pain control (opiate dependency is well recognized), treatment of malabsorption with manipulation of diet to maintain calorie intake (with associated increased caries risk) whilst reducing fat and control of diabetes mellitus (p. 505).

HAEMATOLOGICAL SYSTEM

Anaemia

Anaemia is defined as a haemoglobin concentration less than the reference range for that age and gender of patient. The normal UK adult value is >12 g/dl (females) and >13 g/dl (males).

Causes • blood loss • reduction in, or impaired, red blood cell formation • haemolysis.

Types

Microcytic anaemia (MCV < 80 fl) (MCV = mean corpuscular volume, fl = femtolitres [10^{-15}].) Commonly iron deficiency (microcytic and hypochromic; low serum iron and high TIBC [total iron-binding capacity]) but also sideroblastic anaemia, thalassaemia, chronic disease. Causes of iron deficiency: inadequate diet, malabsorption, blood loss (menorrhagia, GI malignancy, ulceration, haemorrhoids, gastritis, inflammatory bowel disease, parasites), achlorhydria, pregnancy and growth spurts.

Normocytic anaemia (80 fl > MCV < 100 fl) Classically the anaemia of chronic disease (e.g. rheumatoid arthritis, infection, malignancy); also haemolytic and aplastic states; combined deficiencies (e.g. iron and folate).

Macrocytic anaemia (MCV > 100 fl) Causes of megaloblastic erythropoiesis: deficiencies of vitamin B_{12}, folate, pyridoxine, thiamine; preleukaemic states.

Causes of normoblastic erythropoiesis: alcoholism, aplastic anaemia, reticulocytosis, marrow infiltration or suppression, hypothyroidism, hypopituitarism, liver disease.

The dental importance of anaemias and haematinic deficiencies lies in the oral mucosal manifestations of these states, e.g. ulceration, glossitis, angular cheilitis. In addition, GA would be inappropriate for someone with significant anaemia – a good reason to perform a full blood count preoperatively.

Haemoglobinopathies

A group of diseases where the structure or production of haemoglobin has been altered in some way. The main types are:

Variation in Hb structure, e.g. HbS (sickle cell) and methaemoglobinaemia.
Defective synthesis of Hb, e.g. thalassaemias.
Persisting fetal haemoglobin HbF.

Sickle cell anaemia is a homozygous inherited disease, chiefly of black Africans, caused by a substituted amino acid residue (glutamine replaced by valine on the beta-globin chain) of the Hb molecule. This results in RBCs forming a 'sickle' shape when deoxygenated. The *heterozygous* sickle cell *trait* is usually asymptomatic and confers resistance to *falciparum* malaria. The major surgical problems are 'sickling' under GA with resultant vascular occlusions (e.g. brain and bone) and haemolytic anaemia. Preoperative investigations include a FBC (film shows sickle-shaped cells), Hb electrophoresis and the *Sickledex™ test* (RBCs sickle when mixed with sodium metabisulphite on a slide). Operative procedures require expert assessment.

Thalassaemias

Inherited disorders in which the rate of synthesis of one or more globin chains is reduced or absent with resultant haemolysis, ineffective erythropoiesis and anaemia. The beta chain is most commonly affected (beta-thalassaemia) and heterozygote and homozygote states exist. Populations from the Middle and Far East, Africa, Asia and the Mediterranean are chiefly affected. Heterozygote form (*minor*) is mild and largely asymptomatic; homozygote form (*major*) leads to severe anaemia, hypersplenism, bossing of the skull (due to expanded marrow cavity) and RBC dysplasia. Dental procedures require expert assessment.

Haematological malignancy

Includes leukaemias (which can present with infections of the head and neck, e.g. herpes; solitary deposits in soft tissues; gingival swellings), myeloproliferative disorders, multiple myeloma and lymphomas (which are subdivided into Hodgkin's and non-Hodgkin's types).

Dental considerations include: • anaemia • bleeding diathesis • head, neck and oral involvement.

Treatment normally involves *cytotoxic chemotherapy* with *radiotherapy* for solitary soft tissue masses, bone pain or total body irradiation (TBI) prior to bone marrow transplantation. Complications of treatment include: • the need for *urgent* dental assessment before therapy with removal of focal dental sepsis (grossly carious and periodontally involved teeth) • bleeding tendency • infection (which may be life-threatening and from an oral source) • immunosuppression (e.g. oropharyngeal candidosis and herpes) • mucositis (which is extremely painful and notoriously difficult to manage).

In the midst of chemotherapy, any emergency dental work should be performed only in consultation with the patient's haematologist and, normally, as an inpatient. Preoperative assessment will include FBC, coagulation screen and the maximization of antibiotic cover.

BLEEDING DISORDERS

Include blood vessel defects, platelet defects (qualitative and quantitative) and coagulation cascade defects (hereditary and acquired).

Blood vessel defects

Hereditary haemorrhagic telangiectasia Autosomal dominant transmission; multiple dilations of small vessels in skin, mucous membranes and other sites (e.g. brain, liver).

Vascular purpuras caused by • drugs (e.g. NSAIDs) • infections (e.g. meningococcus, infective endocarditis) • Henoch–Schönlein • metabolic (e.g. liver failure, uraemia) • scurvy (vitamin C deficiency).

Often, problems are only highlighted after surgery or routine dentistry when significant bruising and non-healing may occur. Such scenarios should be investigated promptly by a physician.

Platelet defects

Decreased platelet count:

Thrombocytopenia
Idiopathic
Secondary • decreased marrow production (marrow infiltration, alcoholism, viral) • decreased platelet survival (ITP, SLE, drugs, e.g. NSAIDs) • increased platelet consumption (DIC, haemolytic–uraemic syndrome, meningococcus) • platelet sequestration (hypersplenism, hypothermia) • platelet loss (haemorrhage).

Increased platelet count:

Thrombocythaemia May be primary (increased platelet production due to a myeloproliferative disorder) or secondary.

Other defects:

Thrombasthenia The platelets are normal in number but defective in function. May be primary (hereditary defects – very rare) or secondary (e.g. to aspirin therapy).

Platelet levels should be $>50–75 \times 10^9/l$ for planned surgery and deep block LA injections. Levels lower than this require platelet transfusion with i.v. antihistamine and hydrocortisone cover. Bleeding following emergency dental treatment should be treated seriously with admission of the patient for assessment of platelet levels and underlying factors. Haemostasis may be achieved with pressure packs, sutures and resorbable mesh placed within sockets.

Coagulation cascade defects

Hereditary • haemophilia A • haemophilia B • von Willebrand's disease.

Acquired • anticoagulant drugs • liver disease • vitamin K deficiency.

Haemophilia A (factor VIII deficiency) A sex-linked recessive disorder affecting males predominantly, but not exclusively. Childhood haemarthroses are the commonest presentation.

Factor VIII_c deficiency is classified as:

factor VIII_c levels	>25%	very mild
factor VIII_c levels	5–25%	mild
factor VIII_c levels	1–5%	moderate
factor VIII_c levels	<1%	severe

Bleeding from skin or mucosa appears to stop normally but bleeding recommences within an hour of trauma or surgery. Dental treatment should be coordinated by specialists in regional centres. Telephone advice to patients should be readily available and many will now have factor VIII concentrate at home for injection (by i.v. route, *never* by i.m. route to prevent muscle bleeds). Repeated administration is required as the half-life of factor VIII is only 8 hours. Desmopressin causes the release of factor VIII_c from storage sites on endothelium and is helpful before surgery; it is given by intranasal spray or by slow i.v. infusion. Oral antifibrinolytics (e.g. tranexamic acid) can reduce the need for administration of factor VIII. Blood-borne viral infections (HBV, HCV and HIV) are common in haemophiliacs, as is addiction to narcotic analgesic drugs.

Haemophilia B (factor IX deficiency; Christmas disease) A sex-linked recessive disorder, ten times less common than haemophilia A. Clinical features are similar to factor VIII deficiency and treatment is by factor IX replacement – prophylactically prior to dental treatment.

von Willebrand's disease An autosomal dominant disorder, affecting males and females. Factor VIII_c levels are low and two other factor VIII subunits (R:Ag – von Willebrand's factor, and R:RCo) are deficient. Bleeding time is also prolonged since factor $VIII_{R:Ag}$ is important for the normal adherence of platelets to vascular endothelium. von Willebrand's disease should be managed in a specialist regional centre because administration of fresh frozen plasma (FFP), cryoprecipitate (cryoPPT), factor VIII concentrate and desmopressin may be required.

Patients with *acquired coagulopathies* may be treated in general practice. With coumarin anticoagulation (warfarin) for prosthetic

TABLE 16.1 Target ranges for International Normalized Ratio (INR) values (UK)

Indication for warfarin	INR target	INR range
Pulmonary embolism	2.5	2.0–3.0
Deep venous thrombosis	2.5	2.0–3.0
Atrial fibrillation	2.5	2.0–3.0
Recurrence of embolism after warfarin stopped	2.5	2.0–3.0
Recurrence of embolism on warfarin	3.5	3.0–4.0
Mechanical prosthetic heart valves	3.5	3.0–4.0
Antiphospholipid syndrome	3.5	3.0–4.0

Source: *BNF.*

heart valves, deep vein thrombosis, etc., the INR (international normalized ratio) is the recognized measurement and is indicative of the patient's prothrombin time : control prothrombin time ratio. The target ranges for various conditions are given in Table 16.1. It is now generally considered unnecessary to alter a patient's INR value for routine dental treatment where the INR value is <4.0 (www.ukmi.nhs.uk/med_info/documents/Dental_Patient_on_Warf arin.pdf). However, the INR value must be a recent one (i.e. within 48 hours of planned dental treatment) and the patient stabilized on warfarin therapy. Any concerns should be discussed with staff at the patient's anticoagulation clinic.

Patients taking warfarin may also require *antibiotic prophylaxis* against endocarditis because of the underlying pathology, e.g. prosthetic heart valve.

RENAL DISEASE
Infections
Can be either pyelonephritis (affecting the kidney) or cystitis (affecting the bladder). They are common in women, with 50% experiencing symptoms of a urinary tract infection at some point in their lifetime. Whilst may be asymptomatic, symptoms include:
• frequency • urgency • dysuria (pain on micturition) • incontinence or retention.

Dental importance lies in the common use of amoxicillin as a first-line drug of choice and the fact that children with recurrent UTIs may be subjected to multiple courses of antibiotics, making resistance to antibiotics prescribed in dentistry likely. Additionally, the use of sugar-free antibiotic preparations (particularly in the liquid form) should be encouraged.

Chronic renal failure (CRF)

This causes increased levels of circulating urea (uraemia) as a result of progressive kidney damage. May be due to diabetes, hypertension, glomerulonephritis, pyelonephritis, reflux or connective tissue disorders. Symptoms include polyuria, nocturia, anorexia, vomiting and itchiness of the skin. Treatment is by extracorporeal haemodialysis, continuous ambulatory peritoneal dialysis (CAPD) or continuous cyclical peritoneal dialysis (CCPD). Ultimately renal transplantation may be required.

The main dental aspects of CRF are: • growth retardation and delayed dental eruption in children • malocclusion and enamel hypoplasia • pallor (due to anaemia) and ulceration of the oral mucosa • salivary gland swelling, xerostomia and altered taste sensation • immunosuppression, which may cause candidosis; serious odontogenic infection (such infections should be dealt with promptly and aggressively) • bony lesions due to renal osteodystrophy (loss of lamina dura, osteolytic changes) • giant cell bony lesions due to secondary hyperparathyroidism • reduced drug excretion, so prescribing should be conducted in consultation with a renal physician • bleeding tendency due to impaired platelet function • arm veins are precious (especially in the non-dominant arm) as arteriovenous (A-V) fistulae may be required for later dialysis • hyperkalaemia is a risk factor for GA.

Haemodialysis, peritoneal dialysis and transplantation

The presence of indwelling A-V fistulae for haemodialysis or peritoneal catheters for CAPD/CCPD may require antibiotic prophylaxis before invasive dental treatment; in the absence of national guidelines, local policy should be discussed with a renal physician. Normally, CAPD/CCPD catheters do not require cover; A-V fistulae may do, with the same regimens as for endocarditis prophylaxis (p. 72). A-V fistulae should never be used for blood sampling or drug administration.

All dialysis patients require sympathetic dental care at times suitable to them since they spend a significant amount of their week performing dialysis. Haemodialysis patients are at risk from bleeding after dialysis due to heparinization and physical trauma to platelets during dialysis, and surgery should be planned accordingly with local haemostatic measures.

Post-transplant, patients will be taking immunosuppressive drugs, will be at increased risk from infection, and may require prophylactic steroid cover. Dental treatment may be complicated by anticoagulant therapy. Be aware of the effects of nephrotoxic drugs (e.g. NSAIDs).

ENDOCRINE DISORDERS
Diabetes mellitus

> **Diabetes mellitus:** persistent hyperglycaemia due to pancreatic islet beta-cell destruction (*Type 1*) or other causes (*Type 2*).

Emergency management of hypo- and hyperglycaemia is discussed on page 524.

Patients with diabetes mellitus (DM) are at increased risk of oral candidosis, burning mouth syndrome and sialosis. Impaired resistance to infection may be due to defects in chemotaxis and phagocytosis by white blood cells. Antibiotics and atraumatic techniques should be employed routinely. Routine dentistry should be performed soon after mealtimes (breakfast or lunch) with the patient on usual drug/diet regimens. Liaison with the patient's diabetologist is important in advance of planned surgery. Arrange for diabetic patients to go first on the operating list.

Management of patients taking insulin to treat DM
Treatment under LA • Maintain carbohydrate intake and insulin doses as normal. • Ensure emergency glucose and drugs to hand. • Prescribe antibiotics and analgesics judiciously. • Remember that trismus may affect oral intake.

Treatment under GA • Arrange for diabetologist to assess patient (U&E, random blood glucose, glycosylated Hb, FBC, ECG). • Arrange for anaesthetist to assess patient. • Admit to ward *at least* the day before surgery and maintain usual carbohydrate/insulin intake until the evening before surgery, unless the diabetologist wishes a reduction in the long-acting or medium-acting insulins. • When the patient starts to fast, commence i.v. infusion of 10% glucose solution with potassium chloride and soluble insulin. Every hospital has its own regimen and this should be discussed with the local diabetologist. • Blood sugar levels (BM) should be assessed every 30 min initially; aim for 6–10 mmol/l during surgery. • Blood K^+ levels determine if more K^+ is required by infusion. • On regaining consciousness, monitor BMs every 1–2 hours and continue above infusion until patient is eating normally. • Regular insulin regimen can be restarted after the patient is seen to be eating normally.

Management of patients not taking insulin to treat DM

Treatment under LA • Maintain oral hypoglycaemic drugs and carbohydrate intake as usual. • Ensure emergency glucose and drugs to hand. • Prescribe antibiotics and analgesics judiciously. • Remember that trismus may affect oral intake.

Treatment under GA • Arrange for diabetologist to assess patient (U&E, random blood glucose, glycosylated Hb, FBC, ECG). • Arrange for anaesthetist to assess patient. • If random blood glucose >15 mmol/l or planned surgery is to be major or prolonged, use insulin regimen as for patient taking insulin (see above). • Otherwise, for patients on oral hypoglycaemic drugs, half the dose should be taken on the day prior to surgery and omit completely on day of surgery. Half dose should be maintained until patient is eating normally, when usual dose can be reintroduced. • BMs should be monitored at regular intervals pre-, peri- and postoperatively; if precipitous blood glucose changes are evident, change over to the insulin regimen noted above.

Thyroid and parathyroid disease

Functioning thyroid tissue may occur anywhere along the developmental path of the thyroid gland. Thus, lingual thyroid may be the sole functioning thyroid tissue and any suspicious lesions must firstly be assessed by a radioactive thyroid scan.

Hyperthyroidism may be caused by autoimmunity (Graves' disease), toxic nodule, adenoma and overdosing with thyroxine. Features are sweating, heat intolerance, weight loss, anxiety, increased appetite, tachycardia, exophthalmos, lid-lag and tremor. Uncontrolled hyperthyroidism may be the only contraindication to the use of an epinephrine-containing LA.

Hypothyroidism may be caused by autoimmunity (Hashimoto's disease), iodine deficiency and may follow radioactive iodine therapy and surgery. Features are weight gain, cold intolerance, tiredness, depression, constipation, myxoedema, bradycardia, hair loss and hoarse voice.

Hyperparathyroidism may be primary (with high levels of parathyroid hormone [PTH] due to parathyroid adenoma, hyperplasia or carcinoma), secondary (with high levels of PTH in response to prolonged hypocalcaemia, e.g. in renal failure) or tertiary (where PTH secretion becomes autonomous). Bone lesions may be evident around the jaws, e.g. brown 'tumour' of hyperparathyroidism.

Hypoparathyroidism may be primary (autoimmune) or secondary (following surgery to the thyroid gland). The resultant low serum calcium may cause perioral paraesthesia and tetany of the facial muscles after tapping over the facial nerve (Chvostek's sign).

Pituitary and adrenal gland disorders

> The anterior pituitary secretes follicle-stimulating hormone (FSH), luteinizing hormone (LH), growth hormone (GH), prolactin, ACTH and thyroid-stimulating hormone (TSH); the posterior pituitary secretes antidiuretic hormone (ADH) and oxytocin.

Hypopituitarism is most commonly due to tumours (primary or metastatic). Diabetes insipidus is the inability to concentrate urine due to deficiency of ADH, which may follow head injury. Pituitary tumours may cause any kind of hormonal disturbance. They may cause visual field defects due to compression of the optic chiasma; also erosion of the pituitary fossa, which may be seen on skull radiographs. Acromegaly results from excess GH production after closure of the bony epiphyses. Oral manifestations include spacing of the teeth, progressive prognathism and tongue enlargement.

Cushing's syndrome results from chronic exposure to high circulating levels of cortisol (endogenous) or steroid medication (exogenous). Cushing's disease is due to high levels of stimulatory ACTH, usually from a pituitary adenoma. Features are acne, skin atrophy, truncal obesity with sparing of the limbs, moon face and buffalo hump (due to redistribution of fat) and osteoporosis.

Corticosteroid prophylaxis

Prolonged use of systemic steroids may exaggerate some of the normal physiological actions of the corticosteroids:

Mineralocorticoid effects include hypertension, sodium/water retention and potassium loss.

Glucocorticoid effects include diabetes, osteoporosis, mental disturbance (suicidal depression or euphoria), muscle wasting and peptic ulceration (due to antiprostaglandin effects).

Prolonged, high doses may cause Cushing's syndrome with moon face, skin striae and acne. In children, steroids may result in growth suppression; in pregnancy, adrenal development in the fetus may be affected.

Modification of the immune response and tissue reactions may result in spread of infection, and diseases such as septicaemia or tuberculosis may reach an advanced stage before being recognized. Particular problems may arise with exposure to measles, chickenpox and shingles (zoster).

Currently there is no good evidence to suggest that topical steroids (which might be prescribed in dental practice) are associated with significant risk of immunosuppression or the problems of adrenal suppression detailed below. However, dental surgeons will frequently encounter patients for routine dental care who are taking systemic steroids for medical conditions (e.g. inflammatory bowel disease, rheumatoid arthritis).

Long-term administration of systemic corticosteroids suppresses the secretion of endogenous cortisol with atrophy of the adrenal cortex; such adrenal atrophy can persist for many years after stopping steroid therapy. Such patients may be at increased risk of adrenal suppression whereby the stress of surgical dentistry could result in acute adrenal insufficiency with collapse and death. Therefore any illness or surgical treatment may, in theory, require temporary *steroid cover* to compensate for the lack of sufficient *stress* adrenocortical response.

Controversy exists as to the perceived need and ideal regimen for steroid cover and historically a number of regimens have been advocated:

- do nothing by way of steroid supplementation
- simply insert a venous cannula *without* giving any steroids before surgery, choosing instead to give i.v. hydrocortisone only if a reduction in blood pressure becomes evident
- give steroid supplementation by 'doubling the normal oral dose' for that patient 2–4 hours before dental surgery
- give steroid supplementation (i.m. or i.v., usually 100 mg hydrocortisone) prior to the commencement of dental surgery.

Notwithstanding that the current medico-legal 'gold standard' of care may still sit most comfortably with oral, i.m. or i.v. steroid administration for prophylaxis, recent research suggests that steroid supplementation may not be required routinely for patients undergoing dental treatment with local anaesthesia, particularly those on regular, high-dose steroids who should have sufficient exogenous steroids on board to allow the body to cope with additional surgical (physiological) stress. However, some concern still exists for those patients on long-term, low-dose steroids. There is also some confusion as to whether or not the degree of surgery affects the need for steroid prophylaxis (e.g. the extraction of two molar teeth may cause more physiological stress than cutting a crown preparation!).

The current literature points towards the following regimens:

- no additional steroid supplementation preoperatively may be necessary; monitor BP at baseline and throughout the procedure; should the diastolic BP fall by >25% of the baseline value, then give 100 mg hydrocortisone i.v.;[1] or
- supplementation may not be required where the daily oral dose of prednisolone is <7.5 mg; above this dose, double the normal daily dose may be taken 'on the day' of dental surgery.[2]

Regardless, the greatest dangers arise during procedures under general anaesthesia when signs of steroid collapse may be masked. Anaesthetists must therefore *always* be informed of patients currently or recently taking steroid medication. Steroid prophylaxis for dental surgery under GA has been suggested as follows:[2]

- minor surgery: 100 mg hydrocortisone i.m. preoperatively
- major surgery: 100 mg hydrocortisone i.v. preoperatively plus 50 mg 8-hourly for 48 hours.

Pregnancy and the menopause

Pregnancy may lead to worsening of gingivitis and development of inflammatory epulides (swellings on the gingivae). It is a time to avoid: • radiographs (unless essential) • general anaesthesia • drugs (except if essential).

Aphthous ulceration often improves or resolves during pregnancy.

Menopause is a time of great physiological and psychological change. Psychogenic orofacial pain syndromes such as burning mouth syndrome are relatively common at this time (p. 473). There is little evidence to suggest that these are directly related to hormonal changes affecting the oral soft tissues.

LOCOMOTOR SYSTEM DISEASE

DEVELOPMENTAL BONE DISEASE
Osteogenesis imperfecta (brittle bone disease)

An autosomal dominant disease characterized by defective Type I collagen. It occurs in four main types (I–IV), making the older terms *congenita* and *tarda* obsolete. All types are characterized by bone fragility, and non-skeletal collagen can also be affected. Bones are often deformed with multiple fractures; blue sclerae are evident; dentinogenesis imperfecta is variably present (p. 193). Conductive hearing loss due to abnormal or fractured auditory ossicles may be present, as may aortic incompetence, rupture of tendons and hypermobility of joints.

Osteopetrosis (Albers–Schönberg or marble bone disease)

Characterized by an increase in bone density, decrease in blood supply and a propensity for fracture and chronic infection. Bone density may render the roots of teeth almost invisible on radiograph. Extractions are notoriously difficult. The mandible is more frequently affected than the maxilla. Dental management, particularly oral surgery, should be carried out in a specialist centre.

Cleidocranial dysostosis

An inherited defect of bone formation. Skull, jaws and clavicles are particularly affected such that clavicles may be absent, allowing the shoulders to be apposed across the patient's chest. Persistence of the entire deciduous dentition may occur due to the secondary teeth being impeded by multiple impactions and supernumerary teeth.

Achondroplasia

An inherited defect in bone formation which is often autosomal dominant but may arise by spontaneous mutation. The common appearance is that of a dwarf with relatively normal size of trunk and head but excessively short limbs. The middle third of the face is often retrusive due to defective growth at the skull base; severe malocclusion is therefore common.

METABOLIC BONE DISEASE

Fibrous dysplasia

A non-inherited bone disease with replacement of bone by fibrous tissue. It occurs in two forms:

Mono-ostotic One bone is affected; more common form
Polyostotic Multiple bones are affected.

Maxilla affected more than the mandible. Characterized by gradually increasing painless swelling of bones. *Albright's syndrome* is a variant of the polyostotic form in females with accompanying melanotic skin pigmentation (*café au lait* spots) and precocious puberty. A similar entity can occur in males without the precocious puberty. The bone lesions tend to 'burn out' in adolescence but surgical removal of swelling may be judiciously considered to reduce deformity.

Cherubism

Considered by some authorities to be a bilateral variant of fibrous dysplasia and, certainly, histology reveals fibrous replacement of bone but multinucleate giant cells are also prominent. The mandible tends to be involved predominantly but lesions may also occur in the maxilla. The cherubimic appearance of a 'chubby' face occurs around 2–4 years and regresses with puberty and early adulthood as bony infill takes place.

Rickets and osteomalacia

Manifestations of the same disease process – rickets occurring prior to epiphyseal closure, osteomalacia after closure. Both conditions result from defective mineralization of bone, usually caused by a deficiency of vitamin D availability or metabolism. Rickets is characterized by frontal skull bossing and progressive bowing and deformity of long bones. Bone pain is prominent in osteomalacia. Myopathies and manifestations of hypocalcaemia may be present in both conditions.

Osteoporosis

Defined as a reduction in bone mass per unit volume. There is loss of bone matrix with secondary loss of bone mineral. Features are bone pain, backache, and fractures of vertebrae, distal radius and neck of femur. Women are predominantly affected. Causes include postmenopausal, endocrine, nutritional and iatrogenic (steroid therapy). Hormone replacement therapy for postmenopausal women should be considered.

Paget's disease of bone

Characterized by excessive osteoclastic resorption together with compensatory but disorganized increase in bone deposition. The clinical features are: • localized bone pain • deformity of affected bones • limb shortening with accompanying osteoarthritis of associated joints • enlargement of skull vault ('cotton-wool' appearance on radiograph) • deafness • warmth and localized tenderness of bones • cardiac failure • cranial nerve compression.

The maxilla is involved more commonly than the mandible; other dental problems include hypercementosis of teeth with ankylosis; extraction sockets prone to infection; derangement of occlusion and denture difficulties; rare transformation to osteogenic sarcoma.

CONNECTIVE TISSUE DISORDERS

These are really a set of vasculitides, the result of inflammation in blood vessels, and are characterized by the presence of circulating autoantibodies.

Systemic lupus erythematosus (SLE)

SLE is an autoimmune disease of unknown aetiology; more common in women (9 : 1) and certain HLA types. It is a multisystem disorder with symptoms and signs of: • fever and malaise • arthralgia, arthritis, myalgia • facial 'butterfly' and other rashes • pancarditis, pleurisy, pulmonary fibrosis • peripheral neuropathies, cranial nerve palsies • jaundice, splenomegaly, lymphadenopathy.

There is a variability in oral lesions (p. 480). Autoimmune serology will aid diagnosis, especially anti-nuclear antibodies and their subsets.

Polymyalgia rheumatica

A relatively common condition in the middle-aged and elderly, particularly women. Symptoms are pain and stiffness in the shoulders, neck and pelvis; fever, weight loss, general malaise and depression may be evident; elevated ESR is confirmatory as is the dramatic response to systemic steroids. Giant cell (temporal) arteritis may complicate polymyalgia rheumatica in about a third of cases but will often stand alone. Giant cell (temporal) arteritis is discussed on page 477.

Other connective tissue disorders include *progressive systemic sclerosis*, *dermatomyositis*, *polymyositis* and *mixed connective tissue disease*. All of these and other diseases, such as *rheumatoid arthritis*, may be associated with Sjögren's syndrome (p. 465).

JOINT DISEASE AND PROSTHETIC JOINTS
Osteoarthritis (OA)

OA is a common age-related disease of joints. 'Wear and tear' is too simplistic: OA has features of destructive, catabolic, anabolic and reparative processes. It is characterized by pain and stiffness, particularly of weight-bearing joints. Changes may be evident radiographically in the TMJs with bone loss of the articular surface of the condyle, bone cysts, erosions, condylar atrophy and osteophytic lipping. NSAIDs, physiotherapy and weight loss are the treatments of choice with the first two being of relevance for OA of the TMJs. It is now recognized that a Sjögren-like condition may accompany some cases of OA – the so-called SOX syndrome.

Rheumatoid arthritis (RA)

RA is a chronic inflammatory, destructive and deforming polyarthropathy with extra-articular systemic manifestations. It is characterized by the presence of circulating autoantibodies (rheumatoid factor). The systemic manifestations are myriad and include: • anorexia, malaise, lethargy, myalgia • vasculitic lesions (e.g. nail bed infarcts) and Raynaud's phenomenon • pancarditis and lung lesions • anaemia • neuropathies • Sjögren's syndrome (p. 465).

The temporomandibular joints are reported to be involved in about 15% of sufferers.

Other joint diseases include:

Ankylosing spondylitis A disfiguring kyphotic condition affecting young men (M : F, 9 : 1) and associated with HLA B27.

Psoriatic arthritis Affects about 7% of psoriatics. Various types exist, including a severely mutilating arthritis. There are no autoantibodies identified.

Systemic-onset juvenile chronic arthritis (Still's disease) Similar to the adult form of rheumatoid arthritis but often much more aggressive and disfiguring. Ankylosis of the TMJ may occur in up to 25% of sufferers.

Gout and pseudogout Due to deposition in joints of uric acid crystals and calcium pyrophosphate crystals, respectively.

Behçet's disease With arthritis, iritis, recurrent oral and genital ulceration (p. 450).

Reiter's syndrome Comprises conjunctivitis, urethritis, seronegative oligoarthritis. The *genital* type occurs after a sexually transmitted disease (such as non-specific urethritis); the *intestinal* type occurs after enteric infection with *Shigella*, *Campylobacter* or *Salmonella*.

Prosthetic joints and antibiotic prophylaxis in dentistry

Any of the above conditions may require prosthetic joint replacement at some point in the disease process. There is currently no conclusive scientific evidence to suggest that prosthetic joints require antibiotic cover for dental procedures. Joint failure is most likely to occur after colonization with skin flora and *not* oral flora. However, immunocompromised patients merit special consideration and research is evolving in this area. Management regimens should be developed locally.

NEUROLOGICAL DISORDERS

Cranial nerves

Examination of the nervous system is a complex and time-consuming process, best left to physicians trained in that area of medicine. However, knowledge of the cranial nerves may be useful in discriminating organic disease from the psychosomatic (Table 16.2). In all cases of doubt, referral to a suitably qualified physician is imperative.

TABLE 16.2 Assessment of the cranial nerves

I	Olfactory	Sense of smell is assessed with a non-pungent substance; test each nostril separately
II	Optic	Assess: • visual acuity in each eye separately • visual fields by confrontation method • fundi (optic discs, retinal vessels, haemorrhages, exudates), N.B. papilloedema is indicative of raised intracranial pressure • pupils (position, size and shape; equal or unequal; regular or irregular; reaction directly and consensually to light and on convergence)
III	Oculomotor	Assess full range of eye movements; look for nystagmus and strabismus; does patient report diplopia ('double vision')?
IV	Trochlear	Lateral rectus muscle – supplied by VI
VI	Abducens	Superior oblique muscle – supplied by IV All other muscles – supplied by III, i.e. $(LR_6 \, SO_4)_3$
V	Trigeminal	Assess sensation to the face in each of the three divisions (not forgetting the conjunctivae). Assess strength in muscles of mastication (motor division)
VII	Facial	Assess movement in the muscles of facial expression
VIII	Vestibulocochlear	Hearing is assessed by tuning fork tests (Rinne and Weber). The vestibular portion is concerned with balance; lesions may produce vertigo and nystagmus; requires specialist assessment
IX	Glossopharyngeal	Ask patient to say 'Ahhh' and watch palatal movement. It should rise well and in the midline. Hoarseness may result from a lesion of the vagus nerve but assessment requires laryngoscopy by an ENT surgeon
X	Vagus	
XI	Accessory	Test trapezius muscle by shrugging shoulder against resistance. Test sternocleidomastoid muscle by turning chin against resistance
XII	Hypoglossal	Ask patient to protrude tongue. Note deviation (to side of lesion), wasting, tremor and fasciculation

Palsy and neuropathy

Many systemic diseases (such as SLE, diabetes and multiple sclerosis [MS]) can cause palsies and neuropathies. The most important palsy for the dental professional is that affecting the facial (VII) nerve (p. 482).

Neuralgia

Trigeminal neuralgia is discussed on page 475.

Headache and migraine

Three common headaches dominate clinical practice: • migraine • mixed headache (migraine plus tension headache) • tension headache (daily continuous headache).

Facial pain syndromes are described on page 473.

There is some evidence to support the use of dental (occlusal) splints in the treatment of tension headache (associated with myofascial pain dysfunction syndrome) and migraine.

The role of the dental professional in headache is to exclude contributory dental disease (such as pulpitis) and, to some degree, maxillary sinusitis although this should really be dealt with by an ENT surgeon. Local organic disease excluded, the patient should be seen by a physician with an interest in headache.

Epilepsy

May be classified according to seizure type:

Partial • simple partial seizures • complex partial seizures • partial evolving to generalized.

Generalized • absence seizures • atypical absence seizures • myoclonic seizures • clonic seizures • tonic seizures • tonic–clonic seizures • atonic seizures.

There are no contraindications to dental treatment for patients with epilepsy but be aware that fasting, drugs and emotional challenges can all precipitate a seizure. The acute management of a seizure is discussed on page 530.

Multiple sclerosis

An inflammatory, demyelinating disorder affecting any part of the CNS in a variable and unpredictable manner. There are estimated to be around 90 000 sufferers in the UK. Its importance for the dental professional lies in the debilitating nature of the disease, making oral hygiene measures difficult for the severely affected patient. Additionally, cranial nerve palsies and neuralgias are relatively common in patients with MS.

Parkinson's disease

Caused by degeneration of the dopaminergic neurones in the substantia nigra in the CNS with resultant: • tremor • rigidity • bradykinesia • disturbed postural reflexes.

Dental management problems include the inability to sit for treatment due to tremor; drooling of saliva.

Myaesthenia gravis

An acquired autoimmune disorder causing skeletal muscle fatigue and weakness due to loss of acetylcholine receptors in the postsynaptic membrane of the neuromuscular junction. This is caused by serum IgG antibodies to the receptors. Such patients undergoing dental treatment should be given early morning appointments for relatively short sessions because muscle fatigue worsens as the day progresses and after activity.

Chronic fatigue syndrome

Previously called postviral syndrome or myalgic encephalomyelitis, this condition is a complex disorder characterized by lassitude. It is the subject of substantial research. Graded exercise programmes and antidepressants (SSRIs) have been shown to be of some benefit in overcoming symptoms. There is no evidence at all to support the claim from some quarters that 'allergy' to dental amalgam or mercury toxicity have any role in the aetiology of this condition.

PSYCHIATRIC DISORDERS

Personality disorders, *neuroses and psychoses* are all part of the broad spectrum of psychiatric disorders. The possibility of such disorders being part of the aetiology of certain conditions (e.g. chronic orofacial pain disorders) must be borne in mind (p. 473). Psychological aspects of patient management are discussed in Chapter 1.

The role of the dental professional in chronic orofacial pain disorders is to exclude contributory dental disease (such as pulpitis) and be supportive and understanding of contributing psychiatric disease. When local dental disease has been excluded, the patient should be referred to a physician with an interest in such disorders – preferably at a combined oral medicine/psychiatry clinic. However, where severe and overt psychiatric disease is evident, early liaison with a psychiatrist, via the general medical practitioner, is essential. Unnecessary and prolonged dental treatment *must* be resisted since this will only add to the patient's problem.

DERMATOLOGY

The facial and perioral manifestations of skin conditions such as psoriasis and dermatitis should be dealt with by a general medical practitioner or dermatologist, as should skin manifestations of systemic diseases (such as pyoderma gangrenosum and erythema nodosum).

MALIGNANT LESIONS

Basal cell carcinoma (or rodent ulcer)

• Is the most common skin cancer and particularly affects the elderly. • Rarely, if ever, metastasizes; locally invasive. • Develops on sun-damaged skin, particularly the face. • Red nodule becomes an ulcer with classical pearly rolled border. • Treated by surgery or radiotherapy; excellent prognosis.

Squamous cell carcinoma

• Unlike its mucosal counterpart, is rarely aggressive. • Occurs on sun-exposed skin or in areas of chronic trauma (e.g. leg ulcers due to venous stasis). • Indurated ('hard') ulcer with raised border. • Metastasizes to local lymph nodes and beyond. • Treated by surgery or radiotherapy.

Malignant melanoma

• Increasing incidence with increasing sun exposure. • Risk is highest in those with fair skin, dysplastic naevi and congenital melanocytic naevi. • F : M ratio 2 : 1. • Be alert to pigmented lesions which change colour, enlarge, bleed or ulcerate. • Types: lentigo maligna, superficial spreading, nodular. • Histological assessment by Breslow or Clark indices. • Treated by surgery, regional node clearance and adjuvant chemotherapy. • Most common intraoral site is the palate.

Mycosis fungoides

• Most likely a T-cell lymphoma. • Occurs in middle-aged, elderly. • Itchy plaque which resembles psoriasis. • Treated by topical steroids, UV light, PUVA or radiotherapy; rarely curative.

PREMALIGNANT LESIONS

Actinic keratosis

• Common scaly, hyperpigmented lesions in the elderly. • Occur on sun-exposed skin and may affect the lips as shallow erosions.

• Require sun-block to prevent further damage. • Treated with local excision, cryotherapy or topical chemotherapy (e.g. 5-fluorouracil).

Bowen's disease (carcinoma in situ)
• Intraepithelial carcinoma which may progress. • Slowly expanding scaly pink plaque which may ulcerate. • Common on the legs of elderly women.

Dysplastic naevi
• Common in patients who go on to develop malignant melanomas (about 30%). • Require whole-body assessment by an experienced dermatologist with photographic records and regular review.
• Excision of 'at-risk' lesions. • Use of sun-block.

IMMUNE SYSTEM DISORDERS

Immune system disorders may be the result of many factors but all are characterized by increased susceptibility to infection.

Congenital (primary) immunodeficiency
Conditions are myriad and include: • B-cell defects (e.g. Bruton's syndrome) • T-cell defects (e.g. DiGeorge's syndrome) • combined B- and T-cell defects (e.g. severe combined immunodeficiency, Wiskott–Aldrich syndrome) • selective immunodeficiencies (e.g. IgA deficiency, complement component deficiencies).

Acquired (secondary) immunodeficiency
Related to diseases or immunosuppressive therapy (iatrogenic). The major entity today is, of course, HIV and AIDS (p. 484) but there are many others including leukaemias and lymphomas, malnutrition, systemic lupus erythematosus, rheumatoid arthritis, chronic active hepatitis, diabetes mellitus, sarcoidosis, Down syndrome, tuberculosis and numerous viral infections such as Epstein–Barr virus.

Immunosuppressive therapy is now extremely common and may be used in the management of connective tissue disorders, dermatological diseases, mucosal diseases and following organ transplant surgery (e.g. heart/lung, kidney, liver, pancreas).

The problems associated with these conditions are many (e.g. likelihood of infection, bleeding diathesis, steroid prophylaxis) and management of dental and oral diseases is best suited to specialist units.

REFERENCES

1. Thomason JM, Girdler NM, Kendall-Taylor P et al 1999 An investigation into the need for supplementary steroids in organ transplant patients undergoing gingival surgery. A double-blind, split-mouth, cross-over study. Journal of Clinical Periodontology 26:577–82
2. Gibson N, Ferguson JW 2004 Steroid cover for dental patients on long-term steroid medication: proposed clinical guidelines based upon a critical review of the literature. British Dental Journal 197:681–5

FURTHER READING

Lockhart PB, Gibson J, Pond SH, Leitch J 2003 Dental management considerations for the patient with an acquired coagulopathy. Part I, Coagulopathies from systemic disease. British Dental Journal 195:439–45

Lockhart PB, Gibson J, Pond SH, Leitch J 2003 Dental management considerations for the patient with an acquired coagulopathy. Part II, Coagulopathies from drugs. British Dental Journal 195:495–501

North West Medicines Information Centre: http://www.ukmi.nhs.uk/med_info/documents/Dental_Patient_on_Warfarin.pdf

CHAPTER 17

EMERGENCIES IN DENTISTRY

Introduction 522

Emergency equipment and drugs 522

Fainting 523

Collapse of diabetic patient 524

Acute chest pain 524

Cardiorespiratory arrest 525

Anaphylactic reactions 527

Adrenal crisis 529

Epilepsy 530

Asthma 530

Inhaled foreign bodies 531

Cerebrovascular accident ('stroke') 531

INTRODUCTION

There is a desire by many experts to simplify the list of emergency drugs and equipment the dental team is required to have available. This is laudable since it allows the dental team to focus on the more common medical emergencies it may encounter – and, indeed, to function well when such problems present. However, this chapter will suggest a fairly comprehensive approach to emergencies in dental practice – the lists of drugs and equipment are therefore somewhat fuller than reality may dictate. It is not implied that dental practices should carry all equipment and drugs listed.

However, the concept of 'team care' is essential in dealing with emergencies confidently and competently in the dental surgery. The dental team (dentist, dental nurse, hygienist, receptionist, technician) should practise emergency procedures regularly and develop predetermined roles (e.g. opening emergency kit, telephoning for assistance).

EMERGENCY EQUIPMENT AND DRUGS

Emergency equipment

- Portable defibrillator
- Potable oxygen delivery system
- Ambu bag (self-inflating with valve and mask)
- Oropharyngeal airways (sizes 1, 2 and 3)
- Cricothyroid puncture needles
- High-volume aspiration with suction catheters and Yankauer sucker
- Disposable syringes (2, 5, 10 and 20 ml sizes)
- Needles (19, 21 and 23 gauge) and butterflies
- Tourniquet, sphygmomanometer and stethoscope
- Venous access cannulae ('venflons' 16 and 22 gauge)
- i.v. infusion sets
- 'BM sticks' (for rapid assessment of blood sugar levels).

Emergency drugs

- Oxygen
- Nitrous oxide (very useful analgesic following MI)
- Epinephrine injection (1 : 1000 or 1 mg/ml)
- Hydrocortisone injection (100 mg)
- Antihistamine tablets and injection (e.g. chlorphenamine tablets 4 mg, injection 10 mg/ml)

- Diazepam emulsion (Diazemuls™ 5 mg/ml)
- Flumazenil injection (100 µg/ml)
- Glucose (50% solution) for injection, and powder for oral use
- Glucagon injection (1 mg)
- Salbutamol inhaler, or 5 mg preparation for nebulization
- Glyceryl trinitrate (GTN) aerosol spray
- Crystalloid or colloid solution for infusion.

FAINTING

Dentistry predisposes to fainting (syncope or vasovagal episode) due to fear, pain, unusual sights and smells, anxiety, fatigue and fasting. It is the most common cause of loss of consciousness in dental practice. It is common in young men. Treat patients supine wherever possible.

Symptoms and signs
• Light-headed feeling (often with nausea) • warm, sweaty feeling • pallor • skin cool and moist to touch • bradycardia (with a thready, low-volume pulse) • loss of consciousness and collapse with resultant rapid, full pulse.

Differential diagnosis
• Hypoglycaemia • steroid insufficiency • drug reaction • cerebrovascular accident • myocardial infarction • heart block or other causes of bradycardia • early epileptic seizure.

Management
- Lie patient flat with head below heart (modern dental chairs are ideal!).
- Determine bradycardia by taking pulse at major vessel.
- Loosen clothing and open windows.
- Establish verbal encouragement of patient and administer glucose.
- Delay dental treatment unless urgent.

If recovery is slow or delayed – reconsider diagnosis.

- Check blood sugar and, if low, administer i.v. glucose.
- Maintain airway and administer oxygen.
- If persistently hypotensive, consider steroid insufficiency and administer i.v. hydrocortisone.
- Seek urgent medical attention.

COLLAPSE OF DIABETIC PATIENT

If a diabetic patient collapses *assume hypoglycaemia* unless you are certain the cause is hyperglycaemia. You will not worsen any hyperglycaemia by giving glucose or glucagon but failure to raise the blood sugar level in hypoglycaemia may be potentially fatal.

Remember that diabetic patients often have severe atherosclerosis and so ischaemic heart disease is common: *the collapse could be due to a myocardial event*.

Hypoglycaemia may result from excess insulin or missing a meal (in the excitement of attending the dentist), stress, or changing insulin requirements (e.g. dental infection).

Symptoms and signs
See Table 17.1.

Management
● If conscious, administer oral glucose.
● Lie patient flat.

If unconscious or uncooperative:

● Obtain venous access.
● Administer 50 ml of 50% glucose i.v. *or* 1 mg glucagon i.m.
● Urgent transfer to hospital.

ACUTE CHEST PAIN

This is usually myocardial (but exclude collapsed lung or pulmonary embolus).

Differential diagnosis
• Angina pectoris. • Myocardial infarction (MI).

TABLE 17.1 Signs and symptoms of hypoglycaemia and hyperglycaemia	
Hypoglycaemia	*Hyperglycaemia*
Blood sugar *low*	Blood sugar *high*
Rapid onset	Slow onset
Aggressive/irritable behaviour	Drowsy and disorientated
Moist skin	Dry skin
Normal or rapid breathing	Deep, laboured breathing

Symptoms and signs
• Severe, crushing retrosternal pain ('heavy, crushing or constricting'). • Radiations to arm, neck or jaw. • Angina normally relieved by GTN tablet or spray. • MI likely if pain is accompanied by: – breathlessness – nausea – vomiting – loss of consciousness – weak/irregular pulse – hypotension.

Management
- Give patient's own anti-angina medication, e.g. GTN spray or tablet sublingually.
- Wait 3 minutes and repeat if necessary; then assume MI.
- Send for medical assistance by telephoning 999 (or the appropriate national emergency number).
- Do not lie flat as this increases feelings of breathlessness and panic. Allow the patient to assume the most comfortable position for him/her.
- Administer nitrous oxide and oxygen (50/50) as pain relief.
- Obtain venous access in case cardiopulmonary resuscitation (CPR) is required.
- Maintain verbal encouragement of patient.
- Administer oral aspirin (150–300 mg) as antiplatelet agent.
- Urgent transfer to hospital.

CARDIORESPIRATORY ARREST

Most commonly caused by ventricular fibrillation (VF) but consider asystole and electromechanical dissociation (EMD).

Signs
• Loss of consciousness. • Absence of central arterial pulses.
• Absence of breath sounds/chest movements.

Management
The European Resuscitation Council has identified a 'Chain of Survival' to maximize positive outcome (European Resuscitation Council Guidelines for Resuscitation 2005. Resuscitation 67 S1:S3–S6) as follows:

- Early recognition and call for help – to prevent cardiac arrest
- Early CPR – to buy time
- Early defibrillation – to restart the heart
- Post-resuscitation care – to restore quality of life.

The European Resuscitation Council Algorithm 2005 for Adult Basic Life Support is shown in Figure 17.1. This figure is reproduced with grateful thanks.

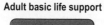

Adult basic life support

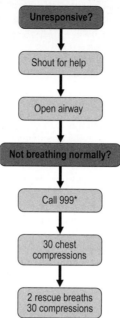

Unresponsive?

Shout for help

Open airway

Not breathing normally?

Call 999*

30 chest
compressions

2 rescue breaths
30 compressions

* or national emergency number

Figure 17.1 Adult Basic Life Support Algorithm. (From Handley AJ, Koster R, Monsieurs K, Perkins GD, Davies S, Bossaert L 2005 European Resuscitation Council Guidelines for Resuscitation 2005. Section 2. Adult Basic Life Support and Use of Automated External Defibrillators. Resuscitation 67(S1):S1–S81. Reproduced with permission of Elsevier.)

Proceed as follows:

- Make sure you, the victim and any bystanders are safe.
- Assess responsiveness by gently shaking the patient's shoulders and asking loudly – 'Are you all right?'
- If there is no response, shout for help and get helper to summon medical assistance by dialling 999 (or the appropriate national emergency number).
- Lie patient flat on the floor on his/her back – soft dental chairs may not be ideal for CPR.
- Open the airway with a gentle head tilt and chin lift.
- Look, listen and feel for normal breathing.

- If the patient is not breathing normally, start chest compressions at a rate of 100 per minute.
- Combine chest compressions with rescue breaths: after 30 compressions, open the airway again using head tilt and chin lift and give two effective breaths.
- Continue compressions and breaths in a ratio of 30:2.
- The same regimen should be used for one- and two-rescuer resuscitation.
- The patient should be turned to the recovery position when he or she shows evidence of recovery with normal breathing – otherwise continue resuscitation until qualified help arrives and takes over or you become exhausted.

ADVANCED CARDIAC LIFE SUPPORT

The European Resuscitation Council Algorithm 2005 for Adult Advanced Life Support is shown in Figure 17.2. This figure is reproduced with grateful thanks.

Following successful resuscitation, the patient should be turned to the recovery position to prevent aspiration of vomitus and airway obstruction.

ANAPHYLACTIC REACTIONS

Anaphylactic reactions show a great deal of variation, from a mild pruritic skin rash to full-blown anaphylactic shock, which is life-threatening. Milder reactions may be managed by withdrawal of the offending drug and use of an oral antihistamine such as chlorphenamine (dose: 4 mg every 4–6 hours). Progressive reactions should be managed under medical supervision as an inpatient: the adage 'better safe than sorry' pertains completely here. Be aware that parenteral routes of drug administration are more likely to produce severe and rapid reactions than the enteral route. *Atopic* individuals are more at risk.

ANAPHYLAXIS
Symptoms and signs
• Facial flushing • itching of the skin • paraesthesia, particularly of the extremities, face and lips • oedema • wheezing • abdominal pain and nausea or vomiting • sense of impending doom, panic with loss of consciousness • facial flushing is replaced by pallor and then by cyanosis • skin becomes cold and clammy • pulse is weak (often

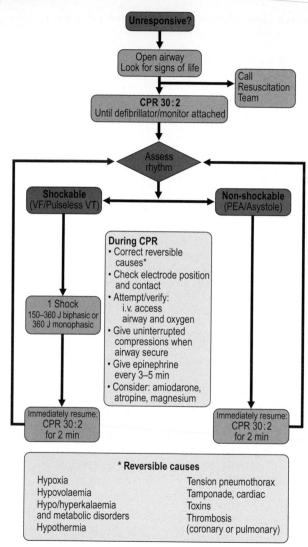

Figure 17.2 Adult Advanced Life Support Cardiac Arrest Algorithm. (From Nolan JP, Deakin CD, Soar J, Böttiger BW, Smith G 2005 European Resuscitation Council Guidelines for Resuscitation 2005. Section 4. Adult Advanced Life Support. Resuscitation 67(S1):S1–S81. Reproduced with permission of Elsevier.)

impalpable) and rapid • blood pressure is low and often unrecordable.

Management
This centres around restoration of blood pressure and circulating blood volume.

- Lay patient flat and raise the legs but be aware that some patients will want to sit in a position more comfortable for them.
- Administer high-flow oxygen (10–15 l/min).
- Administer i.m. epinephrine at a dose of 0.5–1.0 mg (i.e. 0.5–1.0 ml of 1 : 1000). This should be repeated at regular intervals (e.g. every 5 minutes) until a pressor response is noted. N.B. i.v. epinephrine should be given only by experienced staff under cardiac monitoring conditions and then in a concentration of 1 : 10 000 or 1 : 100 000.
- Establish i.v. access and administer:
  — chlorphenamine 10–20 mg diluted in a syringe with 10–20 ml of blood or saline; slowly i.v. over no less than 60 seconds
  — hydrocortisone 100–200 mg i.v.
  — fluid as a plasma expander; 1 litre rapid i.v.
- Endotracheal intubation or tracheotomy, if required.
- If cardiorespiratory arrest occurs, proceed with CPR.
- Urgent transfer to hospital. *All* patients with such reactions *must* be admitted under medical supervision for 8–24 hours because relapse is common.

ADRENAL CRISIS

May be precipitated where dental surgical procedures are not covered by exogenous corticosteroids in susceptible individuals (e.g. long-term steroid users for asthma, inflammatory bowel disease, rheumatic disease, etc.) where suppression of the hypothalamic–pituitary–adrenal axis has occurred.

Corticosteroid prophylaxis is discussed on page 508.

Symptoms and signs
• Rapid loss of consciousness • pallor of skin • rapid, weak pulse • hypotension.

Management
- Lay patient flat and raise the legs.
- Administer high-flow oxygen.
- Establish i.v. access and administer 100–200 mg of hydrocortisone i.v.

- Urgent transfer to hospital.
- Assess for other causes of collapse, e.g. MI.

EPILEPSY

May present in many different forms. Properly controlled, patients with epilepsy present no management problems to the dental surgeon. However, stress, fasting, hypoglycaemia and fainting can all cause a fit in the surgery. Patients who are not well controlled, who state that 'things are not quite right', or who are changing medication should have venous access established prior to commencing dental treatment.

Tonic–clonic seizures are often preceded by an aura, followed rapidly by loss of consciousness and a rigid, extended body (tonic phase) and jerking or flailing movements (clonic phase). Postictal drowsiness and the desire to sleep follow. Most fits last less than 5 minutes and require no intervention except protecting the patient from self-inflicted damage. Where the fit is prolonged or repeated, status epilepticus results and intervention is required to prevent brain hypoxia.

Management
- Administer diazepam emulsion (Diazemuls™), normally at a dose of 10–20 mg i.v. slowly, to abort the attack.
- Administer high-flow oxygen.
- Check blood sugar (to exclude hypoglycaemia as precipitant; correct if evident).
- Urgent transfer to hospital.

ASTHMA

May be predisposed to by anxiety. The underlying problem is that of respiratory tract hyper-reactivity with resultant bronchospasm.

Symptoms and signs
• Breathlessness • wheezing • panic and fear • if severe, inability to speak.

Management
- Give reassurance but don't crowd the patient.
- Allow the patient to use his/her own inhaler or supply a salbutamol inhaler.
- The patient should assume the most comfortable position (usually erect).

- Give nebulized salbutamol (5 mg) if a portable nebulizer is available. Otherwise use high-flow oxygen and deliver salbutamol (6–8 actuations) into the oxygen mask and allow the patient to breathe this mixture.
- Continue high-flow oxygen and repeat the above.
- Obtain i.v. access and give hydrocortisone 200 mg i.v.
- Urgent transfer to hospital.

INHALED FOREIGN BODIES

Inhaled foreign bodies are a hazard of supine dentistry but, with appropriate precautions, are entirely preventable. (For a fuller handling of this topic, see Handley AJ, Koster R, Monsieurs K, Perkins GD, Davies S, Bossaert L 2005 European Resuscitation Council Guidelines for Resuscitation 2005. Section 2. Adult Basic Life Support and Use of Automated External Defibrillators. Resuscitation 67(S1):S1–S81.)

It is important to ask the patient if he or she is genuinely choking. Then, if simple coughing does not dislodge the offending article, give up to five sharp blows between the shoulder blades with the heel of the hand. If this is unsuccessful, use up to five abdominal thrusts as follows: encircle the patient with your arms from behind at the level of the lower border of the rib cage; give a sudden forceful squeeze by pulling your arms together between the umbilicus and the xiphisternum with the hands directed upwards towards the chest. If relief of the obstruction is not evident, alternate five back blows with five abdominal thrusts. Where the article is lying at the laryngeal inlet, a cricothyrotomy may allow breathing until the obstruction can be physically dislodged. In all cases, a follow-up chest radiograph is mandatory.

The above actions are suitable for children over 1 year of age but with very young children, gently swinging the patient around by the legs may be sufficient to dislodge the article.

CEREBROVASCULAR ACCIDENT ('STROKE')

Cerebrovascular accidents are uncommon dental emergencies and unrelated to treatment. The patient may lose consciousness with weakness of one side of the body.

Management
- Maintain the airway.
- Administer oxygen
- Urgent transfer to hospital.

APPENDICES

Appendix A: Further reading   534

Appendix B: Useful Websites   537

Appendix C: Average dates of mineralization and eruption   540

Appendix D: Tooth notation   542

Appendix E: Infection control   542

Appendix F: Normal laboratory values of relevance to medicine   544

APPENDIX A FURTHER READING

PSYCHOLOGICAL ASPECTS OF DENTAL CARE

Kent GG, Croucher R 1998 Achieving Oral Health: The Social Context Of Dental Care, 3rd edn. Wright, Oxford

DENTAL RADIOLOGY

Brocklebank L 1997 Dental Radiology – Understanding the X-ray Image. Oxford University Press, Oxford
FGDP (UK)-RCS 1998 Selection Criteria for Dental Radiography. FGDP (UK)-RCS
Guidance Notes for Dental Practitioners on the Safe Use of X-ray Equipment 2001. HMSO, London
NRPB Guidelines on Radiology Standards for Primary Dental Care. 1994 Doc. NRPB, 5, No 3
Whaites E 2003 Essentials of Dental Radiography and Radiology, 3rd edn. Churchill Livingstone, Edinburgh

DRUG PRESCRIBING AND THERAPEUTICS

Cawson RA, Spector RG, Skelly AM 1995 Basic Pharmacology and Clinical Drug Use in Dentistry, 6th edn. Churchill Livingstone, Edinburgh
Seymour RA, Meechan JG, Yates MS 1999 Pharmacology and Dental Therapeutics, 3rd edn. Oxford University Press, Oxford

ANALGESIA, SEDATION AND GENERAL ANAESTHESIA

Aitkenhead AR, Rowbotham DJ, Smith G 2001 Textbook of Anaesthesia, 4th edn. Churchill Livingstone, Edinburgh
General Dental Council 2005 Standards for Dental Professionals. General Dental Council, London
Meechan JG 2002 Practical Dental Local Anaesthesia. Quintessence, London
Meechan JG, Robb ND, Seymour RA 1998 Pain and Anxiety Control for the Conscious Dental Patient. Oxford University Press, Oxford
Robinson PD, Pitt Ford TR, McDonald F 2000 Local Anaesthesia in Dentistry. Wright, Oxford

DENTAL MATERIALS

Eley BM 1998 The Future of Dental Amalgam: a Review of the Literature. British Dental Association, London

McCabe JF, Walls AWG 1998 Applied Dental Materials, 8th edn. Blackwell Science, Oxford

Van Noort R 2002 Introduction to Dental Materials, 2nd edn. Mosby, Edinburgh

PREVENTIVE DENTISTRY

Murray JJ, Nunn JH, Steele JG 2003 Prevention of Oral Disease. Oxford University Press, Oxford

Pine CM 2005 Community Oral Health. Quintessence, London

PAEDIATRIC DENTISTRY

Chadwick BL, Hosey MT 2003 Child Taming, How to Manage Children in Dental Practice. Quintessence, London

Curzon MEJ, Roberts JF, Kennedy DB 1996 Kennedy's Paediatric Operative Dentistry, 4th edn. Wright, Oxford

Welbury RR, Duggal MS, Hosey MT 2005 Paediatric Dentistry, 3rd edn. Oxford University Press, Oxford

PERIODONTOLOGY

Jenkins WMM, Allan CJ 1999 Periodontics: a Synopsis. Wright, Oxford

Lindhe J, Karring T, Lang NP 2003 Clinical Periodontology and Implant Dentistry, 4th edn. Blackwell-Munksgaard, Oxford

Manson JD, Eley BM 2000 Outline of Periodontics, 4th edn. Wright, Oxford

Palmer RM, Floyd PD 2003 A Clinical Guide to Periodontology, 2nd edn. BDJ Books, Edinburgh

OPERATIVE DENTISTRY

Brunton PA 2002 Decision Making in Operative Dentistry. Quintessence, London.

Ibbetson R, Eder A 2000 Tooth Surface Loss. BDJ Books, London

Kidd EAM 2005 Essentials of Dental Caries: the Disease and Its Management, 3rd edn. Oxford University Press, Oxford

Kidd EAM, Smith BGN, Watson TF 2003 Pickard's Manual of Operative Dentistry, 8th edn. Oxford University Press, Oxford

Smith BGN 1998 Planning and Making Crowns and Bridges. Martin Dunitz, London

Stock CJR, Nehammer CF 1990 Endodontics in Practice, 2nd edn. British Dental Association, London

Whitworth JM 2002 Rational Root Canal Treatment in Practice. Quintessence, London.

REMOVABLE PROSTHODONTICS

Allen PF, McCarthy S 2003 Complete Dentures from Planning to Problem Solving. Quintessence, London

Barnes I, Walls A 1994 Gerodontology. Wright, Oxford

Bartlett DW, Fisher NF 2004 Clinical Problem Solving in Prosthodontics. Churchill Livingstone, Edinburgh

Davenport JC, Basker RM, Heath JR, Ralph JP, Glantz P-O 2000 A Clinical Guide to Removable Partial Dentures. British Dental Association, London

Gray RJM, Davies SJ, Quayle AA 1999 A Clinical Guide to Temporomandibular Disorders. British Dental Association, London

McCord JF, Grant AA 2000 A Clinical Guide to Complete Denture Prosthetics. BDJ Books, London

Palmer R 2000 A Clinical Guide to Implants in Dentistry. BDJ Books, London

Weinberg LA 2003 Atlas of Tooth and Implant Supported Prosthodontics. Quintessence, London.

ORTHODONTICS

Jones ML, Oliver RG 2000 Walther and Houston's Orthodontic Notes, 6th edn. Wright, Oxford

Mitchell L, Carter N, and Doubleday B 2001 Introduction to Orthodontics. Open University Press, Oxford.

ORAL AND MAXILLOFACIAL SURGERY

Banks P, Brown A 2001 Fractures of the Facial Skeleton. Wright, Oxford

Booth PW, Schendel SA, Hausamen JE 1999 Maxillofacial Surgery Vols I and II. Churchill Livingstone, Edinburgh

Harris M, Reynolds IR 1991 Fundamentals of Orthognathic Surgery. WB Saunders, London

Soames JV, Southam JC 2005 Oral Pathology, 4th edn. Oxford University Press, Oxford

ORAL MEDICINE

Field EA, Longman L 2003 Tyldsley's Oral Medicine, 5th edn. Oxford University Press, Oxford

Scully C 2004 Oral and Maxillofacial Medicine, The Basis of Diagnosis and Treatment. Wright, Edinburgh

Scully C, Felix DH 2005 Oral medicine – update for the dental practitioner. British Dental Journal 199:763–70

Wray D, Lowe GDO, Dagg JH, Felix DH, Scully C 1999 Textbook of General and Oral Medicine. Churchill Livingstone, Edinburgh

GENERAL MEDICINE OF RELEVANCE TO DENTISTRY

Scully S, Cawson RA 2005 Medical Problems in Dentistry, 5th edn. Elsevier, Edinburgh

Wray D, Lowe GDO, Dagg JH, Felix DH, Scully C 1999 Textbook of General and Oral Medicine. Churchill Livingstone, Edinburgh

EMERGENCIES IN DENTISTRY

European Resuscitation Council 2005 European Resuscitation Council Guidelines 2005 Resuscitation 76(Suppl 1):1–181

National Dental Advisory Committee 1999 Emergency Dental Drugs. Scottish Office. Department of Health, Edinburgh

APPENDIX B USEFUL WEBSITES

The emergence and the expansion of the Internet has provided a vast repository of information for both oral health care professionals, patients and the general public. Some useful websites are listed below.

Organization	URL
American Academy of Periodontology	www.perio.org
American College of Prosthodontics	www.prosthodontics.org

American Dental Association	www.ada.org
Association of Consultants and Specialists in Restorative Dentistry	www.restdent.org.uk
British Association for the Study of Community Dentistry	www.bascd.org
British Association of Dental Nurses	www.badn.org.uk
British Association of Dental Therapists	www.badt.org.uk
British Association of Oral and Maxillofacial Surgeons	www.baoms.org.uk
British Dental Association	www.bda-dentistry.org.uk
British Dental Health Foundation	www.dentalhealth.org.uk
British Dental Hygienists Association	www.bdha.org.uk
British National Formulary	www.bnf.org
British Orthodontic Society	www.bos.org.uk
British Society for Oral Medicine	www.bsom.org.uk
British Society for Restorative Dentistry	www.bsrd.org
British Society for the Study of Prosthetic Dentistry	www.bsspd.org
British Society of Paediatric Dentistry	www.bspd.co.uk
British Society of Periodontology	www.bsperio.org.uk
Centre for Evidence-Based Dentistry	www.cebd.org
Cochrane Collaboration	www.cochrane.co.uk
Committee of Postgraduate Dental Deans and Directors	www.copdend.org.uk
Committee on Safety of Medicines	www.mrha.gov.uk
Dental Practice Board	www.dpb.nhs.uk
Dental Sedation Teachers Group	www.dstg.co.uk
Dental Systematic Reviews from the Cochrane Collaboration	www.cochrane-oral.man.ac.uk
Dental Vocational Training Authority	www.dvta.nhs.uk
DERweb (Dental Educational Resources on the web)	www.derweb.co.uk
European Resuscitation Council	www.erc.edu/new
Faculty of General Dental Practice	www.fgdp.org.uk
General Dental Council	www.gdc-uk.org

National Electronic Library for Health (NeLH)	www.nelh.nhs.uk
National Electronic Library for Health – Oral Branch	www.nelh.nhs.uk/oralhealth
National Institute for Health and Clinical Excellence	www.nice.org.uk
National Institute of Dental and Craniofacial Research	www.nidcr.nih.gov
NHS Direct	www.nhsdirect.nhs.uk
NHS Education for Scotland	www.nes.scot.nhs.uk/dentistry
PubMed	www.pubmedcentral.nih.gov
Royal College of Physicians and Surgeons, Glasgow	www.rcpsglasg.ac.uk
Royal College of Surgeons of Edinburgh	www.rcsed.ac.uk
Royal College of Surgeons of England	www.rcseng.ac.uk
Society for Advancement of Anaesthesia in Dentistry	www.saaduk.org
Scottish Intercollegiate Guidelines Network	www.sign.ac.uk

APPENDIX C AVERAGE DATES OF MINERALIZATION AND ERUPTION

AVERAGE DATES OF MINERALIZATION AND ERUPTION OF THE PRIMARY DENTITION

Tooth	Mineralization begins	Amount of enamel formed at birth	Enamel completed	Root completed	Eruption
Upper					
Central incisor	4 months in utero	Five-sixths	1½ months	1½ years	7½ months
Lateral incisor	4½ months in utero	Two-thirds	2½ months	2 years	9 months
Canine	5 months in utero	One-third	9 months	3½ years	18 months
First molar	5 months in utero	Cusps united	6 months	2½ years	14 months
Second molar	6 months in utero	Cusps still isolated	11 months	3 years	24 months
Lower					
Central incisor	4½ months in utero	Three-fifths	2½ months	1½ years	6 months
Lateral incisor	4½ months in utero	Three-fifths	3 months	1¾ years	7 months
Canine	5 months in utero	One-third	9 months	3¼ years	16 months
First molar	5 months in utero	Cusps united	5½ months	2¼ years	12 months
Second molar	6 months in utero	Cusps still isolated	10 months	3 years	20 months

It should be remembered that there can be marked individual variation in mineralization and eruption times. The sequence is more important than precise time of eruption.

AVERAGE DATES OF MINERALIZATION AND ERUPTION OF THE PERMANENT DENTITION

Tooth	Mineralization begins	Amount of enamel formed at birth	Enamel completed	Root completed	Eruption
Upper					
Central incisor	3–4 months	—	4–5 years	10 years	7–8 years
Lateral incisor	10–12 months	·	4–5 years	11 years	8–9 years
Canine	4–5 months	—	6–7 years	13–15 years	11–12 years
First premolar	1½–1¾ years	—	5–6 years	12–13 years	10–11 years
Second premolar	2–2¼ years	—	6–7 years	12–14 years	10–12 years
First molar	At birth	Sometimes a trace	2½–3 years	9–10 years	6–7 years
Second molar	2½–3 years	—	7–8 years	14–16 years	12–13 years
Third molar	7–9 years	—	12–16 years	18–25 years	17–21 years
Lower					
Central incisor	3–4 months	—	4–5 years	9–10 years	6–7 years
Lateral incisor	3–4 months	—	4–5 years	10 years	7–8 years
Canine	4–5 months	—	6–7 years	12–14 years	9–10 years
First premolar	1¾–2 years	—	5–6 years	12–13 years	10–12 years
Second premolar	2¼–2¾ years	—	6–7 years	13–14 years	11–12 years
First molar	At birth	Sometimes a trace	2½–3 years	9–10 years	6–7 years
Second molar	2½–3 years	—	7–8 years	14–15 years	11–13 years
Third molar	8–10 years	—	12–16 years	18–25 years	17–21 years

APPENDIX D TOOTH NOTATION

Several notations are available. The two most commonly used are
that devised by the Fédération Dentaire Internationale (FDI) and
the Zsigmondy–Palmer system.

FDI
Permanent teeth

Right

18 17 16 15 14 13 12 11	21 22 23 24 25 26 27 28

Left

48 47 46 45 44 43 42 41	31 32 33 34 35 36 37 38

Thus, upper left first molar is written as: **26**

Deciduous teeth

Right

55 54 53 52 51	61 62 63 64 65

Left

85 84 83 82 81	71 72 73 74 75

Thus, upper left first deciduous molar is written: **64**

ZSIGMONDY–PALMER
Permanent teeth

Right

8 7 6 5 4 3 2 1	1 2 3 4 5 6 7 8

Left

8 7 6 5 4 3 2 1	1 2 3 4 5 6 7 8

e.g. upper left first molar is written as: $\lfloor 6$

Deciduous teeth

Right

e d c b a	a b c d e

Left

e d c b a	a b c d e

e.g. upper left first deciduous molar is written $\lfloor \mathbf{d}$

APPENDIX E INFECTION CONTROL

Adequate precautions should be in place at all times to prevent
infection and protect both patients and staff. Implementing safe
and realistic infection control procedures requires the full

compliance of the whole dental team. Thus adequate training is required and an infection control policy should be in place. Actions can be summarized as a series of *do's* and *do not's*.

Do
- Follow universal infection control procedures.
- Treat all patients as potentially infectious.
- Always use sterilized or disposable instruments.
- Wear operating gloves for all clinical procedures and when clearing contaminated instruments.
- Wear a mask and eye protection when undertaking work likely to produce an aerosol.
- Limit aerosols by efficient aspiration.
- Work in an organized and tidy fashion – place instruments only on the bracket table.
- Ensure appropriate cleaning and disinfection of surgery surfaces between patients.
- Dispose of sharps in a dedicated container.
- Ensure regulations relating to safe disposal of clinical waste are followed.
- Use appropriate cleaning techniques if spillage of body fluids occurs.
- Disinfect impressions and appliances before transfer to the laboratory.
- Ensure all clinical staff are appropriately immunized (especially hepatitis B).

Do not
- Re-cap needles with a two-handed technique.
- Wear gloves and masks in non-clinical areas, when answering the telephone, writing up notes, etc. Remember, hands are the most common source of contamination.
- Use sharp needles for irrigation.
- Leave burs in unattended handpieces.

In the event of a needle-stick or sharps injury
- Encourage the wound to bleed freely.
- Wash thoroughly in running water but do not scrub.
- Cover wound with appropriate dressing.
- Establish hepatitis antibody status of injured party.
- Contact Occupational Health Service or consultant in communicable disease/consultant microbiologist for advice on follow-up. This may include a request to the patient for assessment of hepatitis virus serology and HIV status.

The British Dental Association has produced a very useful advice sheet (A12) which provides guidance on Infection Control in Dentistry.

APPENDIX F NORMAL LABORATORY VALUES OF RELEVANCE TO MEDICINE

It should be noted that some values may vary from laboratory to laboratory.

HAEMATOLOGY

Hb	Male 13–18 g/dl Female 12–16 g/dl
Packed red cell volume (PCV)	Male 40–54% Female 37–47%
Red cell count	$4.6–6.2 \times 10^{12}$/l
Mean corpuscular volume (MCV)	80–100 fl
Mean corpuscular Hb (MCH)	27–32 pg
Mean corpuscular Hb concentration (MCHC)	32–38 g/dl
Total blood volume	70 ± 10 ml/kg
White cell count	$4.0–11.0 \times 10^9$/l
Neutrophils	$2.5–7.5 \times 10^9$/l
Lymphocytes	$1.5–3.5 \times 10^9$/l
Monocytes	$0.2–0.8 \times 10^9$/l
Eosinophils	$0.04–0.44 \times 10^9$/l
Basophils	$0.015–0.1 \times 10^9$/l
Platelets	$150–400 \times 10^9$/l
Bleeding and clotting times are always measured against a laboratory control and reported as such	
Serum iron	Male 14–31 μmol/l Female 11–29 μmol/l
Total iron binding capacity (TIBC)	45–72 μmol/l
Serum ferritin	25–300 μg/l

(cont'd)

Serum vitamin B_{12}	150–900 ng/l
Serum folate	3–20 µg/l
Red cell folate	160–640 µg/l

Erythrocyte sedimentation rate (ESR) varies according to age and gender.

BIOCHEMISTRY

Albumin	35–50 g/l
Alkaline phosphatase (adult)	30–300 iu/l
Aspartate–amino transferase (AST)	5–40 iu/l
Bilirubin	3–17 µmol/l
Bicarbonate	25–33 mmol/l
Calcium	2.2–2.65 mmol/l
Chloride	97–107 mmol/l
Creatinine	40–130 µmol/l
Gammaglutamyl transferase (γGT)	7–51 iu/l
Glucose	3.5–6.0 mmol/l
Phosphate	0.65–1.45 mmol/l
Potassium	3.5–5.0 mmol/l
Protein (total)	60–80 g/l
Sodium	135–145 mmol/l
Urea	2.5–7.5 mmol/l
Uric acid	Male 210–480 µmol/l Female 150–390 µmol/l
IgG	7.2–19 g/l
IgA	0.8–5.0 g/l
IgM	0.5–2.0 g/l
Arterial blood gases pH	7.36–7.44
Carbon dioxide ($PaCO_2$)	4.7–6.0 kPa
Oxygen (PaO_2)	10.7–13.3 kPa

INDEX

Abducens nerve, 514
Abfraction, 280
Abrasion
  cavity preparation, 253
  polishing, 146–7
  tooth wear, 279
  see also Microabrasion
Abscess
  apical, 401
  patterns of spread, 402
  see also Dental abscess; Periapical
    abscess; Periodontal abscess
Absorbed dose, 36
Absorbent pads, 174
Abutment teeth
  Ante's law, 272
  care of, 323
  definition, 270
  dome or thimble shaped, 323
  fixed bridges, 270–1, 274
  fixed–movable bridges, 275
  overdentures, 322, 323
  selection, 323
Access cavities see Cavities
Accessory nerve, 514
Acetylcysteine, 66
Achalasia, 494
Achondroplasia, 510
Aciclovir, 79–80, 445, 446, 454
Acid etch splints, 190
Acid etching, 127
Acid reflux, 495
Acid regurgitation, 279
Acinic cell carcinoma, 468
Acquired coagulopathies, 502
Acquired (secondary)
  immunodeficiency, 518
Acromegaly, 507
Acrylic
  allergy, 314
  antimicrobial fibres/gel, 227
  baseplates, 371
  dentures, 319, 326
  high impact, 142
  relines, 326
  splints, 190, 229
  teeth, 147
ACTH see Adrenocorticotrophic
  hormone

Actinic keratosis, 517–18
Actinobacillus
  actinomycetemcomitans, 201
Acupuncture, 329, 330
Acute chest pain, 524–5
Acute necrotizing periodontitis,
  486
Acute necrotizing ulcerative
  gingivitis (ANUG), 75, 202, 204,
  224–5, 486
Acute pancreatitis, 498
Acute viral hepatitis, 497
Adam's clasp, 190, 336, 370
Addition silicones, 135
Additions, 327
Adenoid cystic carcinoma, 469
Adenolymphoma, 468
Adenomas
  monomorphic, 468
  pleomorphic, 467–8, 469
ADH (antidiuretic hormone)
  deficiency, 507
Adhesion, 126–7, 148
  achieving, 126–7
  factors promoting, 127
  micromechanical, 126
  molecular attraction, 126
Adhesive bridges
  anterior, 277
  case selection, 277
  clinical tips, 277–8
  design, 277
  lifespan, 278
  posterior, 277
  recementing, 278
Adhesive/dentine bonded crowns,
  266–7
Adhesives, dentine, 249
Adolescence
  dental caries, 159
  occult caries, 153
  orthognathic surgery, 379
Adrenal crisis, 529–30
Adrenal gland disorders, 507
Adrenaline see Epinephrine
Adrenocorticotrophic hormone
  (ACTH), 493, 507
Adult Basic Life Support algorithm,
  526

Adult Dental Health Survey (1998), 151
Advanced cardiac life support, 527
Advanced Life Support Cardiac Arrest Algorithm, 528
Aerosols, infection control, 543
Aesthetics
  bridgework, 271
  crowns, 138–9, 256
  dentures, 300, 308, 313, 318, 321, 324
  IOTN, 350
  orthognathic surgery, 432
  veneers, 263, 265
Agar hydrocolloids, 134
Agranulocytosis, 70
AIDS see HIV-positive patient
Air abrasion, 253
Airway
  maxillofacial emergency action, 423
  stroke, 531
ALARP principle, 39
Albers–Schönberg disease (osteopetrosis), 510
Albright's syndrome, 510
Alcohol abuse
  erosion, 279
  general anaesthesia, 112
  hepatitis, 497
  mouth cancer, 462
  pancreatitis, 498
Alginate hydrocolloids, 134
Allergies
  oral dysaesthesia, 474
  orofacial granulomatosis, 481
  recurrent aphthous stomatitis, 449
  to:
    acrylic, 314
    amalgam, 121, 516
    cephalosporins, 77
    local anaesthesia, 100
    methacrylate, 142
    nickel, 141
    penicillin, 77
  see also Hypersensitivity
Allografts, 437
Allopurinol, 471

Alloys
  cobalt–chromium, 140–1
  dental gold, 140
  metal properties, altering, 139–40
  nickel–chromium, 141
  steel, 141
  titanium, 145
  types, 139
Altered cast impression technique, 319
Aluminium oxide, 145
Aluminous porcelain, 137
Alveolar bone graft, 379
Alveolar cleft, 379
Alveolar osteitis (dry socket), 75, 76, 387–8
Alveolar ridge
  architecture problems, 419
  contouring of crest, 297
  resorption, 301, 419–20
  see also Implants
Alzheimer's disease, 321
Amalgam, 119–21
  allergy, 121, 516
  alloy formation, 120
  basic properties, 119
  biocompatibility, 120–1
  chronic fatigue syndrome, 516
  components and metallurgy, 119
  disposal, 121
  post crowns, 260
  primary teeth, 178
  safety, 120–1
  setting reaction, 119–20
  tattoo, 460
'Amalgam free mouth', 148
Ameloblastic fibromas, 410
Ameloblastomas, 409
Amelodentinal junction, caries removal, 243
Amelogenesis imperfecta, 179, 193
Amide link, 92
Amitriptyline, 84, 475
Amoxicillin (amoxycillin), 71, 72, 75, 76, 90, 226, 227, 495, 503
Amphotericin, 77, 78, 444
Ampicillin, 76

Anaemia, 498–9
  causes, 499
  definition, 483, 498
  iron deficiency, 499
  macrocytic, 499
  microcytic, 499
  normocytic, 499
  oral features, 483
  primary sideropenic, 462, 481,
    483, 494
  sickle cell, 499
Anaesthesia
  examination under (EUA), 411
  see also General anaesthesia;
    Local anaesthesia
Analgesics, 62–3, 65–6
Anaphylactic shock, 70, 84, 527–9
Anchorage
  baseplates, 371
  definition, 358
  loss, 373
  orthodontic treatment plan, 358
Angina bullosa haemorrhagica
  (localized oral purpura), 451–2
Angina pectoris, 492, 494, 524
Angio-oedema, 70, 407
Angiography, 49
Angiotensin-converting (ACE)
  inhibitors, 492
Angle's classification, 349
Angular cheilitis, 77, 79, 87, 88, 443,
  483, 494
Ankylosing spondylitis, 513
Ankylosis, 430
Annealing, 140
Anorexia nervosa, 470, 494
Anterior crowns, 256–8
Anterior disc displacement
  acute, without reduction, 472
  chronic, without reduction, 473
  with reduction, 472
Anterior palatal bar, 315
Anterior pituitary, 507
Anterior/posterior relationship, 352,
  353, 356, 363, 365, 367
Ante's law, 272
Anticholinergic agents, 471
Anticoagulants, 64, 89
Anticonvulsants, 81, 461

Antidepressants, 83–4, 465
  epinephrine and, 93
  see also individual drugs;
    Monoamine oxidase
    inhibitors; Tricyclic
    antidepressants
Anti-epileptics, 194
Antifibrinolytics, 502
Antifungal agents, 77–8, 444
Antihistamines, 84–5, 465, 471, 501,
  522
Antihypertensives, 465
  oral effects, 492
  see also Beta blockers
Antimalarials, 461, 471
Antimicrobials, 68, 215, 226,
  227–8
Anti-Parkinsonian agents, 471
Antiplatelet agents, 525
Anti-snoring appliances, 325
Antithyroid agents, 470, 471
Antiviral agents, 79–80
Antibiotic prophylaxis
  cardiac murmurs, 492
  dialysis patients, 504
  infective endocarditis, 70–1, 75,
    76
  prosthetic joints, 513
  warfarinized patients, 503
Antibiotic-associated colitis (AAC),
  70, 77, 497
Antibiotics, 68–70
  antagonism, 69
  bacterial resistance, 69–70
  bacterial sialadenitis, 470
  bacteriocidal/bacteriostatic, 68
  commonly used, 74–7
  definition, 68
  in dentistry, 70–7
  peptic ulcers, 495
  periodontal abscess, 75
  periodontal disease, 227–8
  pulpotomy, 181
  resistance, 215, 228
  side effects, 70
  spectrum of activity, 69
  synergism, 69
ANUG see Acute necrotizing
  ulcerative gingivitis

Anxiety, 7–8
  asthma, 493
  atypical facial pain, 475
  dental, 168, 171
  measuring, 8
  oesophageal spasm, 494
  and pain, 10, 234
  recurrent aphthous stomatitis, 448
  reducing, 8–9, 81, 105
  xerostomia, 465
Anxiolytics, 80–2, 104
Apexification (calcific bridge), 184
Apical curettage, 397
Apicectomy, 396–8
  definition, 295
  indications, 295, 396–7
  technique, 397–8
Apices, open, 183–4
Arachidonic acid, 63
Archwires, 374–5
Arrested caries, 153, 269
Arrhythmias, 95
Arteriovenous (A-V) fistulae, 504
Arthritis
  psoriatic, 513
  rheumatoid, 473, 512–13, 518
  systematic-onset juvenile, 513
  see also Osteoarthritis
Articaine, + epinephrine, 94
Articulation paper, 241, 311
Articulators, 242, 302
Aspirator, high-volume, 174
Aspirin, 63–4, 471, 525
Astemizole, 85
Asthma, 493, 530–1
Asthmatic drugs, 64
Asystole, 525
Atopy, 527
Atracurium, 110
Atraumatic restorative treatment, 178
Atrophic glossitis, 441, 483
Atropine, 109, 465, 471
Attachment, 374
Attachments
  fixed appliances, 374–5
  overdentures, 323
  precision, 321

Attrition, 279
Atypical facial pain, 51, 62, 234, 475
Atypical odontalgia, 475
Audit cycle, 26
Auricular (ear) prostheses, 337
Auscultation, 406
Auxiliaries, 375
Avulsion, 189
Azathioprine, 450, 453, 479

B-cell defects, 518
Backings, 266
Baclofen, 476
Bacterial infections, 440–1
  periodontal disease, 201
  sialadenitis, 469–70
Bacterial resistance, antibiotics, 69–70
Bactericidal drugs, 68
Bacteriostatic drugs, 68
Balanced articulation, complete dentures, 308
Balanced force technique, 290–1
Balancing extraction, 360
Bands, 374
Barbiturates, 454, 471
Bars, 321
Basal cell carcinoma (rodent ulcer), 409, 517
Baseplates, 371
Bases, 128–30
Basic Periodontal Examination (BPE), 206, 208–10
Battle's sign, 424
Beclometasone dipropionate, 87, 450, 479
Behaviour modification, 4–7
  change model, 5–6
  children, 170–2
  craniomandibular disorders, 329
  health locus of control, 6–7
  maintaining, 7
  relapse, 7
  targets, 6
Behçet's disease, 513
Behçet's syndrome, 450–1
Bell's palsy, 80, 482–3

Benign migratory glossitis, 464
Bennett angle, 239
Bennett shift, 239
Benzatropine, 471
Benzhexol, 471
Benzodiazepines, 81–3, 109
    pharmacokinetics, 104–5
    sedation, 102
Benzydamine hydrochloride, 88,
    450, 479
Benzylpenicillin, 74
Beta-blockers, 471, 477
    see also Antihypertensives
Betamethasone, 87, 144, 292, 450,
    479
Betel chewing, 459, 462
Bilateral free end saddle dentures,
    315, 319
Bimaxillary proclination, 363
Biochemistry values, 545
Biocompatibility, 118
Biopsy, 16
    definition, 398
    excisional, 398
    incisional, 399
    labial gland, 466
    punch, 399
    technique, 399
    white/red lesions, 459
BIS-GMA resin, 122, 146, 176
Bis-phenol A, 122
Bisecting angle technique, 43
Bite planes, 369, 371
Biteguard, 229
Bitewing radiographs, 37, 38, 43–4,
    52, 154, 234
Black hairy tongue, 460
Bladder infections, 503
Bleach 'walking', 286
Bleaching
    gel, 284
    non-vital teeth, 285–6
    splints, 325
    vital teeth, 283–5
Bleeding
    disorders, 64, 501–3
    on probing, 206, 210, 224
    see also Haemorrhage
Blood loss, chronic, 494, 496

Blood tests, 16
Blood vessel defects, 501
Bonding agents, 127, 128, 144
Bone
    developmental disease, 509–10
    fractures, radiographs, 186
    grafting, 335, 379, 422
    healing, 383
    implant success, 421–2
    infection, 405
    irregularities, 419–20
    metabolic disease, 510–11
    osteoporosis, 511
    Paget's disease, 511
    pathology, 193, 407
    removal, extractions, 391
    resorption, 301, 419–20
    scans, 49, 50
    substitutes, 437
    thermal injury avoidance, 421
Bone cysts (non-epithelial)
    aneurysmal, 407, 413
    solitary, 413
    Stafne's, 413
Bony exostoses, 481
Bottle brushes (interproximal), 214
Bowen's disease (carcinoma in situ),
    411, 458, 518
Bows, 371
BPE see Basic Periodontal
    Examination
Brachytherapy, 411
Bracing, 318
Brackets, 374
Bradykinesia, 516
Bradykinin, 63
Branchial cyst, 407
Breastfeeding, drugs, 62
    aciclovir, 80
    benzodiazepines, 83
    cautionary note, 89
    dihydrocodeine tartrate, 67
    fluconazole, 79
Bridges
    natural teeth to implant, 335
    porcelain, 137
    spring cantilever, 276
    see also Adhesive bridges; Fixed
        bridges

British Approved Names (BAN), 90

British Dental Association (BDA), 345

British National Formulary (BNF), 60, 89, 161

British Standards Institute's Incisor Classification, 348

Brittle bone disease (osteogenesis imperfecta), 509

Brittleness, 116

Broaches, 288

Bronchial carcinoma, 493

Brown Kelly–Paterson syndrome (Plummer–Vinson syndrome), 462, 481, 483, 494

Brown spot lesions, 152

Brushite, 205

Bruton's syndrome, 518

Bruxism, 113, 228, 271, 279, 281

Buccal bar, 316

Buccal fat pad transfer, 418

Buccal flaps, 393, 416–17

Buccal nerve block, 97, 98

Buccal segment relationship, 344, 353, 363, 365, 367

Buccolingual relationship see Crossbite

Bulimia nervosa, 279, 470, 495

Bulk alumina slabs, 137

Bulk sweeteners, 158

Bullous pemphigoid, 452, 453–4

Bupivacaine, 94

Bupropion, 164

Burning mouth syndrome (oral dysaesthesia), 473–5, 483, 509

Burns, chemical, 456

Burs, 175, 391, 393

Butt joint, 254, 266

Butterfly rash, 512

CAD-CAM technology, 137, 269

Café au lait spots, 510

Calcific bridge, 184

Calcifying epithelial odontogenic tumour, 409

Calcium channel blockers, 471, 477, 492

Calcium hydroxide, 129, 251–2, 292
  non-setting, 144
  sealer, 143

Calculus
  removal, 216
  subgingival, 206, 216
  supragingival, 205

Callus, 383

Camphorated monochlorophenol, 144

Cancer see Mouth cancer; Neoplasia; Tumours

Cancrum oris/noma, 404

Candida spp., 77, 442, 462, 474
  see also Oral candidosis

Candidal leukoplakia see Leukoplakia

Canines
  cavity preparation, 289
  early loss of deciduous, 359
  ectopic upper, 192
  eruption, 173, 540, 541
  exposure/removal of maxillary, 395–6
  extraction technique, 385
  lateral movement guided, 241
  mineralization, 540, 541
  spread of abscess, 402

Cantilever fixed bridges, 275

Capacity, 22

Captopril, 474

Carbamazepine, 67–8, 454, 471, 476

Carbon dioxide laser, 400–1

Carbonated drinks, 159, 279, 281

Carcinoma in situ, 411, 458, 518

Carcinomas, 409, 464
  see also specific carcinomas

Cardiac disorders, 194
  dosulepin, 84
  epinephrine, 93, 94
  local anaesthesia, 95
  see also Infective endocarditis; Ischaemic heart disease; Myocardial infarction

Cardiac failure, 492

Cardiac murmurs, 492

Cardiac pacemakers, 73

Carding wax, 145

Cardiorespiratory arrest, 525–7

Cardiovascular disorders, 491–2
Cardiovascular system, local anaesthesia, 93, 95, 100
Caries, 152–62
　abutment teeth, 322
　aetiology, 152
　arrested, 153, 269
　atraumatic restorative treatment, 178
　cavity preparation, 243
　cervical, 248
　changing levels, 152
　chemocanical removal, 179
　dentine, 153
　diagnosis, 50–2, 153–4
　diet, 156–9
　DMFT index, 154–5
　dyes, 154
　electronic detector, 154
　enamel, 152
　examination, 236, 301
　fibreoptic transillumination (FOTI), 154
　fissure, 153
　fluoride, 160–2
　impacted third molars, 391
　microbiology, 156
　nursing bottle, 153, 169
　occult, 153
　orthodontics, 345, 346–7
　rampant, 153
　recurrent, 153
　restoration, primary teeth, 177–9
　risk, 155
　root, 153, 224
　secondary, 153
　special needs children, 194
　sugar, 157
　see also Deep carious lesions
Carious exposures, 182, 252
Carisolv, 179
Carmellose sodium, 88
Casts/casting
　alloys, 139–41, 148
　surveying, 302
　try-in of, 274
Causation, 21
Cavernous sinus thrombosis, 404
Cavitation effect, 217

Cavities
　Black's classification, 244
　cavosurface angle, 243
　class I, 177, 178, 244–5
　class II, 177–8, 178, 245–6
　class III, 178, 246–7
　class IV, 178, 247–8
　class V, 178, 248
　composite layering technique, 247
　enamel margin finishing, 243
Cavity preparation
　air abrasion, 253
　basic principles, 242–3
　cavity toilet, 243
　enamel margin finishing, 243
　objective, 242
　outline form, 243
　remaining caries, 243
　resistance form, 243
　retention form, 243
　root canal therapy, 289
　sonic preparation, 252–3
　stages, 243
Cavity toilet, 243
Cavity varnishes, 130
Cavosurface angle, 243
Cefadrine (cephadrine), 90
Cefalexin (cephalexin), 77, 90
Cementation
　adhesive bridges, 278
　crowns, 255–6, 260
　fixed-fixed bridges, 275
　inlays, 268, 269
　veneers, 264–5
Cementifying fibromas, 410
Cements
　adhesive bridges, 278
　EBA, 129
　luting, 128–30, 268
　temporary, 130–1
Cementum
　abnormal, 193
　removal, 216
Central giant cell tumour, 407
Central nervous system
　amalgam, 121
　local anaesthesia, 93
Centreline relationship, 344, 353

Cephalometrics, 354–5
  analysis of lateral cephalogram, 355 6
  ANB angle and skeletal values, 356, 357
  definition, 354
  values, 357
Cephalosporins, 77
Ceramic palatal veneers, 266
Ceramics, 116, 136–7
  CAD-CAM, 137, 269
  injection moulded, 137, 257, 262
Cerebellopontine angle tumours, 482
Cerebral palsy, 113, 194
Cerebrospinal fluid (CSF) leak, 424
Cerebrovascular accident (stroke), 430, 531
Cermets, 125
Cervical plexus, 438
Cetirizine, 85
Cetrimide, 86
Chain of Survival, 525
Chairside bleaching, 285–6
Chamfers, 254, 266
Chance HLOC, 7
Chancre, 441
Change model, 5–6
Chemical burns, 456
Chemical etching, 277
Chemical plaque control, 215–16
Chemomechanical caries removal, 179
Chemotherapy, 486, 500
Cherubism, 407, 510–11
Chest pain, acute, 524–5
Chewing
  betel, 459, 462
  endocarditis, 71
  pencil/finger nail, 228
  tooth wear, 279
Chewing gum, saliva stimulant, 159, 466
Chickenpox (varicella zoster), 445–6
Child Dental Health Survey (2003), 185

Children
  aims of treating, 168
  behaviour modification, 170–2
  bone pathology, 193
  dentition development, 172–4
  drugs
    aspirin, 64
    chlorphenamine maleate, 85
    doses, 61
    fluconazole, 79
    ibuprofen, 65
    paracetamol, 65
  examination, 168
  fluoride toothpastes, 160–1
  general anaesthesia, 108, 109, 113
  hard tissue pathology, 190–3
  history, 168
  local anaesthesia, 95
  operating field management, 174–5
  pit/fissure sealants, 176
  preventive regimen, 169
  preventive vs. restorative care, 169
  pulp therapy, 180–2
  restoration of carious primary teeth, 177–9
  role of parents or carers, 169–70
  soft tissue disease, 193
  special needs, 193–5
  tooth form abnormalities, 191
  tooth number abnormalities, 190–1
  tooth position abnormalities, 191–2
  tooth structure abnormalities, 192–3
  trauma
    aetiology, 185
    classification, 185
    examination, 186
    history, 185–6
    predisposing factors, 185
    prevalence, 185
    treatment, 187–90
  treatment planning, 168–9
Chisel (push) scaler, 217, 218
Chlorhexidine, 71, 85–6, 215–16, 224, 226, 228, 388, 395, 402, 450, 471, 479

+ cetrimide (Savlon), 86

Chloroquine, 471

Chlorphenamine (chlorpheniramine) maleate, 85, 90, 522, 529

Choline salicylate, 88

Christmas disease (haemophilia B), 502

Chroma, 138

Chronic acid reflux, 495

Chronic discoid lupus erythematosus (CDLE), 480

Chronic erythematous candidosis (denture stomatitis), 79, 443, 444

Chronic fatigue syndrome, 516

Chronic hepatitis, 497, 518

Chronic hyperplastic candidosis (candidal leukoplakia), 443, 444, 459, 462

Chronic liver disease, 497–8

Chronic obstructive pulmonary disease (COPD), 83, 493

Chronic pancreatitis, 498

Chronic renal failure (CRF), 504

Chvostek's sign, 506

Ciclosporin, 471

Cingulum rests, 319

Circulatory collapse, maxillofacial trauma, 424

Cirrhosis, 470

Clasps
Adam's, 190, 336, 370
design, 317–18
retention, 327
Southend, 370
stainless steel, 141

Cleft lip and palate, 336–7, 377–9
aetiology, 377
anatomy, 435
associated problems, 377–8
classification, 377
incidence, 377
management, 378–9
surgery, 433–6

Cleidocranial dysostosis, 510

Clenching see Bruxism

Clindamycin, 72, 77, 497

Clinical audit, 25, 26–8

Clinical effectiveness, 28–9

Clinical governance, 25–6

Clinical guidelines, 28

Clinical records, 22, 24–5, 29

Close bite, 325

Clostridium difficile, 70, 497

Cluster headache (periodic migrainous neuralgia), 477

CMD *see* Craniomandibular disorders

Coagulation cascade defects, 502–3

Cobalt–chromium
alloys, 140–1
bonding to, 142
dentures, 319, 326
undercut depth, 318

Cocaine, 93

Codeine, 66, 495

Codes for Periodontal Treatment Assessment, 210

Coeliac disease, 448, 449, 495–6

Colchicine, 450

Cold sores (herpes labialis, secondary herpes simplex), 80, 445

Colitis
antibiotic-associated, 70, 77, 497
ulcerative, 448, 481, 496

Collagen, 382, 437

Collagenase, 201

Collapse
diabetic patient, 524
steroid, 509
see also Anaphylactic shock

Colloids, emergency, 523

Colorectal cancer, 497

Colour washout, 138

Committee on Safety of Medicines (CSM), 60

Communication, 3–4
non-verbal, 4, 171
pain control, 10

Community Periodontal Index of Treatment Need (CPITN), 208–9

Compactors, 288

Compensating extraction, 360

Complaints, 30–1

Complement deficiencies, 518

Complete dentures
aims, 304
common problems, 313

Complete dentures (*cont'd*)
 design features, 307–8
 impressions, 308–10, 312
 insertion, 311–12
 jaw registration, 310–11
 maximal extension, 307
 muscle balance, 305–7, 313
 occlusal balance, 307, 313
 occlusal pivots, 312
 retention, 305, 313
 review, 312
 stability, 307
 support, 305, 306, 313
 trial, 311
Compomers (poly-acid modified
  composites), 126, 178
Composite materials, 116
 adhesive bridges, 278
 inlays, 268–9
 primary teeth restoration, 178
 veneers, 265
 see also Resin composites
Compton scatter, 35
Computed tomography (CT), 48,
  416, 425, 476
Condensation silicones, 136
Condylar hyperplasia, 50, 51
Condylar neck, 430
Condyle
 radiographs, 45–7
 terminal hinge axis, 242
 see also Mandible
Condyloma acuminatum, 447
Confidentiality, 22
Congenital (primary)
  immunodeficiency, 518
Congenital syphilis, 441
Congenital TMJ disorders, 431
Connective tissue disorders,
  511–12
Connectors, 315–16
 minor, 318
Conroy obturator, 336
Consent, 22, 102, 112
Contact points
 crown cementation, 255–6
 inlays, 268
 poor, 256
 premature, 207

Continuing professional
  development (CPD), 25, 29–30
Continuous ambulatory peritoneal
  dialysis (CAPD), 504
Continuous clasp, and lingual bar,
  316
Continuous cyclical peritoneal
  dialysis (CCPD), 504
Contour materials, 437
Contractual consideration, 22–3
Contrast techniques, 49–50
Controlled areas, radiation, 42
Controlled drugs (CD), 60, 61
Conventional tomography, 48
Cooling, 140
Copper, 119, 120, 140
Copy dentures, 321–2
Core restorations, 248–50
Corrosion, 117, 259
Corticosteroid prophylaxis, 507–9
Corticosteroid-antibiotic paste, 252
Corticosteroids
 lichen planus, 479
 shingles, 446
Cortisol, 507
Cotton-wool rolls, 174
Coumarin, 64, 502
Coupland's elevator, 390
Coxsackie viruses
 hand, foot and mouth disease,
  446
 herpangina, 446
CPITN *see* Community Periodontal
  Index of Treatment Need
Crack propagation, 137
Cranial implants, 421
Cranial nerves, 513–14
 assessment, 514
 palsies, 515
Craniofacial prostheses, 337
Craniomandibular disorders,
  327–30
 diagnosis, 328
 fixed prosthodontics/endodontics,
  235
 management, 328–30
 orthodontics, 346, 347
 prosthodontics, 300
 treatment, 471

Craniomandibular disorders (*cont'd*)
  see also Myofascial pain dysfunction syndrome
Cricothyrotomy, 531
Crohn's disease, 448, 480–1, 496
Cross infections, 100
Crossbite, 346
  bilateral, 362
  correction, 369
  examination, 353
  lingual, 365
  local, 362
  segmental, 362
  treatment of posterior, 361
  unilateral
    with associated displacement, 362
    with no displacement, 362
Crowding
  Class I occlusions, 361–2
  see also Spacing
Crown:root ratio, 207
Crowns
  adhesive/dentine bonded, 266–7
  anterior, 256–8
  assessment of teeth, 253
  cementing, 255
  definition, 253
  faults
    negative margin, 256
    overhanging margin, 256
    persistent debonding, 256
    poor aesthetics, 256
    poor contact point, 256
    poor gingival emergence angle, 256
  metal–ceramic, 137–9, 256–7, 261
  milled, 274, 319
  partial denture design, 297
  porcelain, 137
  post retained, 258–61
  posterior, 261–2
  preformed acetate, 187–8
  preformed metal, 179
  preparation, 253
  surgical lengthening, 297
  temporization, 147, 254
  types, 253

Cryoanalgesia, 401
Cryoneurectomy, 401
Cryosurgery, 401, 486
Crypts, abnormal position, 192
Crystals (grains), 139
Curettes, 217, 218
Curing
  cold, 142
  heat, 142
  stages, 142
Cushing's disease, 507
Cushing's syndrome, 507
Cyclic neutropenia, 203, 448, 484
Cystic fibrosis, 494
Cystitis, 503
Cysts
  classification, 413
  definition, 412
  enucleation and primary closure, 414
  marsupialization, 414–15
  mucous extravasation, 469
  mucous retention, 469
  orthograde root canal therapy, 413
  pathogenesis, 413
  see also Bone cysts; *specific cysts*
Cytokines, 201
Cytotoxic chemotherapy, 500
Cytotoxic drugs, 471

Dapsone, 450, 453
Darier's disease (follicular keratosis), 456
Data collection and retention, 31
Data Protection Act (1988), 25
Debonding, 256, 259, 271, 347
Debris index, 208
Deciduous (primary) dentition
  development, 173
  early loss, 359
  eruption, 540
  mineralization, 540
  notation, 542
  orthodontics, 344, 359–60
  pulp therapy, 180–2
  restoration, 177–9
  trauma, 187

Deep carious lesions, 250–2
Deep tissue tumours, 411
Deformation, 116
Dehydration, dry mouth, 465
Dens-in-dente, 191
Dental abscess
  antibiotics, 75, 76
  infection, 401
  radiographs, 51
Dental Anxiety Scale, 8
Dental arch
  assessment, 352–4
  interarch variation, 344
  shortened, 337–8
  treatment plan, 357
Dental attendance, 164–5
Dental care
  clinical audit, 26–8
  clinical effectiveness, 28–9
  clinical governance, 25–6
  ethical and medico-legal
    considerations, 20–5
  evidence-based, 28
  need v. demand, 2
  professionals, 165–6
  psychological aspects, 2–10
  quality, 25
Dental caries see Caries
Dental disease
  aetiology, 2
  changing levels, 151–2
  special needs children, 194
Dental floss, 214
Dental floss threader, 214
Dental health component (IOTN),
  350–1
Dental health educator, 166
Dental hygienist, 166, 334
Dental materials
  biocompatibility properties, 118
  chemical properties, 117–18
  current growth areas, 147–8
  mechanical properties, 116
  molecular form, 116
  physical properties, 117
  setting properties, 119
  storage, 118
  testing, 118–19
Dental nurse, 166

Dental phobia, 109, 113, 168, 172
Dental Practitioner's Formulary, 60
Dental recalls, 165
Dental tape, 214
Dental teams
  communication within, 4
  registration requirement, 20
Dental technician, 166, 338–9
Dental therapist, 166
Dentigerous (follicular) cysts, 391,
  413
Dentine
  abnormal, 193
  adhesives, 249
  bonding, 127, 144
  caries, 153
  fractures, 187–8
  hypersensitivity, 224, 229, 265
  pins, 249
  reparative formation, 252
Dentinogenesis imperfecta, 179, 193
Dentist Help Support Trust, 31
Dentists Act (1984), 20
Dentition
  late changes, 174
  management of developing,
    358–9
  orthodontic intervention, 344
  pre-teeth, 172–3
  see also Deciduous (primary)
    dentition; Mixed dentition;
    Permanent (secondary)
    dentition
Dentoalveolar surgery
  apicectomy, 396–8
  chlorhexidine, 86
  extractions, 388–91
  impacted third molars, 391–5
  maxillary canine
    exposure/removal, 395–6
Denture space
  definition, 304
  impression technique, 312
Dentures
  additions, 327
  aesthetics, 300, 308, 318, 321, 324
  appearance problems, 313
  base materials, 141–2
  care, elderly patients, 165

Dentures (cont'd)
cleaning, 339–40
coping with new, 339
diagnosis
edentulous patients, 302–3
partially dentate patients, 303
discomfort with new, 339
eating with new, 339
examination, 236, 300–2
fracture, 325
history, 300
hyperplasia, 407, 420, 421
immediate, 324, 340
looseness, 339
management, 303–4
oral dysaesthesia, 474
overextended, 301
patient advice, 339–40
precision attachments, 321
prescription to technicians, 338–9
relines, 326–7
repairs, 325–6
speaking with new, 339
stomatitis, 79, 443, 444
teeth materials, 147
underextended, 301
unrealistic expectations, 313
see also Complete dentures; Copy
   dentures; Immediate dentures;
   Implant-borne prostheses;
   Partial dentures
Depression, 465, 474, 475
see also Antidepressants
Dermatitis herpetiformis, 452, 455
Dermatology, 517–18
see also Skin
Dermatomyositis, 512
Desensitization, 172, 314
Desmopressin, 502
Desquamative gingivitis, 235
Deterministic effects, 37
Detersive foodstuffs, 159
Devitalizing paste, 181
Diabetes insipidus, 507
Diabetes mellitus, 498, 505–6, 518
definition, 505
dry mouth, 465
NSAIDS, 63–4
oral candidosis, 443

oral dysaesthesia, 474
patient collapse, 524
periodontitis, 203
sialosis, 470
spreading infection, 404
treatment under GA, 505–6
treatment under LA, 505–6
Diagnosis, 16
Diagnostic wax-up, 241, 253, 302,
   334
Diaphragm, 261
Diarrhoea, 70
Diastemas, 190, 229
labial veneers, 263
Diazemuls, 105
Diazepam, 81, 82, 83, 105, 523, 530
Diet
caries, 156–9
cariogenicity, 157
diary, 157
elderly patients, 165
erosion, 279
irritable bowel syndrome, 496
mouth cancer, 462
special needs children, 194
tooth wear prevention, 281
DiGeorge syndrome, 518
Digital imaging, 47
Digital photography, 302, 324, 334
Dihydrocodeine tartrate, 67
Dilaceration, 191
Diltiazem, 471
Dimethylchlortetracycline paste,
   292
Dimethylsiloxane, 135, 136
Diplopia (double vision), 514
Disability, 193–4
Disclosing agents, 212
Dislocations
metal crystal imperfections, 139
temporomandibular joint, 430
Displacement injuries, treatment,
   188–9
Distraction, 10, 172
Diuretics, 471, 492
Diving mouthpiece, 325
DMFT index, 154–5
Dolder bar, 422
Doppler imaging, 49

Dosulepin (dothiepin), 84, 90, 473, 475
Down syndrome, 113, 194, 203, 518
Doxycycline hyclate (doxycycline hydrochloride), 75, 76–7, 90, 228
Drinks, carbonated, 159, 279, 281
Drug abuse, 112
Drugs
  craniomandibular disorders, 329
  effects on teeth, oral mucosa and salivary glands, 471
  emergency, 522–3
  erythema multiforme, 454
  interactions, 89
  melanin pigmentation, 461
  nomenclature, 89, 90
  oral dysaesthesia, 474
  prescribing principles, 60–2
  sialosis, 470
  special needs children, 194
  vascular pupuras, 501
  xerostomia, 465
  Yellow Card Scheme, 89
Dry mouth see Xerostomia
Dry socket (focal alveolar osteitis), 75, 76, 387–8
Ductility, 116
Duodenal ulcers, 64, 495
Duty of care, 21
Dyes, 154
Dyskeratosis congenita, 456
Dysphagia, 494–5
Dysplastic naevi, 518

Ear (auricular) prostheses, 337
EBA cements, 129
Edentulous spaces, Kennedy classification, 315
EDTA see Ethylenediamine tetra-acetic acid
Effective dose, 36
Elastase, 201
Elastic deformation, 116
Elastic impression materials, 133–6
Elastic modulus, 116
Elastics, 371, 375
Elastin, 382
Elastomers, 134–6

Elderly patients
  cleft lip and palate, 337
  copy dentures, 321
  denture care, 165
  diet, 165
  drug prescribing, 61, 64, 65, 68, 81, 82
  healing, 383
  history taking, 13
  local anaesthesia, 95
  mouth cancer, 463
  pemphigus, 453
  plaque control, 165
  polypharmacy, 62, 165
  prevention, 165
  root caries, 153
Electrical conductivity, 117
Electrolytic etching, 277
Electromechanical dissociation (EMD), 525
Electronic apex locators, 289
Electronic caries detector, 154
Electrotherapy (TENS), 329
Elevators, surgical extraction, 389–91
Emergencies
  drugs, 522–3
  equipment, 522
Enamel
  abnormal, 192
  bonding, 127
  caries, 152
  damage, 347
  fracture, 187–8
  hypomineralization, 192–3
  hypoplasia, 179, 192
  margin finishing, 243
  mottled, 162, 288
Endo-perio lesions, 297
Endocarditis see Infective endocarditis
Endocrine disorders, 461, 505–9
Endodontic lesions, 297
Endodontic status, examination, 236, 301
Endodontics
  diagnosis, 237
  instrument colour coding, 288
  management, 237–9

Endodontics (cont'd)
  materials, 143–4
  pulpal damage, 287
  surgical, 295–6
  treatment planning, 235–7
Endotracheal intubation, 423
Enhancing control, 171
Epidermolysis bullosa, 454
Epilepsy, 67, 515, 530
Epimine polymers, 147
Epinephrine (adrenaline), 90, 93
  + articaine, 94
  + lidocaine, 94, 95
  + prilocaine, 94
  cardiac disorders, 93, 94, 95
  emergency use, 522, 529
  hyperthyroidism, 506
  systemic effects, 94
Epithelial cysts, 413
Epithelial dysplasia, 458, 459
Epithelial odontogenic tumours, 409
Epithelium
  junctional, 199
  oral, 198
  sulcular, 198
Epstein–Barr virus (EBV), 485, 497, 518
Epulides, 509
Equivalent dose, 36
Erosion, 280–1
Eruption
  average dates, 540–1
  order and timing, 172
Erythema
  gingival, 206
  linear gingival, 486
  migrans, 464
  multiforme, 454, 471
Erythematous candidosis, 442, 444, 484
Erythroplakia, 458
Erythromycin, 75
Etch-retained metal splints, 229
Etchants, 127
Etching, 140
  acid, 127
  chemical, 277
  electrolytic, 277
Ethanol, 136, 142

Ethical guidance, 20–1
Ethylenediamine tetra-acetic acid (EDTA), 143
  + sodium hypochlorite, 292
  + urea peroxide, 143, 292
European Resuscitation Council guidelines, 525, 526
Evidence-based dentistry, 28
Examinations, 15
Excisional biopsy, 398
Exercise therapy, 329, 516
Extractions
  balancing, 360
  changes following, 304
  compensating, 360
  complications, 384–5
  forceps application, 386
  local anaesthesia, 384
  malocclusion, 368
  perioperative, 386–7
  postoperative, 387
  preoperative, 386
  radiography before, 53
  socket healing, 383
  surgical removal, 388–91
  technique, 384, 385
Extraoral examinations, 15
Extrinsic sugars, 156
Extrusion, 189, 369
Eye (ocular) prostheses, 337

Facebow mounting, 241, 302
Facial arthromyalgia see Myofascial pain dysfunction syndrome
Facial asymmetry, 431
Facial bone, radiographs, 55
Facial cellulitis, 404
Facial changes, following extraction, 304
Facial contours, 300
Facial deformity, 378, 432
  classification of surgery, 433
Facial implants, 421
Facial lacerations, 424, 425–7
Facial nerve
  assessment, 514
  palsy, 464, 482, 494
  paralysis, 468

Facial pain, 473–5
    atypical (persistent idiopathic),
        51, 62, 234, 475
Facial paralysis, 101
Facial plane, 356
Facial skeleton fractures, 71, 427–8,
    429
Facial skin, 425–6
Facial stereotyping, 346
Facial swellings, 51, 405–6, 406–7
Facial trauma, 108
Facings see Inlays
Factor VIII deficiency (haemophilia
    A), 502
Factor IX deficiency (haemophilia
    B), 502
Fainting (syncope, vasovagal
    episode), 100, 523
Falciparum malaria, 499
False pocket, 210
Famciclovir, 80, 445, 446
Fatigue (dental materials), 116
FDI notation, 542
Feathered incisal porcelain laminate
    veneers, 263, 264
Felypressin, 93–4
    + prilocaine, 94
Ferguson's gag, 113
Ferric sulphate vital pulpotomy, 181
Ferritin deficiency, 443, 449, 494
Fetal haemoglobin, persisting, 499
Fibreoptic transillumination
    (FOTI), 154
Fibroblasts, 201, 202, 382
Fibromas
    ameloblastic, 410
    cementifying, 410
    ossifying, 407
Fibrous dysplasia, 407, 510
Files, 218, 288, 291
Fine-needle aspiration, 49
A First Class Service Quality in the
    New NHS, 25
Fissure caries, 153
Fissure sealants, 145–6, 176
Fissured tongue (scrotal tongue),
    464
Fixation
    components, 370

external, 427
facial fractures, 427
internal, 437
Fixed appliances
    advantages/disadvantages, 375
    components, 374–5
    contraindications, 375
    definition, 374
    indications, 375
    malocclusion, 366, 368
    orthodontics, 358, 364
Fixed bridges
    Ante's law, 272
    cantilever, 275
    complications, 271
    components, 271
    conventional fixed–fixed, 274–5
    definitions, 270
    disadvantages, 270
    fixed–movable, 275–6
    general considerations, 270–1
    indications for, 270
    pontic design, 272, 273
    retainers, 272, 274
    saddles, 270
Fixed prosthodontics
    diagnosis, 237
    management, 237–9
    occlusion, 239, 242
    treatment planning, 235–7
Flanges, 309, 320, 324, 325, 326
Flaps, 221–2
    axial pattern, 436
    buccal, 393, 416–17
    extractions, 388–9, 393, 396
    free, 436–7
    labial, 396
    laterally repositioned, 223
    lingual, 393
    mucoperiosteal, 230, 388, 397
    palatal, 396
    palatal rotation, 417
    random pattern, 436
    replaced, 221–2
    repositioned, 222–3
Floss see Dental floss; Superfloss
Flucloxacillin, 76, 470
Fluconazole, 79, 444
Flumazenil, 81, 106, 107, 523

Fluoride
  caries, 160
  drops and tablets, 161, 162
  foams, 162
  gels, 161–2
  milk/fruit juices, 161
  modes of action, 159–60
  mouthwash, 162, 375
  safety, 162
  salt, 161
  tooth wear prevention, 281
  toothpaste, 159, 160–1, 162, 169
  varnishes, 162
  water, 160
Fluorosis, 162
Fluoxetine, 475
Focal epithelial hyperplasia (Heck's disease), 447
Foil splints, 190
Folate deficiency, 443, 449, 474
Folic acid deficiency, 494
Follicular keratosis (Darier's disease), 456
Food
  cariogenicity, 157
  detersive, 159
  see also Diet; Nutritional deficiencies; Sugars
Forceps extraction, 386
Foreign bodies
  inhaled, 531
  oral mucosa, 460
Formaldehyde containing sealers, 144
Formocresol, 181
Fractures
  bone, radiographs, 186
  dentine, 187–8
  dentures, 325
  enamel, 187–8
  facial skeleton, 71, 427–8, 429
  maxillary tuberosity, 419
  post crowns, 259
  radiographs, 425
  root, 186, 188, 418
  temporomandibular joint, 430
Fraena, 307
Fraenectomy, 223
Fraenula, 420

Frankfort plane, 352, 356
Free end saddles, 315, 316, 319
Free gingival grafts, 223
Freedom of Information Act, 25
Freeway space, 301, 308
Frey's syndrome, 438
Frictional keratosis, 457
Full coverage palatal plate, 316
Full-veneer crown, 261, 262
Functional appliances
  advantages, 376
  case selection, 376
  classification, 376
  definition, 376
  disadvantages, 377
  malocclusion, 368
  mode of action, 376
  orthodontics, 358, 364, 366
Functional occlusal plane (FOP), 356
Fungal infections, 442–4
Furcation lesions, 206, 210
  definition, 229
  treatment, 229–30
Furcation-plasty, 229
Fusobacteria spp., 201

Gabapentin, 476
Gallium, 148
Gamma-amino butyric acid (GABA), 81, 105
Gardner's syndrome, 481–2
Gastric carcinoma, 495
Gastritis, 495
Gastro-oesophageal reflux disease (GORD), 495
Gastrointestinal disorders, 494–8
  antibiotics, 70
  oral manifestations, 480–2
  tooth wear, 279
Gate Theory of Pain, 9
General anaesthesia, 107–13
  consent, 22
  GDC guidance, 108–9
  inpatient, 109–11
  outpatient, 111–13
  postoperative pain, 67
  premedication, 109, 112
  steroid collapse, 509

General Dental Council (GDC), 20, 22
  continuing professional development, 29–30
  general anaesthesia, 108–9
  sedation definition, 102
General dental practitioner (GDP), 343, 344, 356, 378
Genial tubercles, 420
Genioplasty, 379, 433, 434
Geographic tongue (benign migratory glossitis), 464
Giant cell arteritis (temporal arteritis), 477
Giant cell lesions, 407
Gingivae
  attached, 223
  erythema, 206
  healthy appearance, 199
  hyperplasia, 194, 206, 471, 492
  inflamed, 199
  periodontal ligament, 199
  recontouring, 225
  structure, 198–9
  see also Oral mucosa
Gingival crevice fractures, 188
Gingival crevicular fluid, 199, 201
Gingival emergence angle, 255, 256
Gingival papilla, 393
Gingival recession, 165, 206
  causes, 211
  free grafts, 223
  pocket chart, 211
  pocket depth, reduced, 219
  tooth brushing, 213
Gingival veneers, 325
Gingivectomy, 221
Gingivitis
  ANUG, 75, 202, 204, 224–5, 486
  children, 193
  definition, 199
  desquamative, 235
  development, 199
  inflamed appearance, 199
  orthodontics, 347
  outcomes, 200
  periodontitis, 200
  plaque-induced, 203, 211
    pregnancy, 509
    smoking, 202
Gingivostomatitis, primary herpetic, 444–5
Glandosane, 89, 466
Glasgow Coma Scale (GCS), 423, 425
Glass ionomers, 123–6, 130, 143
  clinical tips, 125
  constituents, 123–4
  primary teeth restoration, 178
  properties, 124
  resin-modified, 125–6, 178
  setting reaction, 124
  tooth surface pretreatment, 124
  uses, 124
Globus, 494
Glossectomy, 337
Glossitis
  atrophic, 441, 483
  benign migratory, 464
  median rhomboid, 443, 444
Glossopharyngeal nerve, 514
Glossopharyngeal neuralgia, 476
Glucagon, 523
Glucose, 523
Glucose deficiency, 443
Gluten hypersensitivity, 455
Glycerine, 466
Glyceryl trinitrate, 492, 523
Glycosolated haemoglobin, 474
Gold
  alloys, 116, 140
  inlays, 267–8
  palatal veneers, 265
  partial-veneer crowns, 261
  undercut depth, 318
Gonorrhoea (Neisseria gonorrhoeae), 440–1
Gore-tex, 230, 437
Gout, 513
Grafts
  allografts, 437
  alloplastic, 437
  autogenous, 437
  free gingival, 223
  heterografts, 437
Grains (crystals), 139
Gram-negative bacteria, 69, 201

Gram-positive bacteria, 69, 77
Granulation tissue, 382
Grave's disease, 506
Greater auricular nerve, 438
Greater palatine nerve block, 97, 99
Grooves, 249, 254
Growth hormone, excess, 507
GTN (glyceryl trinitrate), 492, 523
Guedel airway, 111
Guidance for Dental Professionals (GDC), 20
Guide planes, 319
Guide-flange prosthesis, 337
Guided-tissue regeneration, 230
Gumshields, 325
Gutta-percha, 131
  cold, 293
  cones, 143, 293
  hot, 143, 293
  lateral condensation, 184
  thermomechanical compaction, 293
  thermoplasticized, 293–4

Habit deterrent appliance, 360, 369
Haemangiomas, 400, 401, 407, 408
Haematinic deficiencies, 450, 494, 497
Haematological disorders, 483–4, 498–503, 500
Haematology values, 544–5
Haematomas, 101, 382
Haemodialysis, 73, 504–5
Haemoglobinopathies, 499–500
Haemophilia, 64, 194, 502
Haemorrhage
  maxillofacial trauma, 423
  nasal, 424
  post extraction, 387
  pulpal, 251
  see also Bleeding
Haemosiderin, 461
Haemostasis, 93, 387, 501
Hairy leukoplakia, 484–5
Halitosis (oral malodour), 487
Hamartomas, 408
Hand, foot and mouth disease, 446–7

Hard tissues
  discrepancy, 433
  orthodontic examination, 352
  pathology, children, 190–3
Hardening, 139, 140
Hardness, 116
Hashimoto's disease, 506
Head
  contrast techniques, 49–50
  infections, 404
Headache, 515
Headgear injury, 347
Healing *see* Tissue healing
Health
  behaviour barriers, 151
  education, 151
  locus of control, 6–7
  promotion, 150–1
  protection, 151
  see also Occupational health; Periodontal health
Health and Safety Executive (HSE), 42
Hearing assessment, 514
Hearing problems, 378
Hearing prostheses, 337
Heart valve disease, 492
Heart valves
  prosthetic, 502
  see also Infective endocarditis
Heat carrier, 293
Heavy metal salts, 460
Heck's disease (focal epithelial hyperplasia), 447
Hedström files, 288, 290
Helicobacter pylori, 495
Hemidesmosomes, 199, 219
Hemifacial microsomia, 431, 432
Hemisection, 230, 296
Henoch–Schönlein purpura, 501
Hepatic disease, 497–8
  drugs, 62
    aspirin, 65
    cautionary note, 89
    dihydrocodeine tartrate, 67
    dosulepin, 84
    paracetamol, 66
  sialosis, 470

Hereditary haemorrhagic telangiectasia, 501
Herpangina, 446
Herpes simplex infection, 79, 80, 444, 454
Herpes virus 8 (HHV8), 486
Herpes zoster (shingles), 79, 80, 446
Heterografts, 437
Highly active anti-retroviral therapy (HAART), 484
Hirschfield files, 218
History taking, 12–15, 232–3, 235, 490–1
HIV-positive patient, 484–7
  ANUG, 486
  candidosis, 484
  classification, 484
  hairy leukoplakia, 484–5
  Kaposi's sarcoma, 485–6
  linear gingival erythema, 486
  non-Hodgkins lymphoma, 486
  periodontitis, 203
    acute necrotizing, 486
  pigmentation, 461
  salivary gland disease, 486–7
Hoarseness, 514
Hodgkin's lymphoma, 500
Hoes, 217, 218
Hollow box obturators, 336
Home bleaching kits, 283
Honesty, 31
Hormone replacement therapy, 511
Host modulatory therapy, 228
'Hot potato' speech, 404
Hue, 138
Human papillomavirus (HPV), 447
Hutchinson's incisors, 441
Hybrid technique, 293
Hydrocolloids, 133–4
Hydrocortisone
  + miconazole, 77, 88
  adrenal crisis, 529
  anaphylactic shock, 529
  asthma, 531
  emergency use, 522
  pellets, 450
  platelet defects, 501
  steroid cover regimens, 508
  topical, 87, 88

Hydrophilic silicone impression materials, 148
5-hydroxytryptamine, 63
Hydroxyapatite, 205, 421
Hygiene phase therapy, 212–14
Hyoscine, 104, 109
Hypercementosis, 193
Hyperglycaemia, 524
Hyperparathyroidism, 407, 506
Hypersensitivity
  antibiotics, 70
  aspirin, 64
  dentine, 224, 229, 265
  gluten, 455
  see also Allergies
Hypertension, 84, 93, 492
Hyperthyroidism, 506
Hypnosis, 10
Hypnotherapy, 102, 113, 281, 314
Hypnotics, 80–2
Hypocementosis, 193
Hypochondriasis, 465
Hypodontia, 191
Hypoglossal nerve, 514
Hypoglycaemia, 524
Hypoglycaemic agents, 471
Hypoparathyroidism, 507
Hypophosphatasia, 193
Hypopituitarism, 507
Hypotension, 106
Hypothyroidism, 506

Ibuprofen, 65, 224, 395
IgA deficiency, 518
Immunodeficiency
  acquired (secondary), 518
  congenital (primary), 518
  spreading infection, 404
Immunosuppressed patients
  antibiotic cover, 513
  healing, 383
  primary herpetic gingivostomatitis, 445
  steroids, 508
Immunosuppression, 404, 462, 500, 518
Impacted teeth *see* Teeth, impacted
Implant borne prostheses, 330–5

Implants, 421–2
  factors influencing success, 421–2
  subperiosteal, 144
  transmandibular, 144
  see also Osseointegrated implants
Impression trays, 309
Impressions
  complete dentures, 308–10
  compound, 132
  fixed bridges, 274
  inlays, 268
  materials, 131–6, 148
  mucofunctional, 319
  overdentures, 323
  partial dentures, 320
  plaster, 132
  veneers, 264
  waxes, 132
  zinc oxide–eugenol, 133
Incisional biopsy, 399
Incisor classification, 348–50
Incisors
  cavity preparation, 289
  classification, 348–50, 353
  early loss of deciduous, 359
  eruption, 173, 540, 541
  extraction technique, 385
  Hutchinson's, 441
  linguo-occlusion, 360
  mineralization, 540, 541
  missing, 191
  spread of abscess, 402
  traumatic loss of upper, 360
Index of Orthodontic Treatment Need, 342, 348, 350–1
Indometacin, 477
Infections
  antibiotics, 73–4
  bacterial, 440–1
  chronic obstructive pulmonary disease, 493
  control, 542–4
  dental origin, 401–4
  fungal, 442–4
  head and neck, 404
  local anaesthesia, 100
  localized, 401–2
  non-dental origin, 404–5

patient assessment, 405
postoperative extractions, 387
pyogenic, 75
recurrent aphthous stomatitis, 449
renal disease, 503
spreading, 402–4
tissue healing, 383
vascular pupuras, 501
viral, 444–7
see also specific infections
Infective endocarditis, prophylaxis, 70–1, 75, 76
Inferior dental nerve
  block, 96, 97–8, 101
  damage, 394
Informed consent, 22
Infra-orbital nerve block, 96, 99
Injection moulded ceramics, 137, 257, 262
Inlays, 145, 267
  composite, 268–9
  gold, 267–8
  porcelain, 269
Inside-outside bleaching, 286
Insulin, 471
Integrated treatment planning, 296–7
Intense sweeteners, 159
Intercuspal position, 239
Internal HLOC, 6
International Normalized Ratio (INR), 502, 503
Interproximal plaque control, 214
Intra-articular steroid injections, 473
Intra-enamel porcelain laminate veneers, 263, 264
Intracanal dressings, 292
Intracanal medicaments, 144
Intracapsular fracture, 430
Intracranial pressure (raised), 514
Intraoral examinations, 15
Intraoral swellings, 406–7
Intraperitoneal catheters, indwelling, 73
Intrinsic sugars, 156
Intrusion, 189
Investigations, 16
Investment materials, 146

Ionising Radiation (Medical Exposure) Regulations (2000), 42–3
IOTN see Index of Orthodontic Treatment Need
Iron, 471
Iron deficiency, 448, 474, 494, 496, 499
Irreversible hydrocolloids, 134
Irreversible pulpitis, 232, 233
Irrigant chlorhexidine gluconate, 86
Irritable bowel syndrome, 496
Ischaemic heart disease, 491–2
Isoniazid, 497
Isoprenaline, 470
Itraconazole, 79, 444

Jaundice, 497
Jaw
    cysts, 412–14
    registration, 268, 310–11, 320
    see also Mandible, Maxilla; Orthognathic surgery
Joint clicking, 235, 300
Joint disease, 512–13
Joint prostheses, 73, 513
Joint surgery, 330
Junctional epithelium, 199

K files, 288, 291
Kaposi's sarcoma, 485–6
Kennedy classification, edentulous spaces, 315
Keratocysts, odontogenic, 413
Keratosis
    actinic, 517–18
    follicular, 456
    frictional, 457
    oral, 457
    smokers', 457
Kidney disease see Renal disease
Koebner phenomenon, 478

Labial flaps, 396
Labial gland biopsy, 466
Labial segment relationship, 353, 357

Labial veneers, 263–4
Lacerations, 424, 425–7
Lactobacilli spp., 155, 156
Laminate veneer preparation, 263–4
Laser doppler, 234
Laser excision, 486
Laser surgery, 400–1
Lateral cephalometric radiographs, 47
Lateral displacement, 189
Lateral movement, 241
Lateral rectus muscle, 514
Le Fort fractures, 427, 428
Le Fort osteotomies, 379, 433, 434
Lead aprons, 41–2
Learning disability, 113, 194
Ledermix, 100, 181
Legislation, 20, 21
Lemon, 466
Leucite-reinforced porcelain, 137
Leucopenia, 70, 483–4
Leukaemias, 483, 500, 518
Leukoplakia
    candidal, 459
    definition, 457–8
    hairy, 484–5
    premalignant, 458
Lichen planus, 87, 478, 479
Lichenoid reactions, 121, 478–9
    drug-related, 471, 492
Lidocaine (lignocaine), 88, 90, 92
    + epinephrine, 94, 95
Lifelong learning, 29–30
Light cures, 122, 130
Light emitting diodes (LEDs), 130
Light (optical properties), 117
Linear gingival erythema, 486
Linear IgA disease, 452, 455
Lingual bar, 316
    and continuous clasp, 316
Lingual flange, 309
Lingual flaps, 393
Lingual nerve
    block, 97
    damage, 393, 394
Lingual plate, 316
Linings, 128–30, 142–3
Lipofuscin, 461
Lipopolysaccharides, 201

Millers Index of tooth mobility, 207
Mineral trioxide aggregate (MTA), 184, 252, 295
Mineralization, 540–1
Minocycline, 76–7
Minor connectors, 318
Mixed connective tissue disease, 512
Mixed dentition
    cleft lip and palate, 378–9
    development, 173
    orthodontics, 344, 360–1
MODCO convention, 350–1, 359
Modelling behaviour, 171
Modelling wax, 145
Modified Bass technique, 212–13
Modified gingival index, 208
Modified ridge lap, 272, 273
Modiolus, 307
Moisture control, 177, 278
    see also Rubber dams
Molars
    cavity preparation, 289
    early loss of deciduous, 359
    eruption, 173
    extraction technique, 385
    first permanent, poor prognosis, 361
    forceps extraction, 386
    impacted, 191–2
    maxillary root, 416
    mulberry, 441
    spread of abscesses, 402
    surgical extraction, 389
    tunnel preparation, 230
    see also Third molar
Moles (pigmented naevi), 408
Molloplast, 326, 336
Mono-ostotic fibrous dysplasia, 510
Monoamine oxidase inhibitors (MAOIs), 83–4, 93, 471
Monochlorophenol, 292
Monocytes, 201
Monomorphic adenomas, 468
MORA see Mandibular orthopaedic repositioning appliances
Mouth cancer, 410–12
    aetiology, 462
    assessment, 410–11
    clinical features, 462
    incidence, 461
    prognosis, 463
    TNM classification, 463
    treatment, 411–12
    verrucous carcinoma, 464
Mouth swellings, 405–6
Mouthpieces, 325
Mouthwashes, 71, 85–6, 162, 215, 375, 450, 479
MRSA (meticillin-resistant Staphylococcus aureus), 69
Mucoceles, 407, 469
Mucocompressive impressions, 309
Mucoepidermoid carcinoma, 468
Mucofunctional impressions, 319
Mucogingival surgery, 223
Mucoperiosteal flaps, 230, 388, 397
Mucosa see Oral mucosa
Mucositis, 500
Mucostatic impressions, 309
Mucous extravasation cysts, 469
Mucous membrane pemphigoid, 452, 453
Mucous retention cysts, 469
Mulberry molars, 441
Multiple myeloma, 500
Multiple sclerosis, 104, 121, 476, 515
Mumps, 470
Munsell colour system, 138
Muscle balance, complete dentures, 305–7, 313
Muscle relaxants, 81, 84, 105, 110, 329
Muscular dystrophy, 194
Muscular function, special needs children, 194
Myaesthenia gravis, 516
Mycobacterium avium-intracellulare, 440
Mycobacterium tuberculosis, 440
Mycosis fungoides, 517
Myeloma, 483, 500
Mylar plastic strips, 241
Mylohyoid ridge, prominent, 307, 420
Myocardial infarction, 84, 524

Myofascial pain dysfunction syndrome (MPDS), 81, 242, 391, 472

Myxomas, odontogenic, 409–10

Naevi
dysplastic, 518
pigmented, 408
white sponge, 455–6
Nasal fractures, 427
Nasal haemorrhage, 424
Nasal prostheses, 337
Nasolabial cysts, 413
Nasopalatine duct cysts, 413
Nasopalatine nerve block, 97, 99–100
Natal teeth, 173, 359
National Institute for Health and Clinical Excellence (NICE), dental recalls, 165
Neck
contrast techniques, 49–50
infections, 404
metastases, 411–12
swellings, 405–6
Necrotizing fasciitis, 404
Needle fracture, 101
Needle phobia, 113
Needle-stick injury, 101, 543
Neoplasia
imaging, 51
malignant melanoma, 461
radiation, 39
salivary gland, 466–9
see also specific conditions; Tumours
Nerve block
buccal nerve, 97, 98
greater palatine, 97, 99
inferior dental, 96, 97–8, 101
infra-orbital, 96, 99
lingual, 97
mental nerve, 96, 98
nasopalatine, 97, 99–100
posterior superior dental, 97
Nerve damage, extractions, 394–5
Neuralgias
glossopharyngeal, 476

period migrainous (cluster headache), 477
trigeminal see Trigeminal neuralgia
Neurological disease, oral manifestations, 482–3
Neurological disorders, 513–16
Neuropathies, 515
Neuroses, 516
Neutrophils, 201, 202
Nickel allergen, 141
Nickel–chromium
alloys, 141
backings, 266
Nickel–titanium files, 291
Nicorandil, 471
Nicotine, 202
Nicotine replacement therapy, 164
Nicotinic stomatitis, 457
Nifedipine, 471
Night guard vital bleaching, 284
Nikolsky sign, 453
Nitrazepam, 82, 83
Nitrous oxide, 102, 104, 110, 112, 401, 522, 525
Non-accidental injury, 185
Non-bacterial tooth surface loss/non-carious tooth surface loss see Tooth wear
Non-Hodgkin's lymphoma, 486, 500
Non-specific plaque hypothesis, 156, 200–1, 215
Non-steroidal anti-inflammatory drugs (NSAIDs), 63–5
asthma, 493
craniomandibular disorders, 329
dental pain, 62
lichenoid reactions, 471
nephrotoxicity, 504
osteoarthritis, 512
peptic ulcers, 495
postoperative extraction, 387
TMJ disorders, 472, 473
vascular purpuras, 501
Non-verbal communication, 4, 171
Non-vital teeth, bleaching, 285–6
Nordiazepam, 83, 105
Normalization, 193
Normocytic anaemia, 499

Nursing bottle caries, 153, 169
Nutritional deficiencies
  immune system disorders, 518
  oral candidosis, 443, 459
  oral dysaesthesia, 474
  recurrent aphthous stomatitis,
    448, 449
  sialosis, 470
  see also Diet; Food
Nylon, 142, 314
Nystagmus, 514
Nystatin, 77, 78, 444

Oblique lateral radiographs, 38, 45
Obturation, 293–4
Obturators, 336
Occipitomental radiographs, 47
Occlusal assessment, 302
Occlusal balance, 307, 313
Occlusal cant, 431
Occlusal disharmony, 228
Occlusal harmony, 239
Occlusal indicator wax, 241
Occlusal indices, 348–50
Occlusal interferences, 239, 241,
  242, 369
Occlusal pivots, 312
Occlusal plane, 356
Occlusal radiographs, 44–5
Occlusal registration, 274
Occlusal rests, 316–17, 318
Occlusal splints, 229
Occlusal therapy, 330
Occlusal trauma, 228
Occlusion
  cleft lip and palate, 378
  definition, 239
  examination, 236, 241–2, 301, 353
  fixed bridges, 271
  fixed prosthodontics, 242
  ideal, 342
  intercuspal position, 239
  mandibular movements, 240, 241,
    255
  normal, 342
  periodontal diseases, 228
  retruded contact position, 239,
    240

  stable, 239, 242
  see also Malocclusion
Occular (eye) prostheses, 337
Occult caries, 153
Occupational health
  heavy metal salts, 460
  mouthpieces, 325
  tooth abrasion, 279
  see also Health and Safety
    Executive
Octacalcium phosphate, 205
Oculomotor nerve, 514
Odontogenic keratocysts, 413
Odontogenic tumours, 409–10
Odontomas (odontomes), 408
Oedema, 407
Oesophageal disorders, 462, 494
Olfactory nerve, 514
Omeprazole, 495
Onlays, 269–70
Openbite
  anterior, 363
  facial/dental asymmetry, 431
  posterior, 363
Opiates, 66–7, 83–4, 109
Optic nerve, 514
Optical properties, 117
Oral candidosis (candidiasis),
  442–4
  anaemia, 483
  angular cheilitis, 443
  antibiotics, 70
  chronic hyperplastic, 443, 444,
    459, 462
  classification, 443
  denture-induced stomatitis, 443
  drug-related, 471
  erythematous, 442, 484
  HIV infection, 484
  investigation and diagnosis, 443,
    444
  medium rhomboid glossitis, 443
  oral dysaesthesia, 474
  predisposing factors, 442
  pseudomembranous, 442, 484
  treatment, 443–4
Oral contraceptives, 461, 471
Oral dysaesthesia (burning mouth
  syndrome), 473–5, 483, 509

Oral epithelium, 198
Oral health
  definition, 2
  national survey (2003), 151
  smoking, 163–4
  social factors, 2–3
Oral hygiene
  aids, 214
  disclosing agents, 212
  instructions, 212
  mouth cancer, 462
  mouthwashes, 215–16
  overdentures, 323
  partial dentures, 315
  periodontal diseases, 205–7
  plaque control, 214, 215–16
  precision attachments, 321
  special needs children, 194
  tooth brushing, 212–14
  tooth wear prevention, 281
Oral malodour (halitosis), 487
Oral mucosa
  atrophy, 494
  effects of drugs on, 471
  fixed prosthodontics/endodontics, 235
  pigmented lesions, 459–61
  prosthodontics, 300
  treatment, 86, 87
Oral purpura, localized, 451–2
Oral sprays, 86
Oral submucous fibrosis, 459
Oral surgery
  analgesia, 67
  antibiotic prophylaxis, 71, 75
  general anaesthesia, 108
  mouthwashes, 85
  radiography before, 53–5
  vasoconstrictors for haemostasis, 93
Oral ulceration
  Behcet's syndrome, 450–1
  causes, 447, 448
  clinical features, 449
  drug-related, 471
  haematinic deficiency, 494
  haematological disease, 483
  orthodontics, 347
  pregnancy, 509

  recurrent aphthous stomatitis, 447–50, 496
  shingles, 446
  treatment, 86, 87, 88
  see also Ulcerative colitis
Oral–antral fistula (OAF), 75, 416
  closure, 71, 416–18
Oralbalance, 89, 466
Orbital wall/floor reconstruction material, 437
Order hardening, 140
Orofacial granulomatosis (OFG), 481
Orofacial pain syndrome, 516
Ortho-ethoxy benzoic acid (EBA), 129
Orthodontic therapists, 166
Orthodontics
  assessment and examination, 352–4
  benefits, 345–6
  classification, 348–52
  craniomandibular disorders, 330
  definition, 342
  developing dentition, 358–9
  diagnostic records, 354
  enamel damage, 347
  fixed appliances, 374–5
  functional appliances, 376–7
  impacted third molars, 391
  practitioners, 343, 344
  presurgical, 379–80
  removable appliances, 368–74
  risks, 346–8
  scope, 344
  timing, 344
  treatment options, 358
  treatment plans, 356–8
Orthognathic surgery
  assessment, 432
  cleft lip and palate, 379
  craniomandibular disorders, 330
  examination, 432–3
  indications, 432
  malocclusion, 364, 366, 368
  orthodontics, 358, 379–80
  procedures, 434
  treatment, 433

Orthopantomogram (OPT/OPG) *see* Panoramic radiographs
Osseointegrated implants, 144–5, 330–5
  case selection, 331–3
  complications, 334
  craniofacial prostheses, 337
  current developments, 334–5
  maintenance, 334
  mechanical components, 331
  planning, 333
  prosthodontic treatment, 334
  radiographs, 333–4
  requirements, 330–1
  temporization, 334
  tooth replacement solutions, 332
Osseointegration, 144, 422
Ossifying fibroma, 407
Osteoarthritis, 512
Osteoarthrosis, 473
Osteoblasts, 383
Osteogenesis imperfecta (brittle bone disease), 509
Osteomalacia, 511
Osteomy, horizontal, 422
Osteomyelitis, 75, 404, 405
Osteopetrosis (Albers–Schönberg or marble bone disease), 510
Osteoporosis, 511
Osteotomies, 108, 379, 422, 433, 434
Otitis media, 482
Outline form, 243
Overbite
  definition, 353
  malocclusion, 363, 365, 367
  measurement, 353
  orthodontics, 346
  reduction, 369
Overdentures, 322–4
  abutment selection, 323
  attachments, 323
  impression techniques, 323
Overjet, 345–6
  definition, 353
  malocclusion, 363, 364, 365, 367
  measurement, 353
  trauma, 345

Overlapping incisal porcelain laminate veneers, 263, 264
Oxcarbazepine, 476
Oxide formation, 118
Oxide layers (metals), 140
Oxygen
  acute chest pain, 525
  adrenal crisis, 529
  asthma, 531
  emergency treatment, 522
  epilepsy, 530
  general anaesthesia, 110, 111
  periodic migrainous neuralgia, 477
  stroke, 531

Pacemakers, 73
Pachyonychia congenita, 456
Paediatric dentistry *see* Children
Paget's disease of bone, 511
Pain
  bridgework causing, 271
  control, 10, 63, 95
  dental, 50, 62, 242
  investigation, 50–1
  nature, 9–10
  postoperative, 67
  psychological approaches to, 10
  salivary gland, 471
  thresholds, 8, 13
  see also Pulpal pain
Palatal bars, 315
Palatal flaps, 396
Palatal horseshoe connector, 316
Palatal lift appliances, 325
Palatal lock, 178
Palatal rotation flaps, 417
Palatal torus, 420
Palatal veneers, 265–6
Palsies, 80, 464, 482–3, 494, 515
Panavia, 249
Pancreatic disease, 498
Panoramic radiographs, 38, 45, 46, 50
Papilloedema, 514
PAR *see* Peer Assessment Rating Index
Paracetamol, 64, 65–6, 224, 495
Paraformaldehyde, 181

Parafunctional forces
  denture fracture, 325
  oral dysaesthesia, 474
  soft relines, 326
  see also Bruxism
Paralleling technique, 43
Parathyroid disease, 506–7
Parkinson's disease, 516
Parotidectomy, 438
Parotitis, suppurative, 405
Partial dentures
  aims, 314–15
  choice of material, 319
  clasp design, 317–18
  clinical stages, 320
  design, 297, 315–17, 339
  disjunct, 320
  guide planes, 319
  hinged flange, 320
  insertion, 320
  jaw registration, 320
  plaque retention, 165
  rests, 318–19
  review, 320
  saddles, 319
  splints, 229
  swinglock, 320
  trial, 320
  two part, 320
Peer Assessment Rating Index, 348, 351
Peer review, 25, 28
Pemphigoid
  bullous, 452, 453–4
  mucous membrane, 452, 453
Pemphigus, 452–4
Pemphigus vegetans, 453
Pemphigus vulgaris, 452–3
Penciclovir, 80, 445
Penicillamine, 471
Penicillin, 68, 72, 74–6, 441, 471
  allergy, 77
Pentobarbitone, 104
Peptic ulcers, 64, 495
Percussion, 233
Perforation, 295, 296
Periapical abscess, 226
  response to analgesics, 63
  tenderness on percussion, 233

Periapical curettage, 296
Periapical periodontitis, 232, 233
Periapical radiography, 43
Pericoronitis, 402
  antibiotic prophylaxis, 75
  irrigant chlorhexidine gluconate, 86
  radiography, 51
  third molar removal, 391
Perio-endo lesions, 207, 225, 227
Periodic migrainous neuralgia (cluster headache), 477
Periodontal abscess
  antibiotics, 75
  definition, 225
  infections, 401
  periapical, differentiated, 226
  predisposing factors, 225
  response to analgesics, 63
  treatment, 226–7
Periodontal assessment, 52–3
Periodontal disease
  antibiotics, 227–8
  bridgework causing, 271
  classification, 203–4
  diagnosis, 204, 205, 207
  examination, 205–7
  impacted third molars, 391
  indices, 208
  occlusion, 228
  oral hygiene, 205–7
  orthodontics, 345, 347
  overdentures, 322
  see also Gingivitis; Periodontitis
Periodontal files, 218
Periodontal health
  fixed prosthodontics/endodontics, 236
  prosthodontics, 301
  see also Oral health
Periodontal ligament
  restitution, 219
  structure, 198, 199
Periodontal pack/dressing, 146
Periodontal pocket, 200
  charts, 210–11
  chlorhexidine, 86, 228
  depths, 202, 206, 210, 219, 225
  false, 210

Periodontal pocket (cont'd)
  metronidazole, 76
  true, 211
Periodontal probe, 206
Periodontal surgery, 220
  care and instruments following,
    223–4
  complications, 224
  flap procedures, 221–2
  gingivectomy, 221
  mucogingival, 223–4
  vasoconstrictors for haemostasis,
    93
Periodontal therapy
  corrective phase, 212
  hygiene phase, 211, 212–14
  reassessment, 211
  recall maintenance, 224
  smokers, 202
  supportive periodontal
    care/maintenance phase, 212
Periodontal tissues, structure, 198–9
Periodontitis
  acute necrotizing, 486
  aggressive, 204
  chronic, 204
  definition, 200
  genetic factors, 202
  gingivitis, 200
  host factors, 201–2
  periapical, 232, 233
  predisposing factors, 200–3
  smoking, 202
  systemic disease, 202–3, 204
  traumatic, 271
Periodontium, 198, 203
  see also Gingivae; Periodontal
    ligament
Periosteal release buccal flap,
  416–17
Peripheral seal, 307, 326
Periradicular surgery, 295–6
Peritoneal dialysis, 504–5
Permanent (secondary) dentition
  cleft lip and palate, 379
  development, 173
  eruption, 541
  mineralization, 541
  notation, 542

  orthodontics, 344
  pulp therapy in immature, 182–4
  trauma, 187–90
Personality disorders, 516
Personnel, ionizing radiation, 43
Pethidine, 67, 84, 104
Peutz–Jeghers syndrome, 461, 482
Pharyngeal pouch, 494
Phenothiazines, 461, 465, 471
Phenoxymethylpenicillin, 74–6
Phenylbutazone, 470
Phenytoin, 454, 471, 476
Photoelectric absorption, 35
Physical disability, 194
Physiotherapy, for TMJ, 472, 512
Pier, 270
Pigmentation, 459–61, 471, 510
Pilocarpine, 466
Pinlays, 274
Pins, dentine, 249
Pit/fissure sealants, 176
Pituitary gland disorders, 507
Placebo effect, 10
Plaque
  control
    chemical, 215–16
    elderly patients, 165
    interproximal, 214
  gingivitis, 203, 211
  index, 208
  non-specific plaque hypothesis,
    156, 200–1, 215
  oral hygiene, 205
  overjet, 345–6
  removal, 216
  smoking, 202
  tooth alignment, 345
  see also Gingivitis; Periodontitis
Plasma curing lights, 130
Plaster, 132
Plastic deformation, 116
Platelet defects, 501
Pleomorphic adenoma, 467–8, 469
Pluggers, 293
Plummer–Vinson (Brown
  Kelly–Paterson) syndrome
  (primary sideropenic anaemia),
  462, 481, 483, 494
Pocket see Periodontal pocket

Point scaler, 217, 218
Polishing
  abrasion, 140, 146–7
  relief, 147
  teeth, 220
Polycarbonates, 142, 314
Polyenes, 77
Polyethers, 134–5
Polyethyl/polybutyl methacrylate, 147
Polyglycolic acid, 400
Polymer denture base materials, 141–2
Polymers, 116, 147
Polymorphonuclear neutrophils (PMNs), 201
Polymyalgia rheumatica, 512
Polymyositis, 512
Polyostotic fibrous dysplasia, 510
Polypharmacy, 62, 89, 165
Polyps, 104, 407
Polysulphides, 135
Polytetrafluoroethylene (PTFE) membrane, 230
Pontics
  cleaning, 214
  definition, 270
  design, 272, 273
Porcelain, 136–7
  aluminous, 137
  bonding, 128
  bridges, 137
  conditioning, 128
  crowns, 137, 257
  inlays, 269
  laminate veneer, 263, 264
  leucite-reinforced, 137
  teeth, 147, 314
Porphyromonas gingivalis, 201
Positive reinforcement, 171–2
Post crowns, 253, 258–61
  clinical tips, 260–1
  problems, 259
  types, 259–60
Post-viral syndrome (chronic fatigue syndrome, ME), 516
Postdam, 307
Posterior composites, 148
Posterior cranial fossa tumour, 476

Posterior crowns, 261–2
  types, 261–2
Posterior dental nerve block, 97
Posterior palatal bar, 315
Posteroanterior jaw radiographs, 45
Postoperative pain, 67
Poswillo Report, 112
Povidone–iodine, 86
Power bleaching, 284
Powerful others HLOC, 6
Pre-adjusted edge-wise appliance, 374
Pre-teeth, 172–3
Precision attachments, 321
Prednisolone, 450, 477, 483
Preformed acetate crowns, 187–8
Preformed metal crowns, 179
Preformed polycarbonate crowns, 147
Preformed root canal fillings, 143
Pregnancy
  amalgam, 121
  drugs, 62
    aciclovir, 80
    aspirin, 65
    benzodiazepines, 83
    cautionary note, 89
    dihydrocodeine tartrate, 67
    felypressin, 94
    fluconazole, 79
  epulides, 509
  general anaesthesia, 112
  gingivitis, 203, 509
  lead aprons, 41–2
  recurrent aphthous stomatitis, 448
  sialosis, 470
Premalignant lesions, 517–18
Premedication, 81, 84, 102, 109, 112
Premolars
  cavity preparation, 289
  eruption, 173, 541
  extraction technique, 385
  maxillary root, 416
  mineralization, 541
  missing, 191
  spread of abscesses, 402
Preprosthetic surgery, 419–21
Prescription writing, 60–1

Prescription-only-medicine (POM), 60
Prevention
  children, 169
  elderly patients, 165
  individual/community basis, 150
  philosophy, 150
  special needs children, 195
Prevotella intermedia, 201
Prilocaine, 92, 94, 100
  + epinephrine, 94
  + felypressin, 94
Primary herpetic gingivostomatitis, 444–5
Probes/probing, 206, 208–9, 210, 233
Professionals, dental care, 165–6
Progressive systemic sclerosis, 512
Proplast, 437
Propofol, 107
Prostaglandins, 63, 64
Prostheses
  appliances, 325
  craniofacial, 337
  heart valves, 502
  implant borne, 330–5
  joint, 73, 513
Prosthodontics *see* Dentures
Prothrombin time, 502
Protocols, 29
Protrusive movement, 241
Pseudobulbar palsy, 494
Pseudogout, 513
Pseudomembranous candidosis, 442, 444, 484
Pseudomembranous colitis, antibiotic-associated, 497
Psoriatic arthritis, 513
Psychiatric disorders, 516
Psychological changes, following extraction, 304
Psychological factors, 2–10, 474, 496
Psychological problems, 378
Psychoses, 516
Puberty
  gingivitis, 203
  precocious, 510
Publication Schedule, 25

Pulmonary tuberculosis, 440, 493
Pulp capping
  deep carious lesion, 251–2
  direct, 183, 251–2
  indirect, 182, 251
  permanent teeth, 188
  primary teeth, 181
Pulp necrosis, 188
Pulp pathology, 180
Pulp therapy
  immature permanent teeth, 182–4
  primary teeth, 180–2
Pulpal damage
  causes, 287
  diagnosis, 287
  orthodontics, 347
Pulpal exposure, 251
  capping, 188, 251
  dentine pins, 249
Pulpal haemorrhage, 251
Pulpal pain
  children, 180
  diagnosis, 180, 232–3
  examination, 233
  special tests, 233–4
  spontaneous, 181
  transient, 180
  types, 232
Pulpectomy
  immature permanent teeth, 183
  primary teeth, 181, 182
Pulpitis, 183, 516
  bridgework causing, 271
  irreversible, 232, 233
  response to analgesics, 63
  reversible, 232, 233
Pulpotomy
  ferric sulphate vital, 181
  multivisit, 181
  permanent teeth, 183, 188
  primary teeth, 181
  single visit, 181
  two-stage desensitizing, 181–2
Pulse oximetry, 106, 113
Punch biopsy, 399
Purpura
  Henoch–Schönlein, 501
  localized oral, 451–2
  vascular, 501

Putties, temporary, 131
Pyelonephritis, 503
Pyostomatitis vegetans, 496

Quantiflex system, 102

Racial pigmentation, 461
Racoon eyes, 424
Radiation
  biological effects, 37–9
  dose levels, 37, 38
  dose limitation, 39–41
  dose measurement, 36–7, 38
  protection, 36–7
  regulations, 42–3
  risks, 37, 38, 39
Radiation Protection Adviser
  (RPA), 42
Radiation Protection Supervisor
  (RPS), 42
Radicular cysts, 413
Radio-opacity, 117, 142
Radiographs, 16
  advanced imaging techniques,
    47–50
  ALARP principle, 39
  caries diagnosis, 50–2, 154
  cavity preparation, 242
  children, 191
  dentures, 301–2
  differential diagnosis, 56–7
  endodontics, 236–7
  equipment, 39–40
  extractions, 53
  extraoral projections, 45–7
    lateral cephalometric view, 47
    oblique lateral, 45
    occipitomental, 47
    panoramic, 38, 45, 46, 50
    posteroanterior jaw, 45
    reverse Towne's, 45–7
    submentovertex, 47
  fixed prosthodontics, 236–7
  guidelines, 50–2
  infection, 405
  interpretation, 56
  intraoral views

bitewing, 37, 38, 43–4, 52, 154,
    234
  occlusal, 44–5
  periapical, 43
lead aprons in pregnancy, 41–2
maxillofacial trauma, 425
mouth, face and neck swellings,
    406
oral surgery, 53–5
orthodontics, 354
osseointegated implants, 333–4
pain investigation, 50–1
periodontal assessment, 52–3
periodontal disease, 207
pulp therapy, 181
pulpal pain, 234
quality assurance, 40–1
root canal therapy, 289
third molar diagnosis, 392–3
trauma, 186
Radionuclide imaging, 49–50
Radiosensitivity, 36
Radiotherapy, 411, 486, 500
Rampant caries, 153
Randomized controlled trials
  (RCTs), 28
Reciprocal bracing arm, 318
Recommended International
  Non-proprietary Names (rINN),
  90
Reconstruction, 436–7
  flaps, 436–7
  grafts, 437
Record keeping, 24–5
Recurrent aphthous stomatitis,
    447–50, 496
Recurrent caries, 153
Recurrent herpetic infection, 445
Red lesions (erythroplakia), 458
Referral, 23
Reimplantation, 189, 296
Reiter's syndrome, 513
Relief areas, 307
Relief polishing, 147
Relines, 326–7
Remineralization, 160, 252
Removable appliances
  active, 368
  advantages/disadvantages, 374

Removable appliances (*cont'd*)
  check visits, 372–3
  components, 370–1
  contraindications, 369–70
  definition, 368
  designing, 372
  fitting, 372
  indications, 369
  malocclusion, 364, 366, 368
  orthodontics, 358
  passive, 368
  problems, 373
Removable prosthodontics *see*
  Dentures
Renal disease, 503–5
  drugs, 62
    aciclovir, 80
    aspirin, 65
    cautionary note, 89
    dihydrocodeine tartrate, 67
    fluconazole, 79
Renal failure
  chronic, 504
  dry mouth, 465
  haemodialysis for, 73
  oral keratosis, 457
  pancreatitis, 498
Renal transplants, 462
Repairs, 325–6
Reparative granuloma, 407
Replica (copy) dentures, 321–2
Research, audit compared with, 27
Resin composites, 121–3
  components, 121–2
  direct, 148
  indirect, 123
  properties, 121
  setting, 122
  types, 122
  uses, 122–3
Resin-modified glass ionomers,
  125–6, 178
Resins
  chemically active, 278
  natural, 130
  sealers, 293
  shellac, 145
Resistance
  form, 243

partial dentures, 316–17
  to antibiotics, 69–70
Resorbable materials, 437
Resorption, 419–20
Resource allocation, 350
Respiratory depression, 106
Respiratory disorders, 104, 493–4
Restorations
  carious primary teeth, 177–9
  core, 248–50
  examination, 236, 301
  root-canal treated tooth, 294
  special needs children, 195
  temporary, 131
  see also Crowns; Inlays; Onlays
Restorative materials, 250
Rests, 318–19
Retainers
  choice, 272
  definition, 270
  labial veneer, 263
  removable, 369
  sprung, 271
Retching, 314
Retention
  clasps to improve, 327
  complete dentures, 305, 313
  form, 243
  grooves/slots, 249, 254
  indirect, 316, 317
  orthodontic treatment plan, 358
  partial dentures, 316, 317
  precisional attachments, 321
Retentive bracing arm, 318
Retractors, 174, 370
Retrograde root filling, 144, 296,
  398
Retruded contact position, 239, 240,
  301, 307–8
Retrusive movement, 241
Reverse Towne's, 45–7
Reversible hydrocolloids, 134
Reversible pulpitis, 232, 233
Reye's syndrome, 64, 65
Rheumatic fever, 492
Rheumatoid arthritis, 473, 512–13,
  518
Rickets, 511
Rigid impression materials, 132–3

Risk assessment, radiation, 42
Risk management, 29
Robert's retractor, 371
Rochette splint, 229
Rodent ulcer, 409, 517
Root amputation, 296
Root canal
  cleansers, 143, 292
  fillings, 143, 144, 258, 398
  sealers, 143–4
Root canal therapy
  access cavity preparation, 289
  aims, 287
  chlorhexidine, 86
  cleansing, 292
  colour coding, 288
  dimensions, 289
  instrumentation, 288
  intracanal dressings, 292
  manual preparation
    with increased taper
      instruments, 291
    with ISO instruments, 290–1
    rotary preparation, 291–2
  obturation, 293–4
  orthograde, 413
  prior restoration, 294
  problems, 294–5
  rubber dam isolation, 289
  single-visit, 294–5
  successful, 294
  working length determination,
    289
Root caries, 153, 224
Root filling
  retrograde, 144, 296, 398
  through and through, 296
Root fractures, 418
  formation, 188
  post crowns, 259
  radiographs, 186
  subgingival, 261
Root perforation, 259
Root planing, 216–20, 230
Root resection, 230
Root resorption, 188, 189, 347
Roots, post-retained crowns, 258–9
Rotary files, 288
Rotary preparation, 291–2

Rubber dam, 174–5
  pulp capping, 251
  pulpotomy, 181
  root canal therapy, 289

Saddles
  anterior, 315
  bounded, 315
  classification of support, 315
  connectors, 315–16
  dentures, 303
  examination, 236
  fixed bridges, 270
  free end
    bilateral, 315
    unilateral, 315
  Kennedy classification, 315
  partial dentures, 315–16, 319
  repairs, 325
Salbutamol, 523, 531
Saline, 226, 529
Saliva
  drooling, 516
  ejector, 174
  erosion, 279
  stimulants, 159, 466
  substitutes, 89
Saliva Orthana, 89, 466
Salivary gland
  bacterial sialadenitis, 469–70
  disorders, 465–6
  effects of drugs on, 471
  enlargement, 494
  HIV disease, 486
  infection, 405
  mucoceles, 469
  neoplasms, 466–9
  radiographs, 55
  surgery, 437–8
Salivix, 89
Salt, fluoridated, 161
Sandblasting, 278
Sanitary pontic (all-gold posterior
    pontic), 272, 273
Sarcoidosis, 464–5, 494, 518
Sarcomas, 409
Savlon, 86
Scalers, 216, 217–18

Scaling, 230
  hand instruments, 216, 217, 218
  healing following, 219
  techniques, 219
  ultrasonic, 217–18
Scanning technology, 335
Scar tissue, 382
Schilder's technique, 293
Schirmer test, 466
Scintigraphy, 466
Scissors bite, 365
Screening, 351
Screws, 371
Scrotal tongue, 464
Scurvy (vitamin C deficiency), 501
Sealants, pit/fissure, 145–6, 176
Sealers, root canal, 143–4, 293
Secondary caries, 153
Sedation
  antihistamines, 84
  conscious, 101–2
  GDC definition, 102
  inhalation, 102–4
    contraindications, 104
    sensory disturbances, 103–4
  intravenous, 81, 104–7
    benzodiazepines, 104–5
    future developments, 107
    midazolam, 105–7
  patient consent, 22, 102
Selective serotonin reuptake
  inhibitors (SSRIs), 83, 475, 516
Self-esteem
  orthodontics, 346
  see also Aesthetics
Sensation assessment, 514
Sensitivity (vitality) tests, 16
  children, 186
  infection, 405
  maxillary sinus, 416
  pulpal pain, 233
  swellings of mouth, face and
    neck, 406
Sensory disability, 194
Serology, 495, 496, 512
Severe combined
  immunodeficiencies, 518
Sevoflurane, 112
Shades, 138–9, 275

Sharpey's fibres, 199
Sharps injury, 543
Sheet casting wax, 145
Shellac resin, 145
Shimstock plastic strips, 241
Shingles (herpes zoster), 79, 80, 446
Sialadenitis, 466, 469–70
Sialogogues, 470
Sialography, 49, 466, 470
Sialolithiasis, 438
Sialosis (sialadenosis), 470, 494
Sickle cell anaemia, 499
Sickledex test, 500
Side-cutting burs, 288
Significant event analysis, 30
Silane coupling, 128
Silicoating, 326
Silicones
  addition, 135
  condensation, 136
Silinization, 121
Silver, 119
Silver points, 143
Sintered alumina, 137, 257, 262, 269
Sinus lift bone grafting, 422
Sinuses see Maxillary sinus
Sinusitis, 51, 75, 233
Sjögren's syndrome, 465–6, 512
  American–European
    classification criteria, 467
  features of primary and
    secondary, 465
Skeletal classification, 349–50
Skeletal discrepancies
  mixed dentition, 361
  orthodontics, 344
Skeletal features
  class II division 1 malocclusion,
    363–4
  class II division 2 malocclusion,
    365
  class III malocclusion, 367
Skeletal pattern
  ANB angle, 356, 357
  classification, 349
  cleft lip and palate, 378
  dental arch relationship, 352
  openbite, 363
  treatment planning, 364

Skin
  disease, oral manifestations,
    478–80
  grafts, 437
  infection, 405
  lacerations, 425–7
  malignant lesions, 457–9, 517
  pigmentation, 459–61, 471, 510
Skull, base of, fracture, 423, 424
Sleep period, 422
Slots, 249, 254
Smell assessment, 514
Smokers' keratosis, 457
Smoking
  early deaths from disease, 493
  melanin pigmentation, 461
  oral health, 163–4
  periodontitis, 202
  recurrent aphthous stomatitis, 449
  see also Tobacco
Snail track ulcers, 441
Snoring, 325
Social history, 13–15
Social response, orthodontics, 346
Socio-economic factors, 151
Socket healing, 383
Socket implants, 334–5
Sodium bisulphate, 92
Sodium hypochlorite, 77, 143
Soft tissues
  crease/wrinkle obliterative
    materials, 437
  discrepancy, 433
  disease, children, 193
  examination, 352–3
  implant success, 421
  problems, 420–1
  surgery, 335
  see also Lips; Tongue
Solubility, 117
Solution hardening, 139
Sonic abrasion, 252–3
Southend clasp, 370
SOX syndrome, 512
Space maintainers, 369
Spacing
  balancing/compensating
    extractions, 360
  Class I malocclusion, 362

mixed to permanent dentition,
    173
  orthodontic treatment plan, 357
  tooth loss, 359
Special needs, 193–5
Special tests, 16
Speech problems
  cleft lip and palate, 378
  denture problems, 313
Spencer Wells (mosquito) forceps,
    101
Spina bifida, 194
Spiral paste fillers, 288
Splints
  acid-etch, 190
  acrylic, 190, 229
  bleaching, 325
  classification, 229
  composite, 190
  direct, 190
  etch-retained metal, 229
  foil, 190
  function, 190
  indirect, 190
  interocclusal, 329
  multistrand, 229
  occlusal, 229
  partial dentures, 229
  provisional, 329
  repositioning, 329
  stabilization, 329
  tension headache, 515
  thermoplastic, 190
  TMJ, 472, 473
  tooth wear prevention, 281
  wire, 229
Spontaneous pain, 181
Spreaders, 288
Spring cantilever bridges, 276
Springs, 370–1, 375
Sprue (vent), 146
Squamous cell carcinoma, 411, 464,
    517
Squamous cell papilloma, 447
SSRIs (selective serotonin reuptake
    inhibitors), 83, 475, 516
Stability, complete dentures, 307
Stability ratio, 370
Stable occlusion, 239, 242

Staff training, radiation protection, 40
Stafne's bone cyst, 413
Staining, causes, 283
Stainless steel, 141
   crowns, 147
   undercuts, 318
Staphylococcus aureus, 77, 443, 469
   meticillin-resistant, 69
Status epilepticus, 530
Steel alloys, 141
Step-back technique, 290
Step-down technique, 290
Stereotyping, facial, 346
Sternocleidomastoid muscle, 514
Steroid cover, 508–9
   Crohn's disease, 496
   ulcerative colitis, 496
Steroid inhalers
   candidal leukoplakia, 459
   localized oral purpura, 452
Steroids
   Behçet's disease, 450
   collapse, 509
   Cushing's syndrome, 507
   drug-related oral effects, 471
   epidermolysis bullosa, 454
   giant cell arteritis, 477
   glucocorticoid effects, 507
   intracanal medicaments, 144
   mineralocorticoid effects, 507
   osteoporosis, 511
   pemphigus, 453
   pulpotomy, 181–2
   systemic, 508
   TMJ, 473
   topical, 507–8
   see also Corticosteroids
Sticky wax, 145
Still's disease (systemic-onset juvenile chronic arthritis), 513
Stochastic effects, 37–9
Stomatitis, 492, 494
   denture-induced, 79, 443, 444
   gangrenosum, 496
   migratory, 464
   nicotinic, 457
   recurrent aphthous, 447–50, 496
Stone, removal of, 438

Stop signal, 171
Strabismus, 514
Strain, 116
Strength, 116
Streptococcus mutans, 155, 156
   and *S. sobrinus*, 156
Streptococcus viridans, 469
Stress, 116
Stress breaker (flexible denture base), 319
Stroke (cerebrovascular accident), 430, 531
Studs, 321
Study casts, 241, 253, 281, 302
Study models, 16, 354
Subcondylar fracture (condylar neck), 430
Subgingival calculus, 206, 216
Sublingual bar, 316
Subluxation, 189
Submandibular gland excision, 438
Submentovertex radiographs, 47
Subperiosteal implants, 144
Sucking habits, 360, 363
Sugar-free preparations, 61
Sugars
   caries, 157
   classification, 156
   consumption frequency, 157, 158
   dietary advice, 157–9
   sweetener substitutes, 158–9
Sulcular epithelium, 198
Sulcus, deepening, 421
Sulphonamides, 68, 454, 471
Sumatriptan, 477
Superfloss, 214
Superinfection, 70
Superior oblique muscle, 514
Supernumerary teeth, 190–1
Supplemental teeth, 190
Support, complete dentures, 305, 306, 313
Supraclavicular lymphadenopathy (Virchow's node), 495
Supragingival calculus, 205
Surgical sieve, 406
Surveying, 302

Suturing
  materials, 400
  techniques, 399–400
Suxamethonium, 110
Swallowing, difficulty, 404, 494–5
Sweeteners
  bulk, 158
  intense, 159
  non-sugar, 158
Sweets, tooth-friendly, 159
Swellings
  facial, 51, 406–7
  incision and drainage, 296
  intraoral, 406–7
  mouth, face and neck, 405–6
  postoperative, 395
  salivary gland, 471
Swinglock partial dentures, 320
Syncope see Fainting
Synergism, 69–70
Syphilis, 441
  mouth cancer, 462
Systematic reviews, 28, 159
Systemic lupus erythematosus
  (SLE), 480, 512, 518
Systemic-onset juvenile chronic
  arthritis (Still's disease), 513

T1 lesions, 411
T2 lesions, 411
T-cell defects, 518
Tacrolimus, 450
Tapers, 254, 261
Tattoo
  amalgam, 460
  laser removal, 400
  recognition, 425
TCAs see Tricyclic antidepressants
Team care, 522
Technetium-99m, 49
Teeth
  abutment see Abutment teeth
  alignment and plaque
    accumulation, 345
  angulated, 261
  anterior, 301, 308
  apicected, 261
  assessment for crowns, 253, 258

cleft lip and palate, 377
conical, 191
crypt position, 192
drug-related discoloration, 471
ectopic, 192, 344
extractions see Extractions
extrusion, 369
form, abnormalities, 191
formation, 172
hypoplastic, 263
impacted, 346
increased length, 224
mobile
  Millers Index, 207
  occlusal examination, 242
  orthodontics, 373, 375
  palpation, 207
  pocket chart, 210
  splints, 229
  treatment plan, 358
natal, 173, 359
national survey (2003), 151
notation, 542
polishing, 220
porcelain, 314
position
  abnormalities, 191–2
  complete dentures, 308
posterior, 261, 301, 308
pretreatment, 124
radiography, trauma, 186
reimplantation, 189, 296
remineralization, 160, 252
root fractures see Root fractures
selection for dentures, 310
supernumerary, 190–1
supplemental, 190
symptomatic, 236
tender to percussion, 51
tilted, 165, 242, 270, 274
tipping, 369
to implant bridges, 335
transplantation, 296
transposed, 192, 344
tuberculate, 191
vital see Vital teeth
see also Canines; Dentition;
  Incisors; Molars; Pre-teeth;
  Premolars

TEGDM (tri-ethylene glycol dimethacrylate), 122
Tell–show–do, 171
Temazepam, 81, 82
Temperature, and NSAIDs, 63
Templates
  radiographic, 333
  surgical, 334
Temporal (giant cell) arteritis, 477
Temporary bridges, 274
Temporary cements, 130–1
Temporary crown materials, 147
Temporary linings, 142–3
Temporary putties, 131
Temporary relines, 326
Temporary repairs, 326
Temporary restorations, 131
Temporary veneers, 264
Temporization, 254, 268, 269, 334
Temporomandibular joint
  acquired conditions, 428
  anatomy, 429
  ankylosis, 430
  anterior disc displacement
    acute, without reduction, 472
    chronic, without reduction, 473
    with reduction, 472
  arthrography, 49
  assessment, 354
  common disorders, 471
  congenital conditions, 431
  dislocation, 430
  fracture, 430
  investigation of pain, 51
  magnetic resonance imaging, 48
  osteoarthritis, 512
  osteoarthrosis, 473
  rare disorders, 471
  rheumatoid arthritis, 473, 513
  seronegative arthritis, 496
  see also Craniomandibular disorders; Myofascial pain dysfunction
TENS (electrotherapy), 329
Tension headache, 515
Terfenadine, 85
Terminal hinge axis, 242
Terms of Service, 23
Tetanus prophylaxis, 427

Tetracyclines, 227, 228, 284, 441, 450, 454, 471
Thalassaemias, 500
Thalidomide, 450
Thermal conductivity, 117
Thermal expansion, 117
Thermoplastic splints, 190
Thiazide diuretics, 454, 492
Third molar
  eruption, 173, 541
  extraction technique, 385
  impacted, 391–5
  mineralization, 541
  radiographs, 54
  removal of impacted, 393–5
  spread of abscess, 402
Thrombasthenia, 501
Thrombocythaemia, 501
Thrombocytopenia, 70, 501
'Through and through' root filling, 296
Thyroid collar, 41
Thyroid disease, 470, 506–7
Thyroid hormones, and aspirin, 64
Tin, 119
Tinnitus, 65, 103
Tissue healing
  bone, 383
  extraction socket, 383
  factors influencing, 383–4
  wounds, 382–3
Titanium
  alloys, 145
  implants, 145, 330, 421
  pure, 145
TMJ see Temporomandibular joint
TNM classification, 463
Tobacco
  black hairy tongue, 460
  candidal leukoplakia, 459
  mouth cancer, 462
  pigmentation, 459, 460
  see also Smoking
Tongue
  black hairy, 460
  cancer, 412
  fissured (scrotal), 464
  geographic, 464
  orthodontic examination, 352–3

Tongue (*cont'd*)
 thrust, 363
 tumours, 411
Tonic–clonic seizures, 530
Tonsillitis, 494
Tooth brushes
 electric, 213, 214
 single tufted, 214
 special needs children, 195
Tooth brushing
 behaviour change, 5–6
 disease prevention, 345
 endocarditis, 71
 technique, 212–14
Tooth grinding, 228, 279
Tooth 'slooth', 234
Tooth wear
 abfraction, 280
 abrasion, 279
 assessment, 280
 attrition, 279
 diagnosis, 280–2
 erosion, 279–80
 examination, 236
 failures, 282
 management, 282
 measurement, 281
 monitoring, 281
 onlays, 269–70
 palatal veneers, 265–6
 prevention, 281
 shortened dental arch, 338
Tooth-friendly sweets, 159
Toothache (odontalgia), 51, 62, 475
Toothpastes
 chlorhexidine, 86
 fluoride, 159, 160–1, 162, 169
 whitening, 283
Topical agents, 85–9
Tori, 407, 419, 420
Training, ionizing radiation, 43
Tranexamic acid, 502
Transillumination, 154, 234, 406
Transmandibular implants, 144
Transplant
 renal, 462, 504–5
 teeth, 296
Transportation (zipping), 295

Transposed teeth, 192, 344
Transverse problems, crossbite, 362
Trapezius muscle, 514
Trauma
 children *see* Children
 facial, 108
 gingival recession, 211
 labial veneers, 263
 maxillofacial, 423–7
 mouth cancer, 462
 occlusal, 228
 ulceration, 449
Treatment, ethical and medico-legal considerations, 24
Treatment planning
 children, 168–9
 dentures, 300–2
 factors which influence, 17
 fixed prosthodontics/endodontics, 235–8
 integrated, 296–7
 orthodontics, 356–8
 purpose, 16–17
Treponema spp., 201
 see also Syphilis
Triamcinolone, 87, 292, 450, 479
Tricyclic antidepressants, 83–4, 93
 craniomandibular disorders, 329
 facial pain, 475
 myofascial pain dysfunction, 472
 tooth wear, 281
 xerostomia, 465, 471
Trigeminal nerve
 assessment, 514
 sensory loss, 482
Trigeminal neuralgia, 475–6
 cryosurgery, 401
 drugs for, 67
 imaging, 51
Trismus, 101, 112, 235, 395, 402
Trochlear nerve, 514
True pocket, 211
Tuberculosis (*Mycobacterium tuberculosis*), 440, 493, 518
Tumours, 408–10
 benign, 408–9
 imaging, 50
 laser removal of sensitive, 400

Tumours (cont'd)
  locally invasive, 409
  malignant, 408, 409
  odontogenic, 409–10
  pituitary, 507
  surgery, 438
  see also Neoplasia; specific
    tumours
Tuning fork tests, 514
Tunnel preparation, 230

Ulcerative colitis, 448, 481, 496
Ultrasonic scalers, 217–18
Ultrasonography, 48–9
Ultrasound, 406
Ultraviolet light, 462
Undercuts
  cobalt–chromium, 318
  gold, 318
  partial dentures, 318
  stainless steel, 318
Underperformance, 31
Unit, 270
Upper motor neurone lesions, 482
Urinary tract infection, 503

Vagus nerve, 514
Valaciclovir, 80, 446
Value, 138
Vapocoolants, 329
Varicella zoster (chicken pox),
  445–6
Varnishes
  cavity, 130
  fluoride, 162
Vascular purpuras, 501
Vasoconstrictors, 93–4
Vecuronium, 110
Veneer crowns, 261–2
Veneers
  clinical stages, 264–5
  definition, 263
  gingival, 325
  labial, 263–4
  palatal, 265–6
Venlafaxine, 475
Vent (sprue), 146

Ventricular fibrillation, 525
Verrill's sign, 106
Verruca vulgaris, 447
Verrucous carcinoma, 464
Vertigo, 514
Vesiculobullous lesions, 451–5
  classification, 451
  immunopathological features,
    452
  types, 451–5
Vestibulocochlear nerve, 514
Vestibuloplasty, 421
Vicryl, 400
Viral infections, 444–7, 518
Virchow's node (supraclavicular
  lymphadenopathy), 495
Visual assessment, 514
Visual disturbance, 101
Vital teeth
  bleaching, 283–5
  restorations, 248–9
Vital tests see Sensitivity tests
Vitamin B deficiency, 443, 448, 449,
  474, 494
Vitamin C deficiency, 501
Vitamin D deficiency, 511
Vitamin E, 454
Von Willebrand's disease, 502–3
Vulcanite, 142

Walking bleach technique, 286
Warfarin, 64, 502, 503
Warwick James elevator, 389–90
Water fluoridation, 160
Waxes, 145
Websites, useful, 537–9
Weight loss, 512
Wetting, 126
White patches, 455–7
  classification, 455
  conditions, 456–7
  renal failure, 457
  see also Hairy leukoplakia;
    Lichen planus; Lupus
    erythematosus; Neoplasia; Oral
    candidosis
White sponge naevus, 455–6
White spot, 152

White strips, 283
Whitlockite, 205
Wickham's striae, 478
Widman flap, 221
Willis bite gauge, 310
Wind instrument mouthpiece, 325
Wire fixation, facial fractures, 427
Wire splints, 229
Wiskott–Aldrich syndrome, 518
Wooden sticks, 214
Working length, 289
Working side, 239
    non, 239
Wound healing
    phases, 382
    primary/secondary intention,
        382–3
Wrought alloys, 139–41

X-rays, 34–5
Xerostomia (dry mouth), 89
    candidosis, 465
    drug-related, 471
    oral dysaesthesia, 474

Yellow Card Scheme, 89

Z-spring, 370
Zinc oxide–eugenol, 129, 130, 132,
    143, 268, 293
Zinc phosphate, 129
Zinc polycarboxylate, 129–30, 131
Zipping (transportation), 295
Zsigmondy–Palmer notation, 542
Zygomatic fractures, 423, 427, 428